Calm Tummy Happy Heart ©

The First Monash Certified LOW FODMAP COOKBOOK From The United States

by

Amy Laura

LOW FODMAP ❤ IBS FRIENDLY ❤ GLUTEN-FREE ❤ DAIRY-FREE

to ease symptoms of
IBS • IBD • Celiac Disease • Crohn's Disease
Ulcerative Colitis and other Digestive Disorders

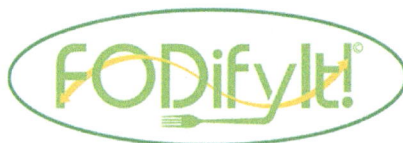

FODify It!®

www.fodifyit.com

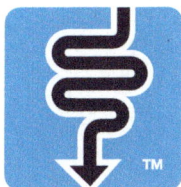

MONASH UNIVERSITY LOW FODMAP CERTIFIED ™

All recipes within this book are Monash University Low FODMAP Certified™. One serving of a meal made in accordance with this recipe can assist with following the Monash University Low FODMAP Diet™. A strict low FODMAP diet should only be commenced under the supervision of a healthcare professional. Monash University Low FODMAP Certified trade marks used under license worldwide by FODify It!.

A low FODMAP diet does not treat a disease but may help to meet nutritional needs with reduced gastrointestinal symptoms. Monash University receives a licence fee for the use of Monash University Low FODMAP Certified trade marks.

Published in the United States by FODify It! LLC

First Edition Printing, 2022

www.fodifyit.com (see contact page)

Ordering Information: Amazon.com and IngramSpark.com

ISBN 979-8-9871139-0-5

Author: Amy Laura

Cover and Book Design: Jim Dodson of Dodson Creative Agency

Editor and Recipe Consultant: Dédé Wilson of FODMAP Everyday

Primary Photography: Amy Laura and Jim Dodson

Monash FODMAP App images on page 24-27 provided by Department of Gastroenterology, Monash University. Images reproduced with permission from Monash University (**monashfodmap.com**).

Licensed Stock Photos by Freepic.com: pages 12, 16, 28, 36, 55, 109, 156, 252, 253, 264

On The Cover:

Classic Beef Tacos Plate - page 178

Flan - page 232

Green Chile Burger - page 172

Pulled Pork Caesar Salad - page 126

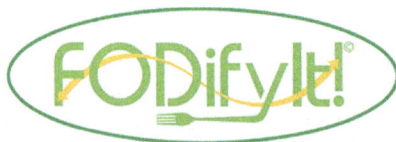

www.fodifyit.com

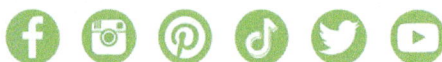

Calm Tummy ❤ Happy Heart

Dear friend,

This disclaimer applies to all content and pages of this cookbook.

The information included in *Calm Tummy ❤ Happy Heart* is intended for educational and informational purposes only. Content provided in this cookbook is not a substitute for professional medical advice, diagnosis or treatment. Always seek the advice of your physician or another qualified healthcare provider before altering your diet, changing your exercise regimen, starting any new lifestyle changes or modifying an existing treatment plan. Never disregard professional medical advice or delay in seeking it because of something you have read in this cookbook. When it comes to your health, consult your GP, GI, and do your research.

Calm Tummy ❤ Happy Heart is a personal journey written by me. I am not a doctor, nutritionist, registered dietitian nor a fitness expert. In this cookbook I am sharing my thirty-year personal experience with IBS, foods in general, the Low FODMAP Diet and personal lessons that changed my life. This is purely my experience and it is not my intention to give you information above or on behalf of your physician or qualified healthcare provider.

I'm also sharing with you my love and passion for the American Southwest. This book has been designed as a resource for calming digestive symptoms, creating delectable recipes, and as a soothing, artful experience with iconic landscape images and details taking you on a journey of the Southwest region that I know and love. I like to think of this book as a meeting where health, great food, the Southwest and art intersect.

The views and opinions expressed in this cookbook belong to the book owner. If I claim or appear to be an expert on certain topics, products or service areas, I will only endorse products or services that I believe in, based on my expertise or knowledge. Any product claim, statistic, quote or other representation about a product or service should be verified with the manufacturer or provider.

All recipes were based on information certified by Monash University at the time of publication.

For questions about this cookbook, please visit **www.fodifyit.com**, contact page.

Thank you and buen provecho!

❤ *Amy*

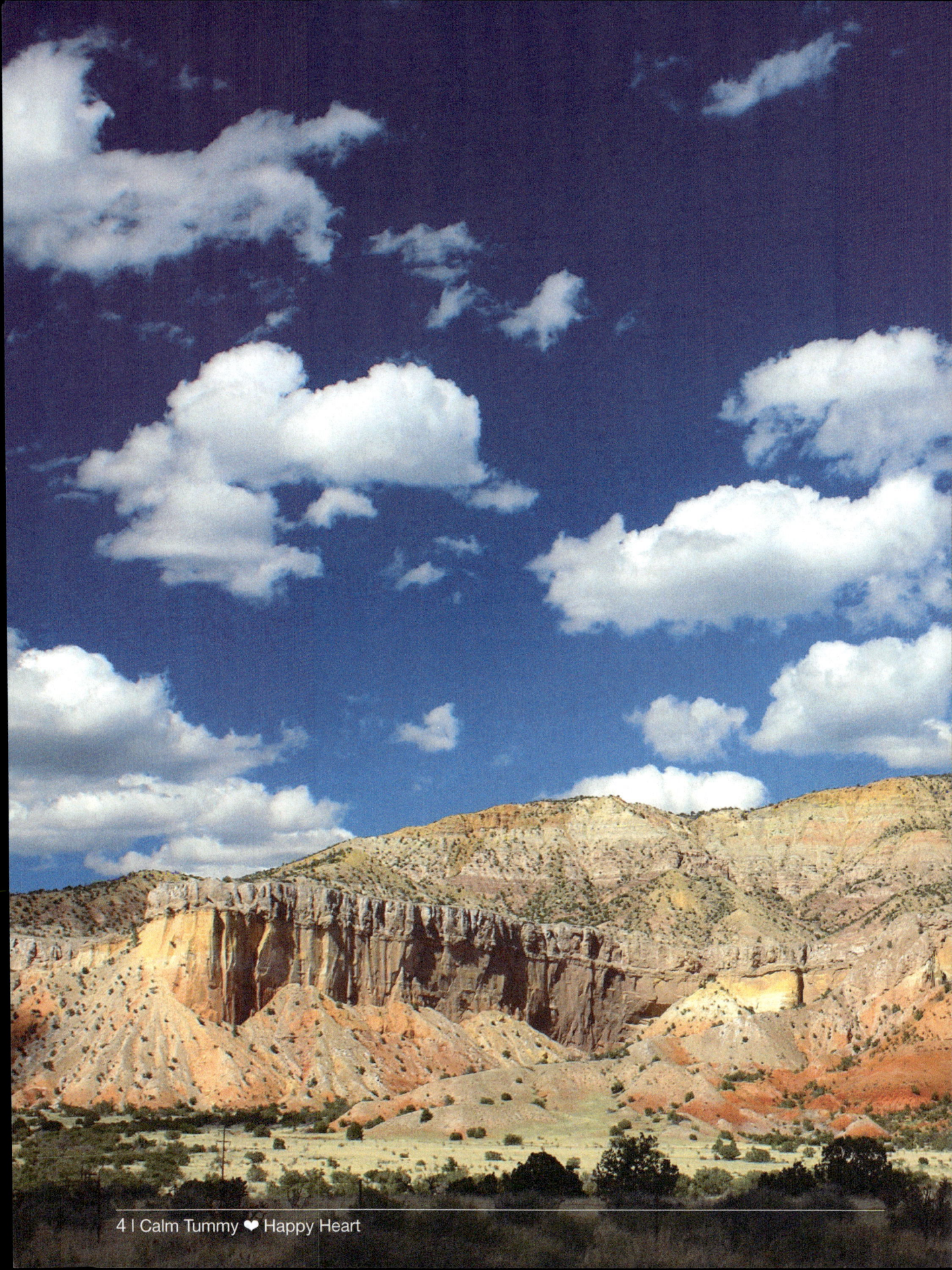

Dedication

To my husband, Jim, who designed this cookbook and stood by me while I searched for answers, thank you for believing in this project. I love you, sugar.

To my family who've encouraged me to cook and create art since I was a little peanut, your support and reassurance to keep up the search for answers made this labor of love possible.

To everyone at Monash FODMAP of Melbourne, Australia who developed this food plan and taught me how to take the guessing out of managing my chronic condition - you are my heroes.

To those who suffer from IBS or chronic digestive distress, may you find joy in cooking meals that calm your tummy, relief that lifts you up, enhances your life, and brings happiness to your heart. *xo Amy*

Banded Cliffs - Abiqui
New Mexico

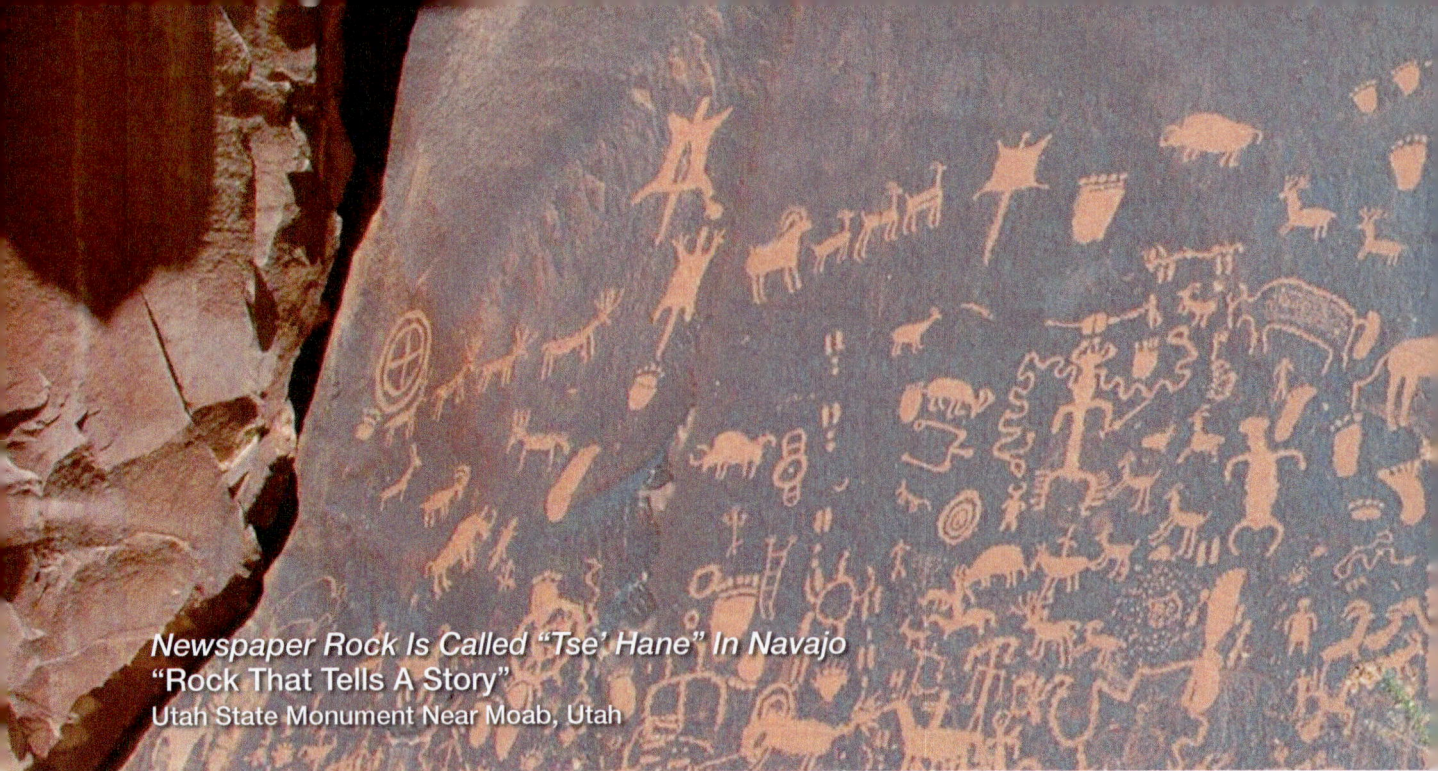

Newspaper Rock Is Called "Tse' Hane" In Navajo
"Rock That Tells A Story"
Utah State Monument Near Moab, Utah

Contents

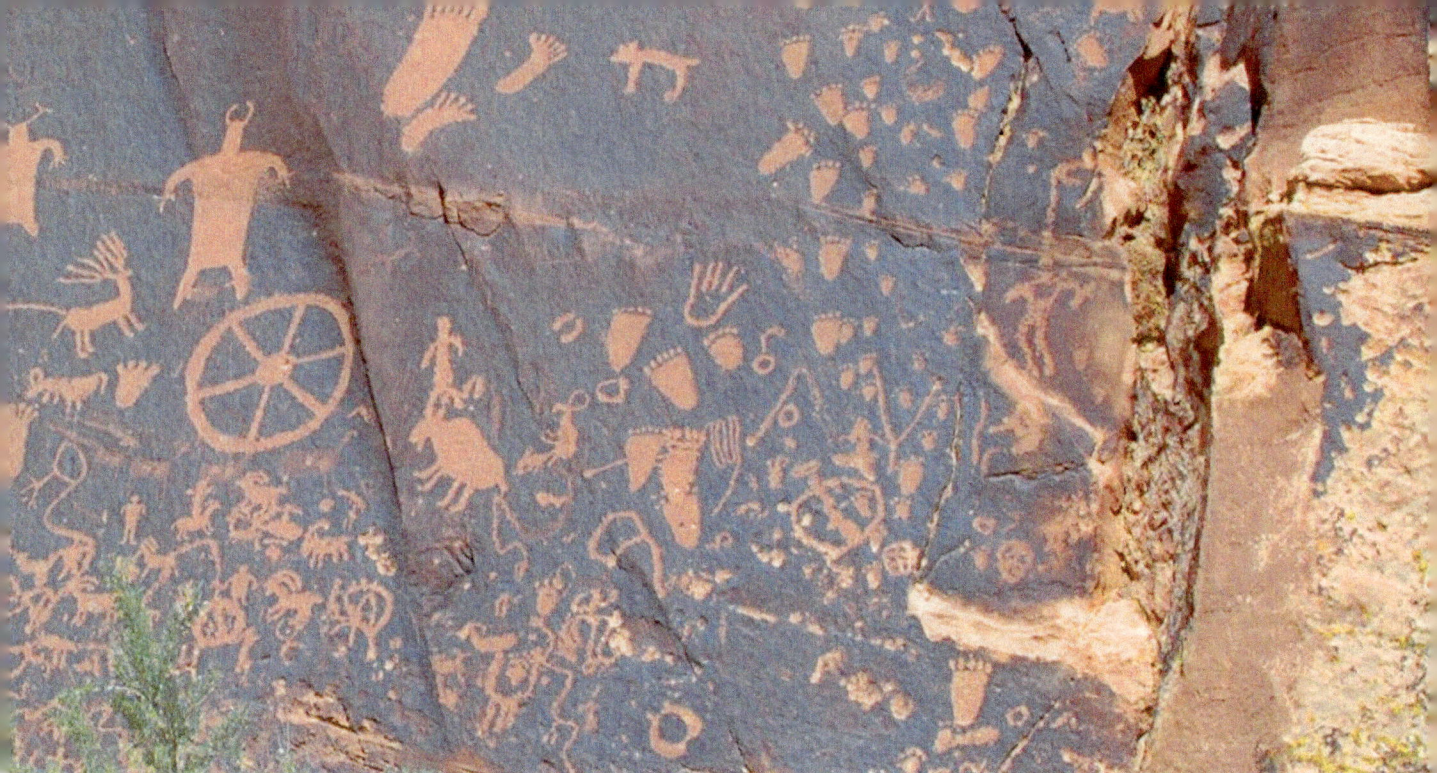

Thank You

The first book I checked out of a library was a children's cookbook. All of my birthday gifts through the years included art and cookbooks, cooking equipment and eventually, inspired by my mother's love of photography, a camera. And yet, not once did I imagine I would write and photograph a cookbook of my own — and about a food regimen that saved my life no less.

First and foremost, this cookbook owes its existence to the Department of Gastroenterology – Monash University FODMAP Team of Melbourne, Australia. To Dr. Peter Gibson, Dr. Jane Muir, Elizabeth Ly, all of the dietitians, lab workers and FODMAP Team members who assessed my recipes, and continue to educate and help millions of people around the world — it has been a privilege collaborating with you.

To Dr. Sue Shepherd, a pioneer of FODMAP development and research, thank you for sharing your scientifically proven findings with IBS sufferers and creating recipes for us to follow. In the early steps of following the low FODMAP plan, your cookbook gave me hope and relief.

Dédé Wilson and Robin Jaffin of FODMAP Everyday, I am so grateful to know you, and proud of the quality of work your editing brought to this book, Dédé. You know the science and are the Martha Stewart of LoFO cooking. Robin, how brilliantly you take care of the business details. Your mindful heart is always in the right place. I admire you both and will always think of you as my cool breeze across a lovely pond.

To Kate Scarlata of For A Digestive Peace Of Mind, it was through reading your blog and relating to your story toward this diet plan that reinforced my decision to try low FODMAP. Thank you a million times over.

Double-handed high fives to the IBS / FODMAP community who share stories, peaks and valleys of managing symptoms, research findings and gut health tips. Your posts led me to this diet, helped me to not feel alone in this, and to learn to laugh about my condition through your humor.

To Norma and Hutch of The Feasting Place, Ohkay Owingeh Pueblo, the Santa Fe School of Cooking, and Chef Lois Ellen Frank – thank you for teaching the traditional techniques of New Mexican and southwest cooking, making it possible for me to share with others.

In honor of the late Diana Kennedy, the Julia Child of Mexican cuisine, I've had her cookbook *The Art of Mexican Cooking: Traditional Mexican Cooking for Aficionados* since I was a teenager. I only wish I'd had the chance to tell her in person how much I treasure her book. Through it, she will continue to be an excellent teacher.

David Rein of Erickson Kernell, your support and professional guidance at the very beginning of this project is something I am eternally grateful for. You are an ace and I look forward to working together on future projects.

To Dr. Paul Bosland of the New Mexico Chile Pepper Institute, Ferrinda Fresh and Queen Victoria Market of Melbourne, Australia – thank you for your help in locating fresh chiles to have tested for FODMAPs. This cookbook would not be complete without those chile peppers.

Dalton Ranch Pottery owner and ceramist Nick Blaisdell, thank you for your beautifully detailed, master artworks. It is impossible for food to look unappetizing on one of your plates.

A huge shout-out is due to the farmers, chile growers, and ranchers of southwest Colorado and the Mesa Verde area, our chile farmer friends in New Mexico, the grocers and carniceria owners and patrons in the check-out lines who offer their knowledge on the best food brands to buy, and my southwest home cook friends who share just enough family recipe tips to not cause your moms and abuelas to disown you.

To my gastroenterologist, chronic illness therapist and general physician, I'm so glad to have found you. It has been a long journey in finding a medical team who knows about and understands my condition.

Mark Stevens, your expertise in writing promotional materials and helping me to view my story objectively is a gift. Thank you for your generosity and support of this book.

To my ranch family – Kate, Rick, Chris, Heather and all of the ranch pups – you make this a place that brings out the best in people. Kate and Rick, I will always be grateful to you for creating this haven of beauty we call home.

My heartfelt thanks goes to my family – Abner (Pa), Sandy (Ma) and Jill. You have always supported my cooking and work in photography. During the making of this book, I realized how all of the classes and training you encouraged me to pursue came together with this project. I don't know what would have become of me without your understanding of my condition and help in seeking answers. I love you all so very much.

Jim, my darling husband, I am the luckiest woman to have you as my best friend and soulmate. You brought your A game brilliance in designing this cookbook. Your kindness, strength and support always lets me know we can solve anything that comes our way – together. Thank you for this, and for never making me feel less than about my condition. You have my love and respect always, forever and then some.

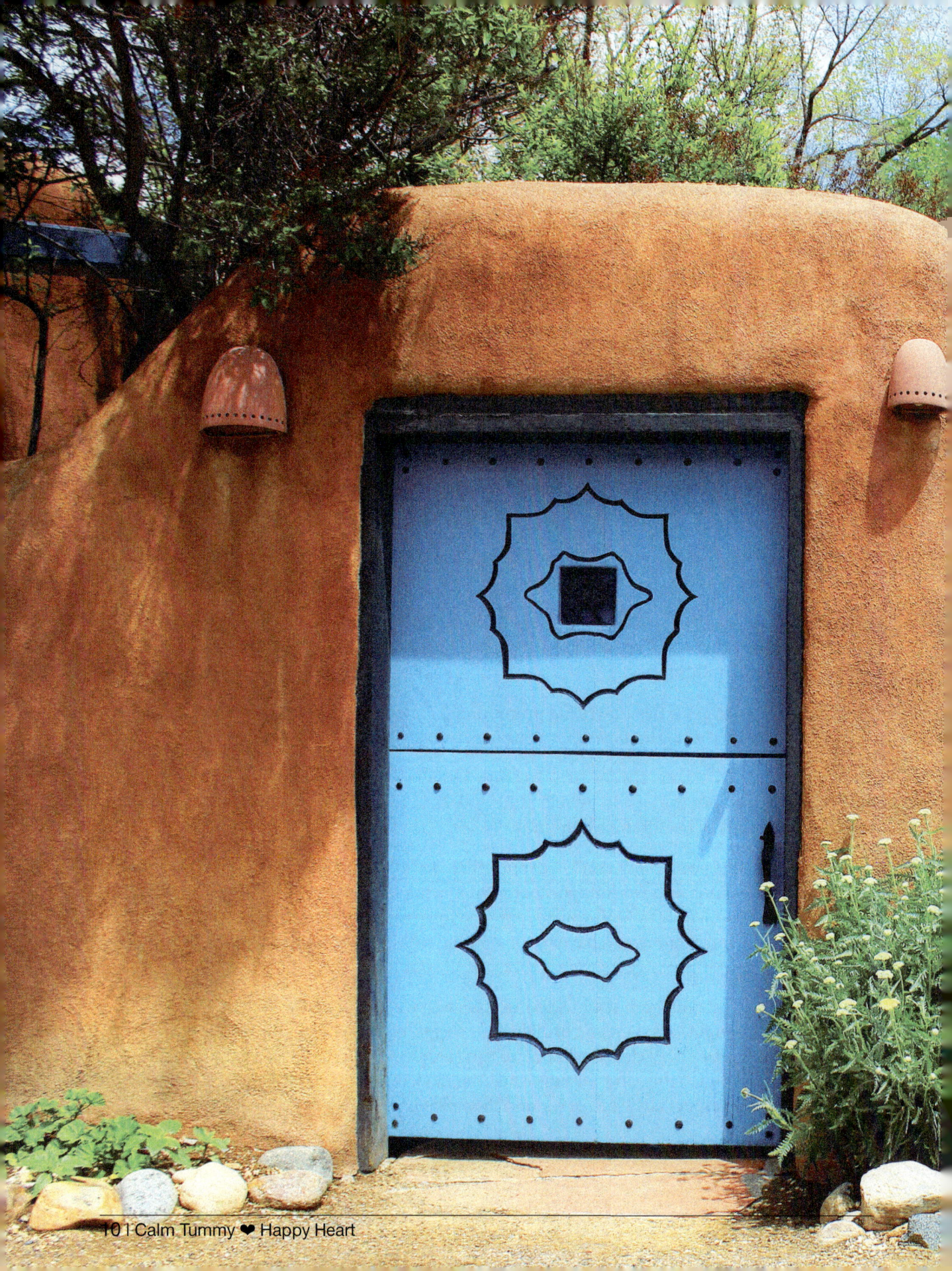

"You're not going to master the rest of your life in one day.
Just relax. Master the day.
Then just keep doing that every day"
Unknown

Santa Fe, New Mexico

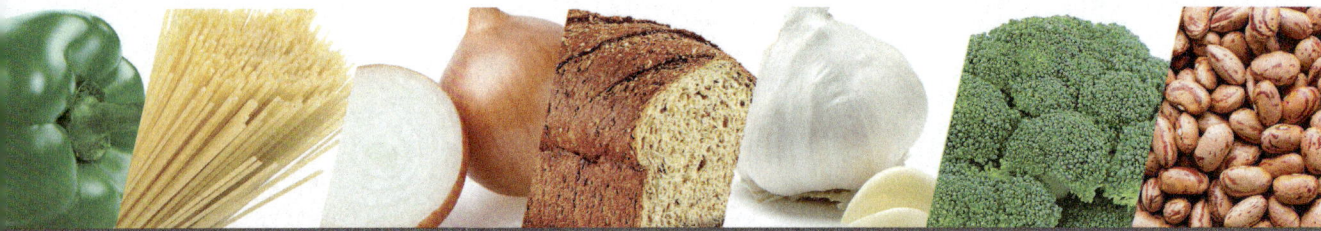

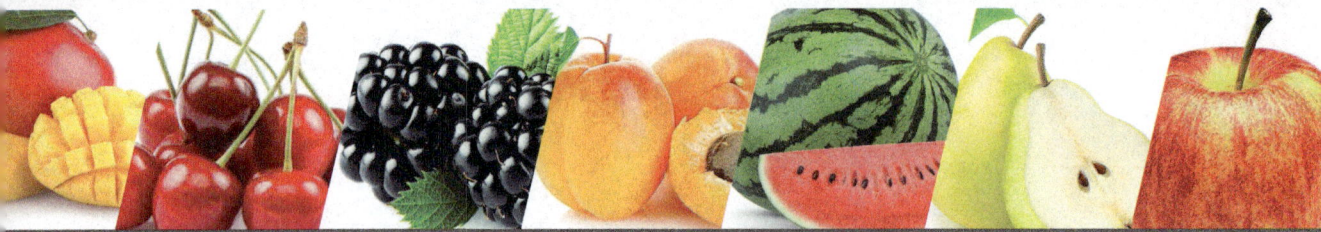

What Are Fodmaps and How Does The Diet Work?

If you are experiencing the telltale reoccurring symptoms of IBS – abdominal cramping and pain, bloating, stomach upsets, diarrhea and/ or constipation, and gas – before beginning any change in your diet or trying a new health-related food plan, it is best to consult with a gastroenterologist first to rule out other conditions that may be causing IBS and digestive upsets. Also, working with a FODMAP registered dietitian will make the process easier for you.

ABOUT MONASH FODMAP

My background is in the arts, photography and American Southwest cooking. I am not a dietitian or medically trained. When I felt the calling to write a low FODMAP cookbook to share my experience and recipes with those who suffer from IBS and chronic digestive conditions, I immediately contacted the FODMAP team at Monash University of Melbourne, Australia. These are the dynamic, progressive doctors and researchers who developed this remarkable food regimen that changed my life.

Through their Recipe Certification Program I had each recipe assessed and approved, which means for the last couple of years I've been collaborating with my heroes to ensure that my cookbook provides proper amounts of low FODMAP ingredient combinations.

The Monash team is continually expanding their research, testing new foods, certifying low FODMAP brands and sharing their findings and advice on the **monashfodmap. com** website, blog, social media and phone app (page 24). They offer a global listing of certified dietitians to work with, and so much more.

This amazing group of people who devote their time and careers to help those with chronic GI illnesses – safe to say that it's unlikely they go to sleep each night questioning if they are living a life of value and purpose.

WHAT ARE FODMAPs?

The best explanation comes from the Monash Team who developed the diet:

"FODMAPs are a group of sugars that are not completely digested or absorbed in our intestines. When FODMAPs reach the small intestine, they move slowly, attracting water. When they pass into the large intestine, FODMAPs are fermented by gut bacteria, producing gas as a result. The extra gas and water cause the intestinal wall to stretch and expand. Because people with IBS have a highly sensitive gut, 'stretching' the intestinal wall causes exaggerated sensations of pain and discomfort."

"Put simply, FODMAPs are a collection of short-chain carbohydrates (sugars) that aren't absorbed properly in the gut, which can trigger symptoms in people with IBS. FODMAPs are found naturally in many foods and food additives."

FODMAP is an acronym for Fermentable Oligosaccharides, Disaccharides, Monosaccharides and Polyols. These are the fermentable carbs (sugars) found in some foods and additives that, when removed from your diet or consumed in moderation can significantly improve the symptoms of IBS.

To learn more about the science behind FODMAPs, **visit www.monashfodmap.com** for explanations and examples of foods containing:

F   Fermentable gas forming foods and additives

O   Oligosaccharides: Fructans + GOS found in wheat, rye, garlic, onions, inulin, legumes, etc

D   Disaccharides: lactose in milk, yogurt, some soft cheeses, etc

M   Monosaccharides: Fructose found in honey, high fructose corn syrup, dried fruits, agave syrup, etc

A   nd

P   Poloyols: sugar alcohols and artificial sweeteners such as sorbitol, mannitol xylitol, some foods such as avocado and watermelon, sugar-free gums

Monash offers an online Patient Course. For a one-time fee they take you through the steps of the plan and offer a wealth of information in learning scientifically proven facts for the best results in detecting your triggers. The course is interactive which makes it fun, and I found that the science was not overwhelming. This is also an excellent source in learning how to use their app, and you will need to have it on hand to complete certain course modules.

The low FODMAP diet has also been proven to relieve IBS-like symptoms associated with Celiac Disease, Inflammatory Bowel Disease (IBD), SIBO, and other digestive disorders.

There is no cure for IBS, but if you discover that your body is sensitive to FODMAPs, you can find relief and learn how to manage your symptoms by following the steps of the diet.

HOW DOES THE LOW FODMAP DIET (LoFO) WORK?

Monash research estimates that 15% of the world's population (1 in 7 people) is affected by IBS. And 75% of these people find relief by eating foods that are low in FODMAPs.

There are 3 steps to the FODMAP diet:
- Elimination Phase
- Reintroduction Phase
- Personalization/Maintenance Phase

Monashfodmap.com offers information on getting started, which low FODMAP foods to eat in proper amounts, high FODMAPs to avoid, new findings, steps to reintroduce foods, with detailed guides, online training and resources.

Please note that Low FODMAP and High FODMAP are oftentimes referred to as LoFO and HiFO in this cookbook.

Following is a brief outline of how it works.

STEP 1 Elimination Phase is a 2 to 6 week step where you are swapping in low FODMAP portions of foods in place of high FODMAP foods.

The best approach is to work with a qualified dietitian and use the Monash University FODMAP Diet Smartphone App that is continually updated with lab tested foods and low FODMAP serving amounts. This takes the guessing out of what to eat and swap out by following the red, yellow and green traffic light system that displays high, moderate and low levels of serving sizes. You can type in an item like mushrooms and get the lowdown on which are LoFO and how much to eat. For example, oyster mushrooms are LoFO in 1 cup (75 g) or less per serving, whereas button mushrooms are HiFO at 1 cup and moderate at 1/2 tablespoon (10 g).

Some people feel relief and a calmness in their digestion in a week's time. I knew in 3 days that it was working (more about that in My Story chapter).

The best advice I can offer is to make every effort to eat LoFO for 2 to 6 weeks and keep a daily food and mood journal to track your progress (page 28). You may also like using the app diary.

It can be confusing and a little complex at first, but the closer you stick with it, the more accurate the results will be in determining your relationship with FODMAPs.

STEP 2 We're all unique cases with different sensitivities. In the Reintroduction Phase, we continue eating LoFO while adding back larger portions of foods with higher FODMAP content one at a time. Monash describes these as Challenges and their Patient Course will walk you through this process. Your dietitian will also be a huge help here.

For quite some time I considered the diet to be dairy-free because my food journal indicated that the lactose in dairy was a trigger. I later learned in Reintro that many cheeses have been tested to contain only trace amounts of FODMAPs, and butter also contains only trace amounts of lactose. Today, I am primarily dairy-free but have made progress with lactose-free dairy products and small amounts of conventional cheeses with no flare-ups! I am also continuously re-testing my relationship with wheat and also with gluten. This is why I chose to present a dairy-free, gluten-free cookbook for you, with a few tips on adding lactose-free and conventional dairy per your personal tolerance.

STEP 3 Personalization/Maintenance is a continuation of expanding your diet and finding your balance. Also, a tolerance can change over time, so reintroducing a trigger HiFO food a few months later may no longer cause a flare-up for you.

For your convenience in navigating the diet, all recipes in this cookbook are low FODMAP compliant for the Elimination Phase. Please see page 268 for a Quick Reference List of swaps. Monashfodmap.com offers a sample foods list- from the source!

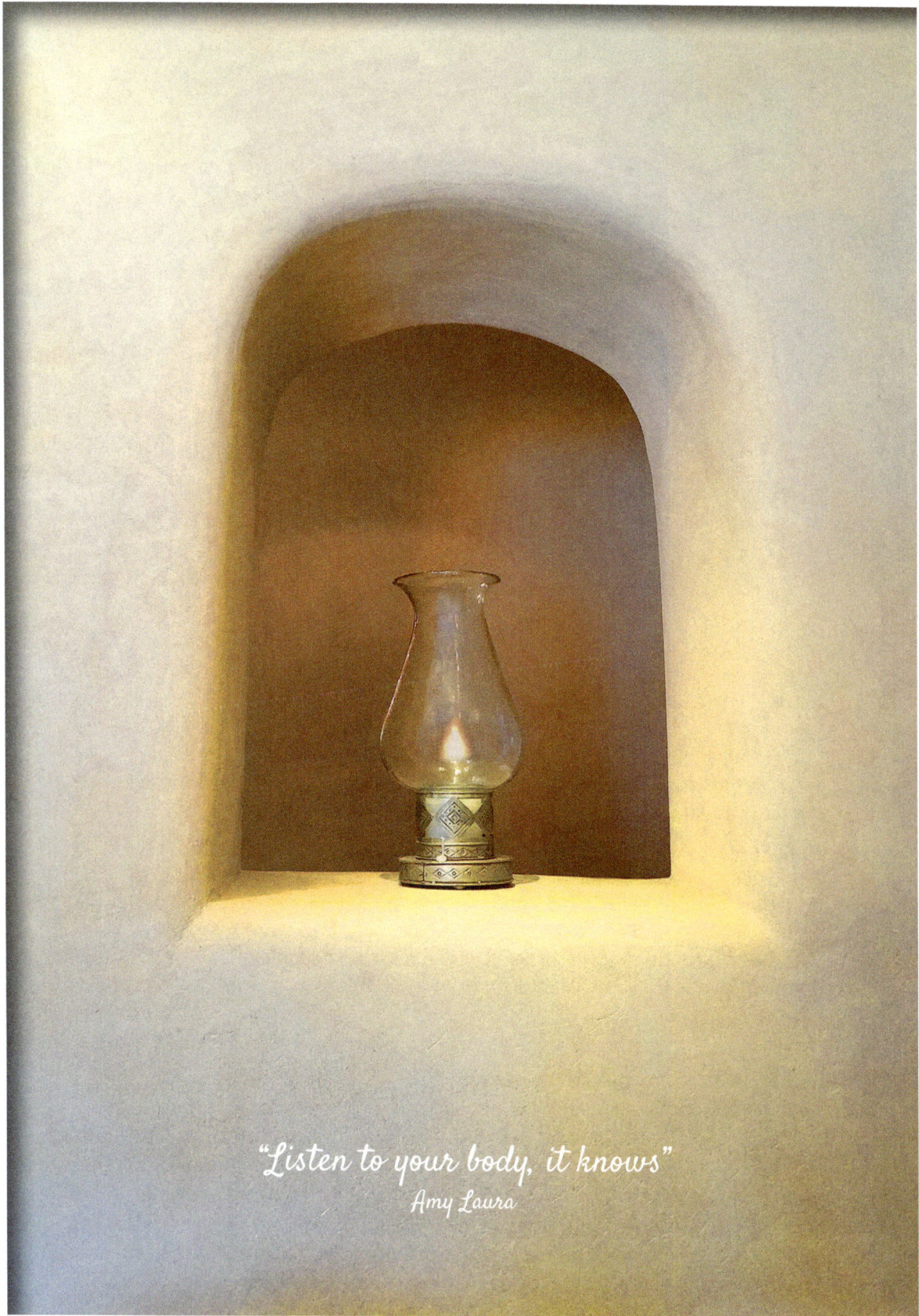

"Listen to your body, it knows"
Amy Laura

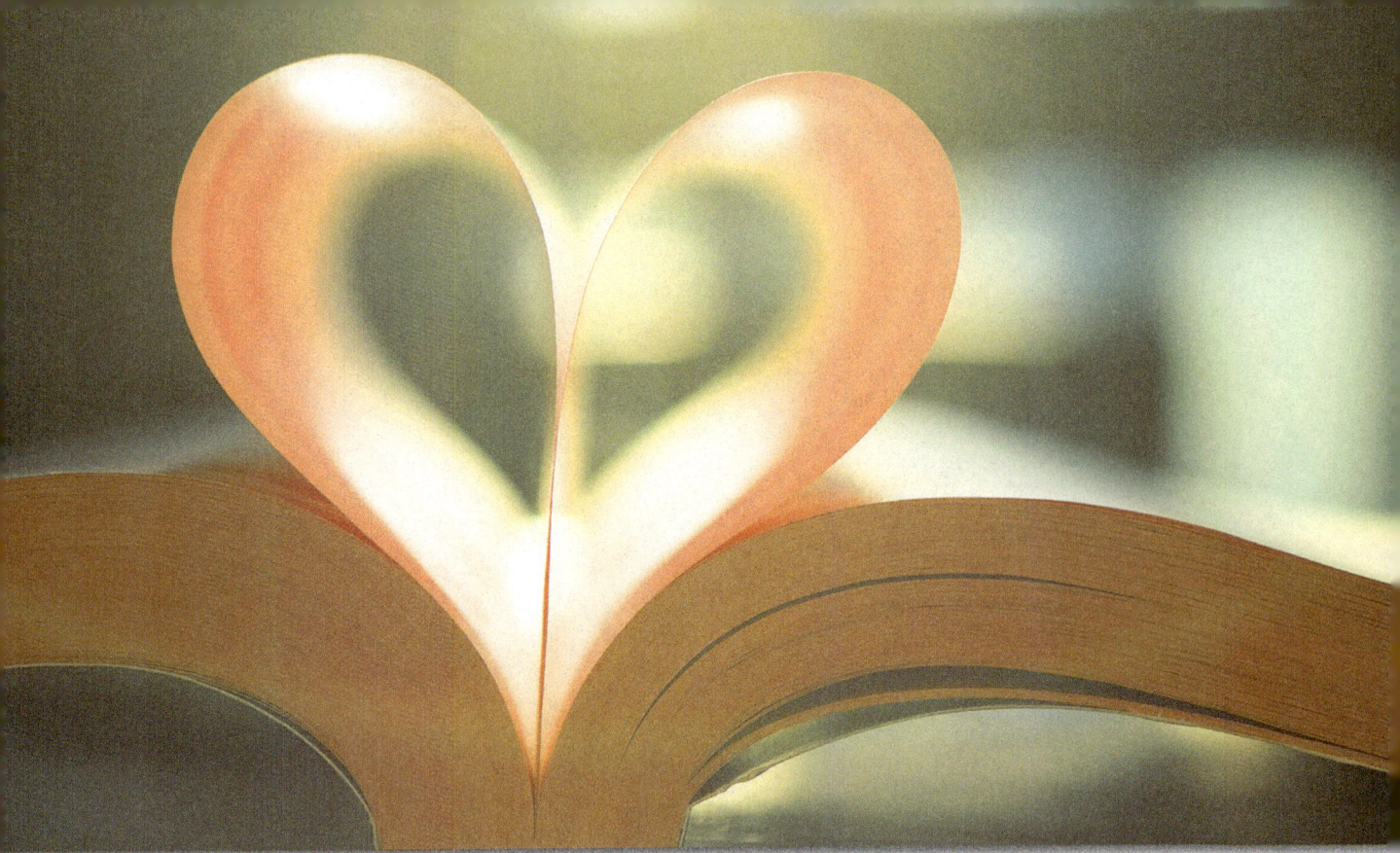

My Story

How eating low FODMAP for 3 days began to calm 30 years of chronic digestive pain …

Hello there. I'm Amy – a travel and lifestyle photographer, national parks enthusiast, historic district fanatic, gluten-free bakery stalker, and avid home cook. I live in Colorado on a ranch with my darling husband Jim, a group of big-hearted people, two dachshunds, and twenty-six dogs who belong to the ranch and think of me as Auntie Cookie. One of my greatest joys is to fill my pockets with doggie treats and walk out into the play yard.

I've written this cookbook because for most of my life I've suffered from unpredictable, misdiagnosed and oftentimes severely painful digestive symptoms due to Irritable Bowel Syndrome (IBS-D). It is my wish to offer help by sharing recipes and my journey in finding answers for relief, because it was through reading about the personal experiences of others that had me nodding my head "I know how that feels, yes, that's me." I believe it's important for us to share our stories because this was the manner in which I discovered the Low FODMAP Diet that has given me the gift of a calm tummy, empowerment in finally knowing how to manage my condition, and comfort that lifts my heart with happiness and hope.

There is no single known cause or cure for IBS. The good news is that it is not contagious and we can find ways to alleviate the symptoms. Mine was a thirty-year process of trial and error to find answers. In the U.S., digestive disorders don't come up in general conversation very often, but more recently the Low FODMAP Diet is finding it's way onto the radar of U.S. health publications, general physicians, gastroenterologists and cookbooks. There are now LoFO meal delivery services and food brands specifically tailored to the diet. This gives me comfort that awareness is building, because 1 in 7 people are affected by IBS and 75% find relief through this food regimen.

This is another reason why I decided to include so many personal details of my search – that is rather lengthy due to 30 years of seeking answers – because if you or someone you know suffers from IBS and relates to even a portion of my story, it is my hope that these examples will lead to ending the discomfort and confusion they are going through. And to not feel so alone in this as I did.

HOW DID I GET IBS?

When I was in school, I shared lunch with a classmate who went home later that day and collapsed from meningitis. She was taken to the hospital and placed in the Intensive Care Unit. Thankfully, she completely recovered. As a precaution, I was quarantined and given heavy doses of medications. I never contracted meningitis, but shortly after this incident my IBS symptoms began with sharp abdominal cramping, random diarrhea upsets, bloating, fatigue, brain fog, gas, feeling overheated and flushed, with fluky bouts of anxiety.

I would later learn that a few members of my family have sensitive digestion, indicating that I was genetically predisposed and the heavy meds triggered my IBS. I also went through a series of dental procedures that

required prolonged use of antibiotics – another IBS instigator.

I have since learned of people who have contracted IBS due to a bad case of food poisoning, a highly stressful moment in their lives, some who've served in the military under extreme pressure, stressful work environments, and intestinal bacterial and viral infections. These are only a handful of other causes.

Early on I remember thinking "what is giving me food poisoning all the time?" And then came to the realization that consuming bad dairy or contaminated foods several times a week was unlikely and not the culprit.

Early on I remember thinking "what is giving me food poisoning all the time?"

My physicians were caring, concerned and baffled about what was happening with my body. Very little was known about IBS when my illness began in the 1980s. It was called spastic colon then, and it would be decades until IBS or FODMAPs were on mine or my doctor's radar.

Before delving further into my story, I want to mention that countless chapters of my life have been positively joyful. Sure, I've missed out on family celebrations, had to cancel plans with friends and missed special events because of my condition. But many times I've felt like my life was and is a great book I've picked up and I cannot wait to turn the next page. I've married the love of my life, found peace in living in the quiet beauty of the U.S. Southwest, and I've been known to laugh in my sleep. My story to find answers was a long, at times maddening maze of hit or miss testing and treatments, but I want to be sure to convey that it hasn't been an entire existence of cheerless bummed-out tummy drama.

ALLERGY & GASTROINTESTINAL TESTING

If you are suffering from the symptoms of IBS it is critical that you go through testing with a gastroenterologist to rule out other conditions that may be the cause, or life threatening. It is important to note that home tests are not reliable or supported by reputable RDs or MDs at this time.

Mine began with allergy panels. Most people who knew about my condition were incredibly encouraging and would say, "It's gotta be a wheat allergy or dairy. Once you're confirmed for one of them, you'll eliminate it and will be out of the woods." I waited for the results with a smile on my face, confident that the scoundrel would be revealed and tah-dah! Poof! I'd be cured! To my surprise and disappointment, all tests came back negative including wheat and dairy. Years later I would learn that the body can have sensitivities to certain foods that do not show up on allergy panels.

Next came a gastrointestinal series of x-rays, colonoscopies and more tests. This time it was not all smiles as I waited for the results. Rather, a bundle of nerves that something serious would be revealed that might require surgery. All came back clear along with the first diagnosis that I needed to meditate and handle my stress better because it was "all in my head." After all, my tests were negative so what else could it be? I feel it's important to lay it on the line that I never believed it was all in my head. Anxiety can be an IBS trigger, but I'd been on vacations that were entirely designed around relaxation.

These were not high adrenaline dune buggy trips in the southern Arizona sand dunes, or jumping out of perfectly good airplanes over the Mojave Desert. While on these rejuvenation trips, my mind was at ease, I was completely removed from daily routines and work stress, and still I had flare-ups and abdominal pain. My gut instinct knew that there was something more to it.

Can meditation, good counseling for anxiety and exercise help to soothe digestive upsets? Absolutely. Anxiety and stress play a part in IBS symptom flare-ups because the gut and brain are always talking to each other. But for me, one who is highly sensitive to FODMAPs, I was still in digestive discomfort because I had no idea about FODifying - modifying the FODMAPs in my diet.

ELIMINATION TESTS

My first food elimination test was with dairy. For one month, aside from a few forgetful moments with cheese on tacos or in a burrito, I stuck with it and kept a food journal (page 28). No change or relief, so I then removed all wheat and gluten containing foods from my diet. Bye-bye flour tortillas! For two months I managed this strict approach, and guess what? I felt a little better! One week into giving up wheat flour tortillas, breads, pizza, pasta – my condition improved with noticeably fewer upsets or abdominal pain.

A glimpse of what it felt like to have a semi-calm belly! Was this the moment of truth I'd been hoping for? Just as I began to feel healthier, hocus-pocus the IBS symptoms mysteriously returned. I later learned that the fructans in wheat make it one of the greatest FODMAP offenders, so it made sense that I would feel a bit of relief. But giving up wheat and going gluten-free alone was not enough for my sensitivities.

BLAND FOODS

My next effort was to try bland foods such as rice, potatoes, oatmeal, flour and corn tortillas, vegetable soups, wheat crackers,

I feel it's important to lay it on the line that I never believed it was all in my head.

puréed vegetables (like homemade baby foods) and minced chicken. Again, no relief. What I didn't know was that along with these foods I was mixing in onion, garlic, stone fruits and other ingredients containing high amounts of FODMAPs.

In order to have a social life, make it to work and have as normal a lifestyle as possible, I managed by taking over-the-counter antacids and other drugstore tablets that semi-calmed my symptoms but merely masked the problem. While taking these pills on a daily basis was not healthy, I was grateful that they helped me to get out into the world because I was living in the fast lane due to the nature of my work in photography, traveling and being on location sets.

Please know that I am not encouraging self-medicating like this. This was something I did just to get by, and not one gastroenterologist I've consulted with has recommended pro-longed use of these drugstore digestive aides.

I was living the life I'd trained for and always wanted – to work in my field, travel to places I'd might never have had the opportunity to explore, and meet interesting people through photography. But there was also the reality that if word got around that I needed to leave the set several times during shooting (due to abdominal pain or a flare-up), and certainly if I was a last-minute cancelation for an assignment, I would be replaced. That was and is the nature of freelance employment in the overnight photo deadline machine.

I couldn't let anyone in the industry know about my condition and kept taking far more doses of drugstore remedies than recommended. Conversations about my condition were reserved for family, a few close friends and my doctors. Occasionally, a friend or someone on a job would look me in the eyes and say," You sound fine but you look so tired. Are you okay?" My response was

"Not getting enough sleep. It's just a phase I'm going through." I also drank coffee all day long (caffeine can be an IBS trigger) to keep my energy up on long work days.

Eventually, I began arranging to work from home and gradually, reluctantly turn down travel assignments. Working in remote off-the-beaten-path locations, climbing to building rooftops for great view situations or just driving to another city in gridlock traffic were risky. Restrooms were not easily accessible, and if a location budget didn't provide an RV, that was panicky. Many people with IBS feel the workplace pressure of limited breaks and long commutes.

Still, I held onto the belief that you are never defeated until you give up, and continued my search to be properly diagnosed. Later came parasite tests, more x-rays, blood tests and consultations with some of the best gastroenterologists in Southern California.

FASTING, JUICING & GARLIC

It took only a matter of days to recognize that, for me, fasting was not a good idea. Multiple daily flare-ups began and I must have been quite desperate to try this because for years I'd known that if my stomach became empty it would growl. Loudly. Just imagine the sounds of handing a metal pie tin full of marbles to a raccoon to play with. I'm only slightly exaggerating here. Then came GI upsets, so fasting was out.

Regarding juice cleanses, I gave up after only a couple days because the juices I used were apple or apple juice-based that are high FODMAP and caused more GI distress.

In the 90s, health magazines began printing articles on foods that were antioxidants and

Still, I held onto the belief that you are never defeated until you give up.

reduced hypertension and cholesterol. Garlic was high on the list, so I would frequent a garlic-themed restaurant that was known for their 40-clove garlic chicken, garlic steamed clams, garlic mashed potatoes, garlic spread breads, and garlic ice cream. Anyone leaving this place smelled like a garlic festival and that was a part of the fun. This was when I began to notice how bloated my stomach could become. I looked like I'd eaten twenty-five pounds of tofu. What a mystery this was. "Was it the clams? Did I eat too much bread? It can't be the garlic. Garlic is healthy." Around this time I began wearing clothes that were two to four sizes larger in order to hide my tummy.

Garlic is one of the first ingredients in virtually every savory recipe I've cooked with. It turns out that garlic (and onion) contain fructans, and if you are sensitive to this FODMAP you need an alternative strategy. The LoFO swap is that we can properly infuse oil with garlic and onion (page 50) to get around the fructans (which are not oil soluble) and still enjoy their pungent, aromatic flavors. More good news is that in the Reintroduction Phase, many people find that they are no longer a digestive trigger.

THE PILLS INCIDENT

I want to preface this next story by noting that there are medications that help people with the symptoms of IBS. The following incident took place twenty years ago and since then there have been improvements in understanding GI conditions and drug research that offer relief. Unfortunately, I had a dicey experience with a medication.

A top gastroenterologist in his field handed a prescription to me for a medication that was "helping thousands of women" with my symptoms. This was a highly recommended Los Angeles doc so I immediately took the pills.

The next day, I left for a travel shoot and began to feel nausea, loss of appetite, abdominal cramping, a flare-up, headaches and brain fog. I stopped taking the pills and once home, went for a follow-up exam. The doc looked at my chart and said "You're not still taking these pills, are you? They've been causing intestinal bleeding." The lesson I learned that day was: no matter who writes the prescription, research the blazes out of it before you take it, and even if it is a supported drug, listen to your body. If it doesn't work for you, advocate for yourself with your GI.

VEGAN, VEGETARIAN & HOLISTIC

I was a vegan for almost two years, then vegetarian for several years and my symptoms during both food phases, to my amazement, worsened. (Don't be worried if you are vegan or veggo. It is possible to FODify your foods and you can find tips and notes at **monashfodmap.com**).

My foods were combinations of HiFO cauliflower steaks, cashew butter, wheat flour tortillas, refried and various beans, salsas with garlic and onion, wheat pasta and breads, lots of corn, white and red onions, lots of chickpeas and garlic hummus, button mushrooms, garlic dressings, and certain vegan soy products that aggravated my digestion. I enjoyed being vegan and was confused when my flare-ups increased. Unbeknownst to me at the time, many of these foods were fructan-rich, and FODMAP stacking was taking place. (More on stacking page 52).

I then joined a sustainable, costly health food delivery program, but no tummy relief. Shortly after, I began reading articles about a new holistic practice that people were raving about. The therapists had been mentored by great healers and used natural remedies that had been proven over thousands of years. It was all about balance, finding your center, calmness and being present. Examination rooms were like softly-lit spas. Layers of incense hovered around as we sat on the floor with poofy pillows. Therapists spoke in sweet soothing voices one uses to calm babies down for naptime. I immediately fell in love with this place. They created tinctures and tea blends for me to drink each day. We meditated together, I spent a small fortune, and when nothing worked we were all puzzled. But at least I had learned new tools for living and communicating through their mindfulness teachings.

THERAPY

I'm a strong believer in psychotherapy as an objective touchstone during difficult times and life changes. When I first began interviewing for the right confidant, I remember that the focus was on anxiety and life experiences, but none knew to ask about my digestive issues and foods, or to pursue the subject when I brought it up. This is why I am elated that today, because of the Monash team and publications of GI related articles that raise awareness for a more open attitude in discussing GI conditions, I have a therapist who specializes in chronic illnesses and anxiety, a general physician who is familiar with the Low FODMAP Diet, and my gastroenterologist is also on the plan. Things in the therapy and GI world have come a long way in 30+ years.

MY BIG MISTAKE

We all make mistakes, and this one became an important life lesson.

Around the 20ish year mark of my IBS onset, I was mentally and physically exhausted. Feeling hopeless, I rejected my mantra that we are never defeated until we give up and discontinued my GI doctor appointments, research and reading, elimination diets – just

flat-out stopped for almost ten years. Again, I took lots of drugstore temporary aides to get by. I could have marked a calendar to take a break for six months and then pick up the search again, but I didn't. This was a big mistake because during this time huge strides were being made in gastrointestinal research, FODMAPs and the gut-brain axis relation to IBS. Had I stuck with my mantra, I would have found relief years earlier.

Then one night while I was getting ready to meet friends for dinner, I collapsed. I had doubled over with abdominal pain before but this one was different. I fell to the floor and could not get up or move out of the fetal position. The pain kept coming in waves. Finally, through breathing, remaining calm, and getting through a bad stomach flare-up, I was able to stand and drink some water. It scared me so much that I'd almost grabbed my phone to call an ambulance. I was sicker than I'd realized.

I canceled the dinner, made an appointment with my doctor, and got online to look up my symptoms again. The same acronym kept popping up – FODMAP. A food program for IBS relief? Food as medicine? I found a few online lists of low FODMAP foods, woke up the next morning, drove to the market and stocked my kitchen with a week's supply of ingredients to test on myself.

We all make mistakes, and this one became an important life lesson.

IT WORKED

Within three days – and I will never forget this – I was sitting in the living room with Jim. We were watching a movie and I suddenly realized that my body had been peaceful all day. I had eaten strictly LoFO foods, my stomach was calm, not at all bloated and I had no discomfort or pain.

After three decades I felt significant relief! I remember smiling that I might be able to trust my body again. "But will this last?" I also wondered.

Two months later, I was on a natural high having gained a huge boost of energy and my digestion was so improved that I woke up each morning with a newfound sense of normalcy and understanding of how to manage my condition.

HOW I'M DOING NOW

When you have a chronic illness and find something that gives you relief of symptoms and pain, you will do anything to maintain that feeling of freedom and bliss. I have followed the Monash plan, am eating according to what works for me, and reintroducing ingredients to find my balance of maintenance through foods and mindfulness.

I follow the Monash and FODMAP community online for updates on research and newly tested foods, to hear their stories, humor, triumphs and setbacks, and am eternally grateful to be a part of this supportive community.

Rather than dwelling on times of hopelessness and feelings that "Life isn't fair," and "Why did I have to go through all of this?" I channel these thoughts into being thankful for where I am now with my health, and how lucky I am to have the knowledge to calm my symptoms.

I am thankful for where I am now with my health.

I am a travel photographer in the Southwestern United States where there are plenty of wide-open spaces. Driving long distances has become much easier and I can enjoy the five hours from Santa Fe to Mesa Verde National Park without worrying "sheesh, what will I do if my stomach starts the marble rumbling thing?"

Taking a personal day off doesn't give me the guilt like it used to. If I do have a flare-up or if my sleep is off, my body will tell me that it needs rest and I'm far more mindful of that now. In the past I would have pushed through to work that day and meet friends for dinner. There are instances in which taking the day off is not possible due to a deadline, and I know now to eat strictly LoFO, drink my peppermint tea and be kind to myself as I would for a friend who is having a bad day.

I still have bouts of anxiety and know the value of a support system in getting through difficult times. But even so, I've never felt so comfortable in my own skin, and the word grateful seems to come up in conversation every day. Grateful for foods as medicine. Grateful for people who share their victories and struggles. Grateful to not feel so alone in all of this. Grateful to not be home bound. Grateful to feel that I can trust my body again. Grateful for the people who developed my food plan and gave me answers.

THE COOKBOOK

The robust cuisines of the Southwestern United States and Southern California are my every-day craveables. When I first realized I had complex food sensitivities (and even beyond FODMAPs from skins of fruits and vegetables, and MSG) I made an assumption that my days of eating dishes like fajitas, gazpacho and creamy caramel flans would be limited. And what about chiles? A life without green chiles would be like a sky without stars. At first I was worried about what I'd have to give up.

So, I flipped through my recipe box and began converting my best efforts with appropriate food swaps. It took no time at all to realize that I did not have to give up the flavors and foods that are a big part of my regional cuisine. I could FODify It! by swapping out certain foods. A few years after this epiphany, I had the makings of a cookbook and began to photograph my favorite classic and updated dishes.

My one concern was that I was not medically trained or a certified low FODMAP dietitian and would need to collaborate with someone who could make absolutely sure that my ingredients and measurements were properly accounted for. Through the Monash Team and their Recipe Certification Program and phone app, I found oodles of ways to test and re-test my recipes. For the past two years, my kitchen has been a fantastic wreck as I assembled batches of recipes to send for certification by the very people who created the 3-Step plan that saved my life.

I want you know that if you are relating to my story, I am sorry. Because I know the pain and disruption this has on your life. I wish I were there to give you a big hug right now. This is why I feel it is my calling to share my story, create cookbooks and offer helpful resources. Once we have answers, we know how to make decisions to improve our health. That's what I wanted and daydreamed about for so long – a scientifically proven method to manage my symptoms without all of the guessing.

I hope you will try the Low FODMAP Diet and find relief. I hope my recipes and resources will help you. I can tell you from experience that working with a physician to first rule out other possible causes of your symptoms, and a Monash Certified dietitian will make the journey easier and you will be far more informed. Stick with your food journal to track which foods are triggers or okay for you, take the online Monash Patient Course, and if for some reason your body does not adapt to the diet, do not give up your search for answers and a proper diagnosis.

If you are already LoFO, I hope you enjoy my recipes and that they help you to never feel deprived of flavorful foods. IBS may be a pain to deal with but it doesn't mean we have to live in frustration or give up the richness of foods we love.

Wishing you a calm tummy and happy heart. 💙 Amy Laura

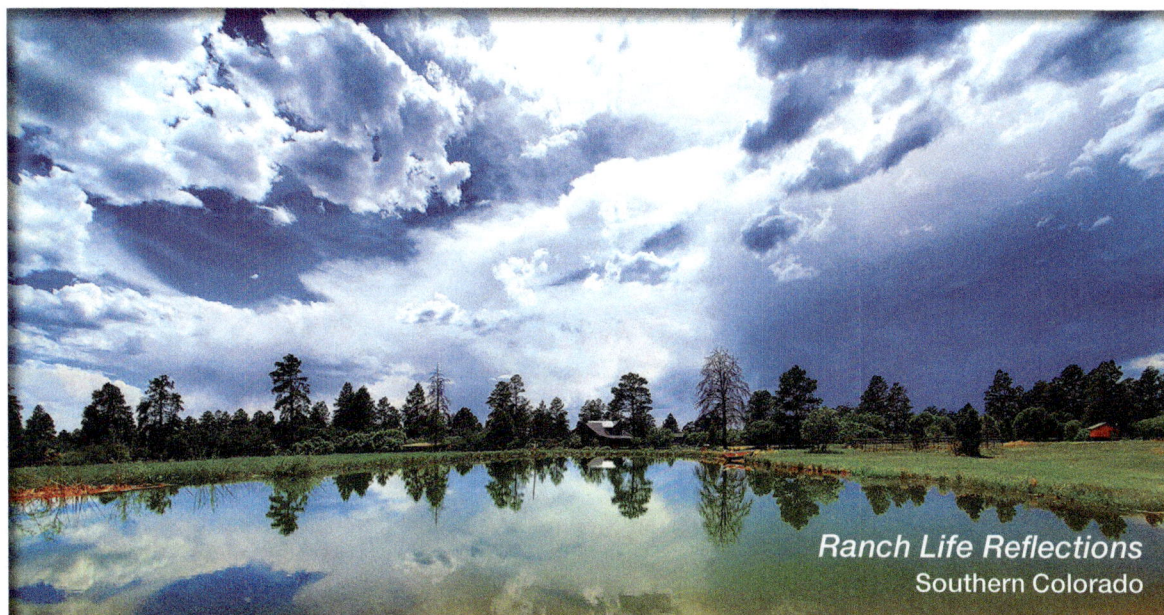

Ranch Life Reflections
Southern Colorado

The Monash University FODMAP Diet Smartphone APP

This app contains the largest database of FODMAP tested foods, additives, dietary supplements and Monash University Low FODMAP Diet™ certified food brands in the world, and so much more. It has been downloaded in over 130 countries, and proceeds from app sales support IBS research projects within the Department of Gastroenterology at Monash University. Following is a brief description of the tools and features offered.

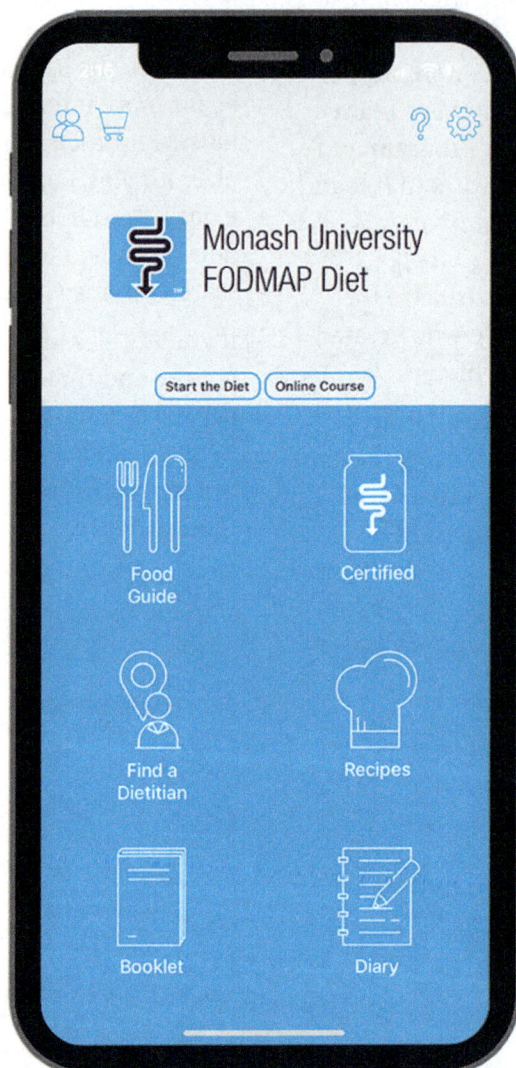

Please note: All tablespoon measurements in this cookbook are U.S. tablespoons that equal 3 teaspoons. Other countries such as Australia and the UK use 4 teaspoons per tablespoon.

When using the app, the tablespoon amount equals 4 teaspoons because Monash is located in Australia.

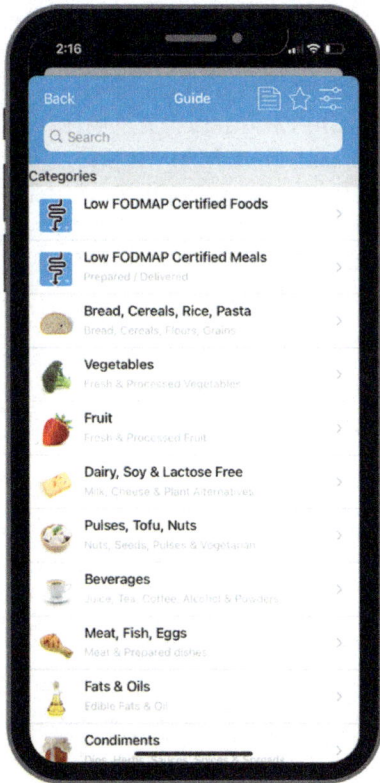

FOOD GUIDE

Continually updated with newly lab tested foods, the app lists foods using Green, Amber (Yellow) and Red traffic lights to indicate if they are Low, Moderate or High in FODMAPs at a particular serving size. You may enter a particular food in the search bar, or view by category: Vegetables, Fruit, Beverages, Condiments, Dairy, Soy & Lactose-Free, etc. This feature takes the guessing out of grocery shopping, and there are more features such as filters to set according to the step you are currently applying to your diet.

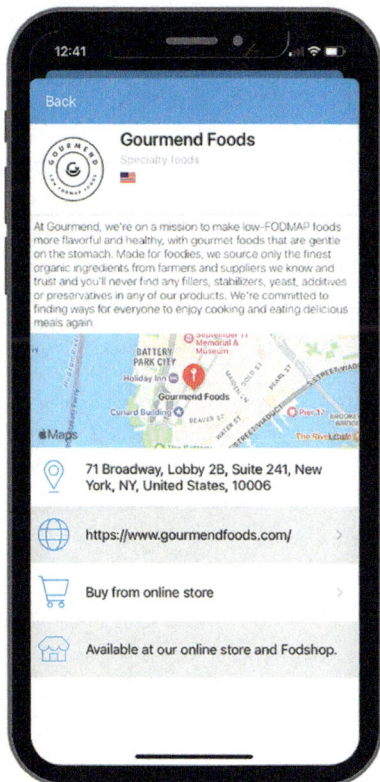

CERTIFIED

Here you will find food brand products that have met the qualifications for low FODMAP certification, and their product's packaging has been approved to display the Monash FODMAP certified logo:

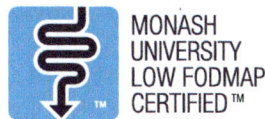

MONASH UNIVERSITY LOW FODMAP CERTIFIED™

Along with company descriptions and where to find their products, links to online shops are listed (when available). This is particularly helpful in introducing new brands to try when you are searching for swaps.

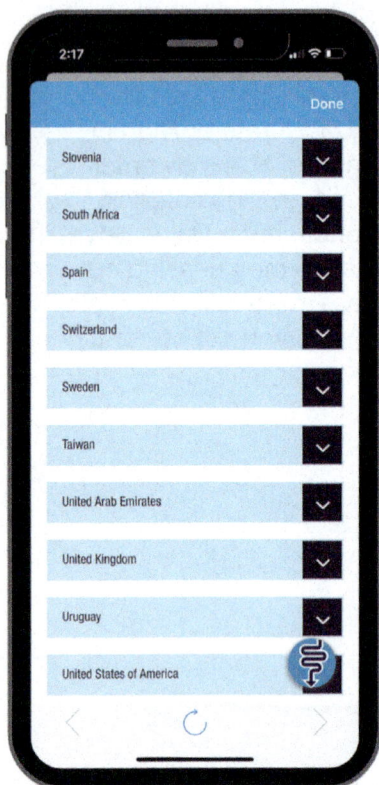

FIND A DIETICIAN

From the get go, it is much easier to follow the three-step program when working with a knowledgeable dietitian. All dietitians listed in this feature are Monash FODMAP trained and have passed the Monash FODMAP online course for dietitians. They are listed by country with email and phone number contact information. At the writing of this cookbook there were over 800 dietitians listed in 51 countries.

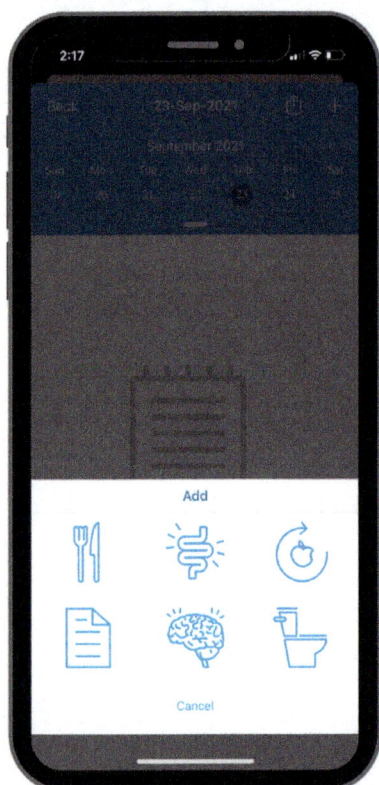

DIARY

The Diary is a helpful tool for day-by-day tracking of your meals, IBS symptoms and discomfort levels, personal notes, rating your stress level, and consistency of bowel movements. Think of it as your food and mood journal app with reports that summarize your progress. The Diary is also a valuable feature for the reintroduction step, allowing you to track the type of FODMAP you want to reintroduce (Lactose, Fructose, etc.) with suggested food options. serving sizes, and your digestive reactions

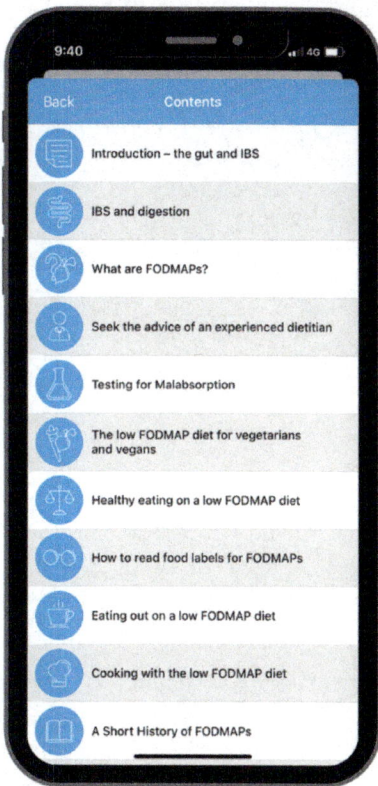

BOOKLET

This is the official Monash University Low FODMAP Diet™ Guide booklet outlining what the diet is all about with clear-cut explanations of: what IBS is, how FODMAPs affect your gut, food recommendations for vegetarians and vegans, cooking and dining out tips, how to read food labels, and more. In the palm of your hand you have the key to better gut health and the science behind it.

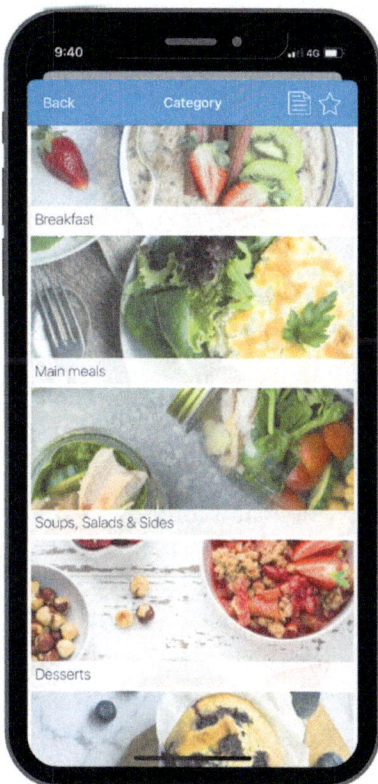

RECIPES

When you're not sure what to cook or are looking for new ideas, this feature offers a delicious collection of low FODMAP recipes with easy to follow ingredient lists and steps. The categories are: Breakfast, Main Meals, Soups, Salads, Sides, Desserts, Snacks, Basic Recipes (vinaigrettes, white sauce, flour mix), and Vegetarian meals. The strawberry icon gives nutrition info for each recipe, you can write and save notes about your GI and palate experiences, and the star icon helps to track and easily access your favorites.

For the complete app explanation, visit
monashfodmap.com
or the Monash FODMAP YouTube channel tutorials.

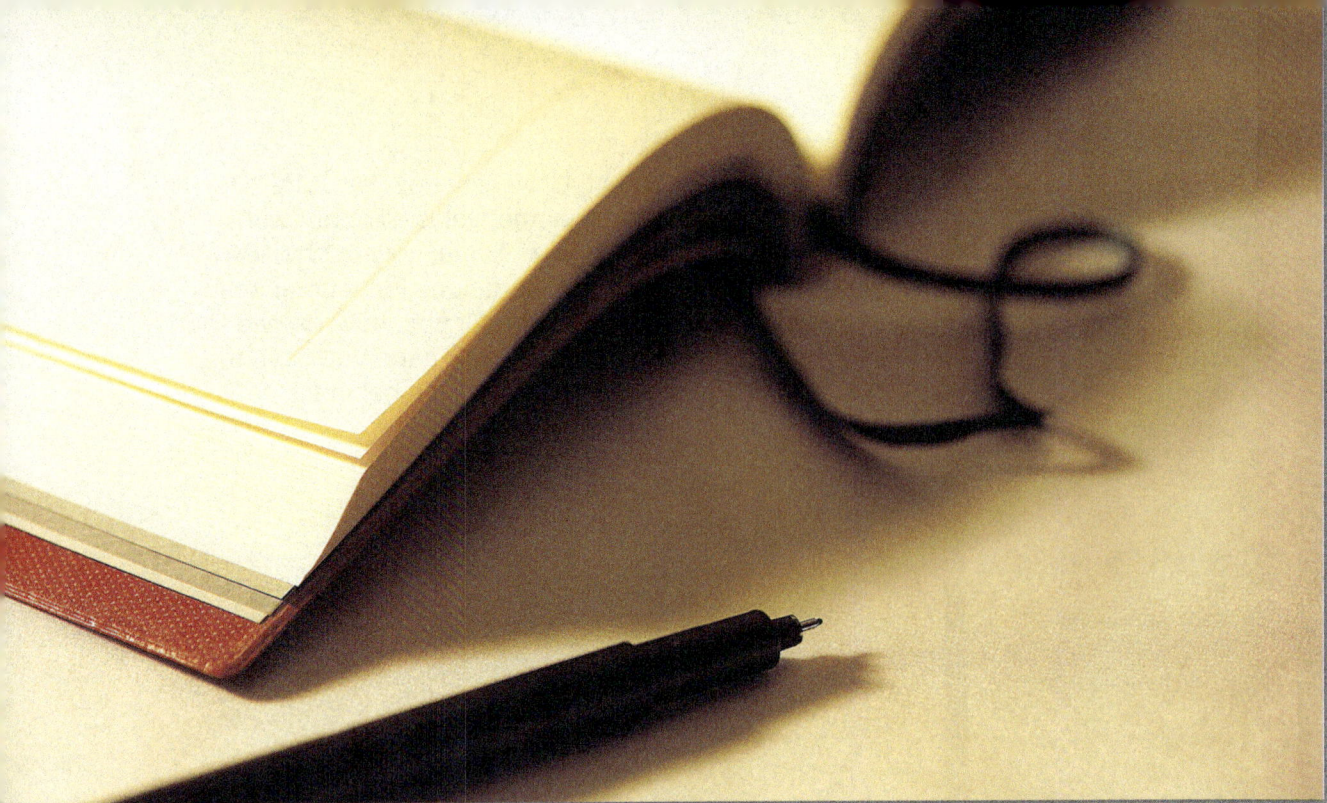

Food & Mood Journal

Have I swapped green tea in place of coffee and how did that go? How are my sleep patterns affecting my digestion? Was I okay with that sweet dairy-free flan and caramel? What helps most after a flare-up? How did reintroducing more avocado to my diet go? This is a lot of information to remember.

Keeping a Food & Mood Journal is a simple way of tracking what you're eating, how you're feeling physically and mentally throughout the day, and digestive reactions. It is also a fantastic reference document to have to show your dietitian, if and when you work with one (which I do highly recommend).

This is how it works:

WHAT I ATE

Record at what time and all of the ingredients you've consumed. Rather than logging in that you had a salad, it's best to list the individual ingredients so you will be able to track what is irritating and what is calming for your tummy. For example, when I FODified my beef chili recipe it worked very well to calm my symptoms. One day I lost count of the recommended amount of pure red chile powder per serving I'd added to the pot and within a few hours after Chili Night the result was a bad flare-up. In looking at my journal, the only possibility was the excess chile powder as all of the other foods from the previous 3 days were low FODMAP proper amounts.

HOW I FEEL PHYSICALLY

Note how you feel physically and in as much detail as best you can. Are you energized or tired from lack of sleep? Do you feel bloated or have abdominal pain? Do you have heartburn or a growling stomach? Did you have a relaxing 45 minute nature walk?

HOW I FEEL MENTALLY

It's a huge help to include why you are feeling this way or that, because our emotions, stress and anxiety play a big part in our digestive health. In this column go notes such as: busy day but feeling great, tired but good, anxiety about tomorrow's work schedule, canceled plans and need to rest tonight, dining out anxiety - my taco plate may have contained gluten, feeling organized, frustrated with a project, best vacay day ever, no time to eat lunch, making great progress with LoFO.

BM/DIGESTION NOTES

With each BM (bowel movement) note the time and result. If it's normal, give yourself a star. If there is diarrhea or constipation, circle it for easy reference that you've had a reaction to something. (Refer to the **monashfodmap.com** blog: What's Normal Bristol Stool Chart).

Also make note of any digestive pain, cramping or discomfort on a scale of 1 (mild) to 10 (severe). When there are changes such as uncomfortable bloating, gas or a flare-up, you'll begin to see a pattern and identify the culprit.

Keeping notes at the bottom of each page are a quick reference for foods and moods to look for, reminders such as to chew your food slowly and not rush, sources of anxiety, and those soothing days when your digestion is happy and you've tracked exactly what foods and moods gave you relief.

If you miss a day or two of food journaling or can't remember exactly what you had for breakfast, it's okay. Don't stress over it. Just write as many details as you can remember and then pick up the tracking again. During a flare when you're not feeling well and are most likely in pain and exhausted, it's more important than ever to log in your foods and moods so you'll know what contributed to it. But really, just do your best and give as many specifics as you can. It can be tedious at times, but stick with it. When you feel relief and calmer digestion, the hopefulness and encouragement that it's working will keep you motivated. And your tummy will thank you.

On the next two pages, I have chosen two entries from my food journal – one as an example of a good day and the other tracks a difficult day with things that factored into a flare-up. You will notice that some foods do not note an amount, in which case I knew it was within a proper LoFO serving. Make notes of serving amounts whenever you can, and instances in which you venture into moderate to high FODMAP amounts need to be noted because they are particularly helpful in the Reintroduction Phase.

"The day I began to think of food as medicine, I'd found my words to eat by."
Amy Laura

FOOD & MOOD JOURNAL

(example: on a good day)

DATE **Jun. 14** DAY **Mon.**

TIME	WHAT I ATE	HOW I FEEL PHYSICALLY	HOW I FEEL MENTALLY	BM / DIGESTION
BREAKFAST 9:30	salsa: cilantro, lime, tomato, scallion greens, 1/4 t. cumin, 1/8 avo, 1 egg, 2 corn tortilla, peppermint tea	good sleep, good energy level	10 min. meditation, feel good, very present	10:00 —normal —pain Ø ✗
SNACK 11:30	sm. just-ripe banana, (green tea) 1 cup		need a little (caffeine)	
LUNCH 1:30	cornmeal meatloaf w/ bokchoy + carrots, lettuce, tomato, oil + vinegar, G-free roll	good — nice walk after lunch	good	
SNACK 4:30	lactose-free yogurt, 2 t. pecans, 1 t. maple syrup		good	
DINNER 7:30	Turkey, arugula, zucchini, carrots, 1/2 c. quinoa, 1/8 cup chopped green chile, 1 radish, oil + vinegar, grapes	good — play time w/ the pups	tired - busy day but overall good	
SNACK 10:00	ginger tea, 2 LoFo gluten-free cookies			

Notes: - swapping green tea for coffee is calming, working.
- try adding corn to salads / re-introduction.
- keep chewing slowly

FOOD & MOOD JOURNAL

DATE **Dec. 8** DAY **Tues.** *(example: on a bad day)*

TIME	WHAT I ATE	HOW I FEEL PHYSICALLY	HOW I FEEL MENTALLY	BM / DIGESTION
BREAKFAST 7:00	1 cup LoFo cereal, strawberries, plain almond milk, Peppermint tea	restless sleep — got @ 4 hours	tired, wanting coffee — some brain fog	9:30 — soft — Pain 0
SNACK 10:00	sm. just-ripe banana	abdominal cramps, pain 2	want caffeine, not drinking it.	— Pain 2 ✗
LUNCH	∅	shoulder phys. therapy, getting stronger, some Pain 2	busy day, probs concentrating on billing	12:00 — Pain 2 ✗
SNACK 4:15	carrot hummus, 6 rice crackers, water	stomach empty, growling	frustrated	
DINNER 6:00 ↓ on	chicken tortilla soup — mostly broth, cilantro, tomato, Peppermint tea	abdominal cramping, bloating, exhausted	canceled plans, need to stay in and rest	5:00 — flare-up ✗ — pain 4–5
SNACK	Peppermint oil Pills, lots of water			

Notes: lack of sleep, busy day, pain, flare-up, stomach empty not good, forgot to meditate, skipped lunch. Go strict 'LoFo for 2 days. This will pass! ♥

FOOD & MOOD JOURNAL

DATE _____ DAY _____

TIME	WHAT I ATE	HOW I FEEL PHYSICALLY	HOW I FEEL MENTALLY	BM / DIGESTION
BREAKFAST				
SNACK				
LUNCH				
SNACK				
DINNER				
SNACK				

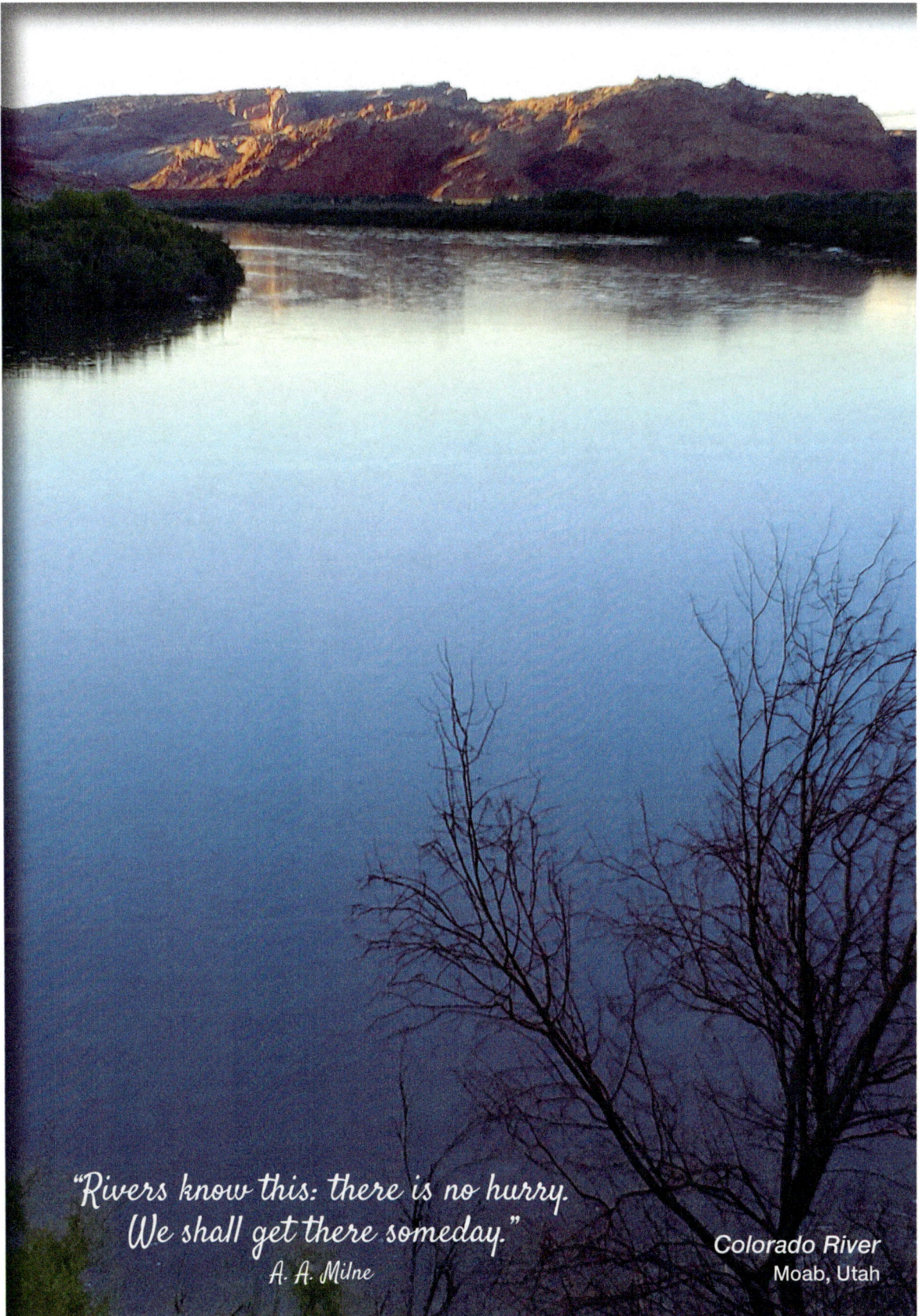

"Rivers know this: there is no hurry.
We shall get there someday."
A. A. Milne

Colorado River
Moab, Utah

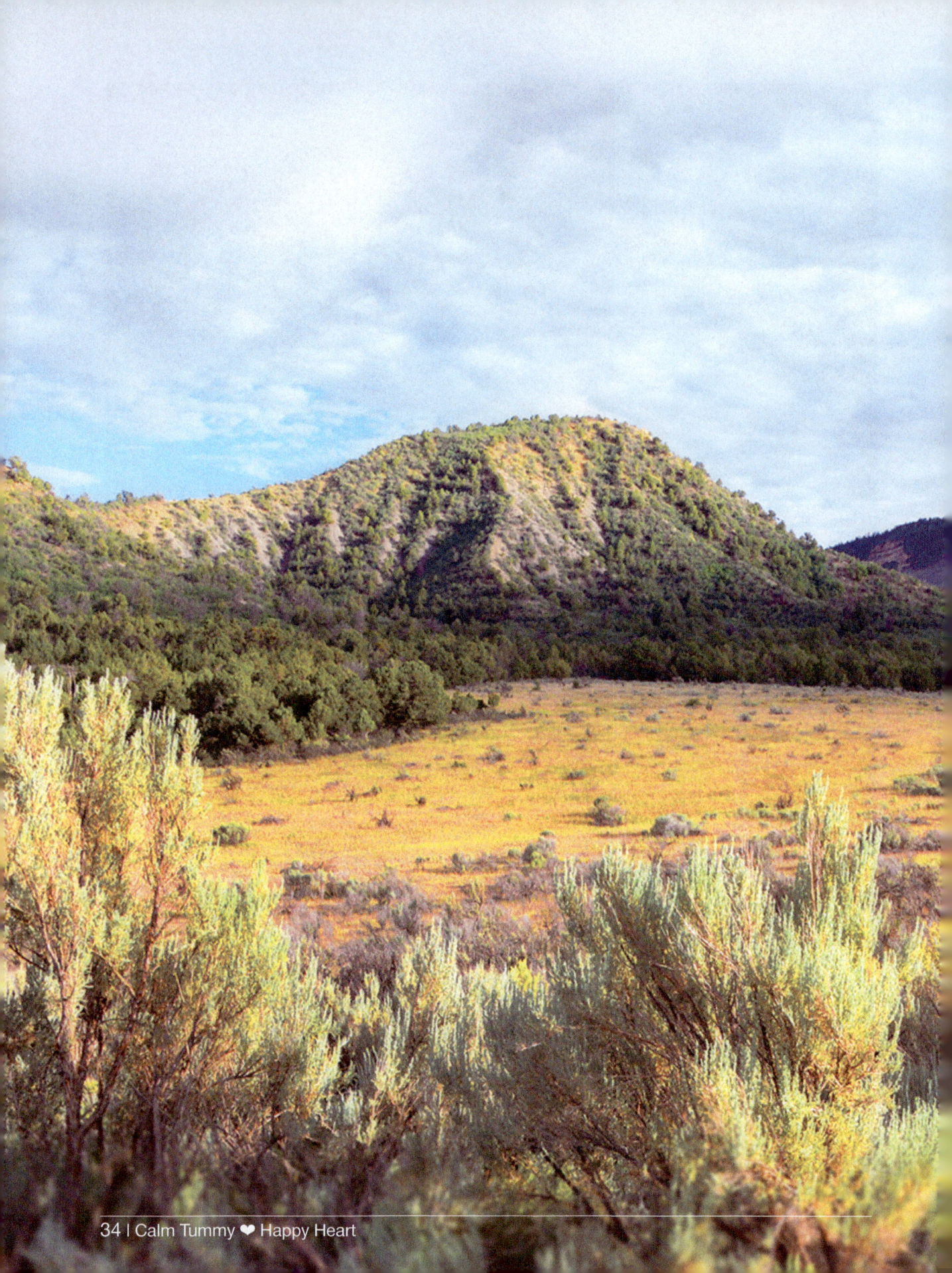

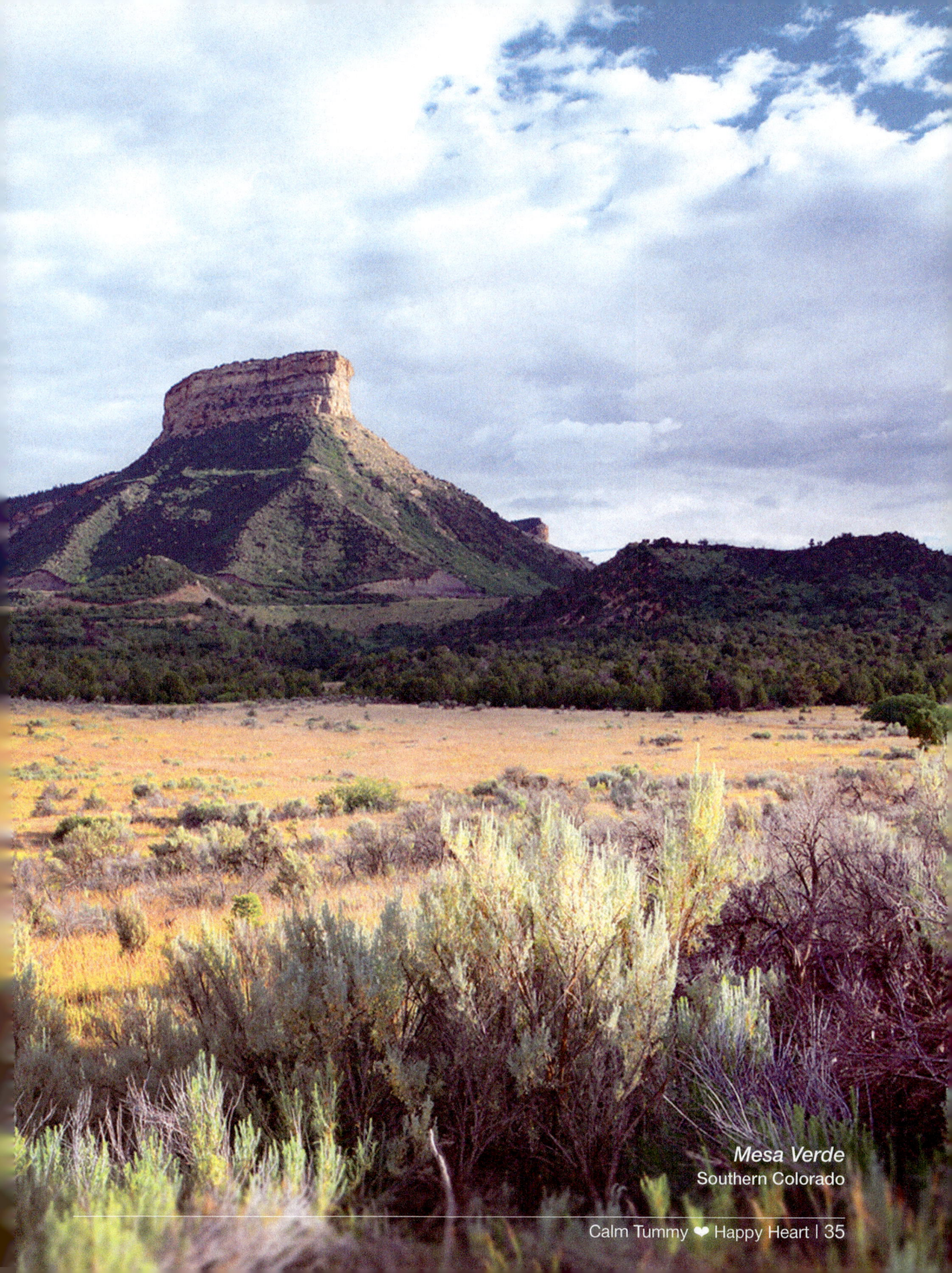

Mesa Verde
Southern Colorado

Always In My Fridge

These are must-have ingredients I use all the time for whipping up delicious frittatas, tacos, scrambled eggs with salsa, salads, snacking and so much more.

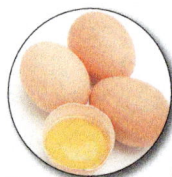
Eggs

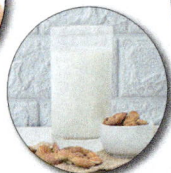
Plain Unsweetened Almond Milk

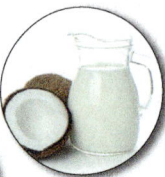
Canned Full-fat Coconut Milk, for Cooking

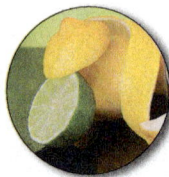
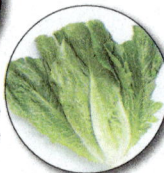
Lemons and Limes

Romaine Lettuce

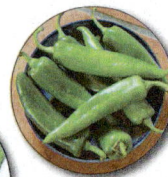
Green Chiles

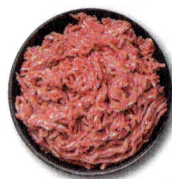
Grass Fed Ground Beef

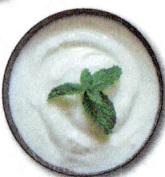
Plain, dairy-free unsweetened coconut yogurt

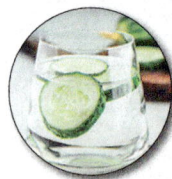
Cucumber Water

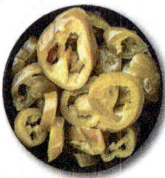
Pickled Jalapeños

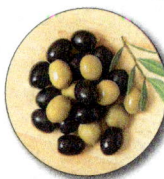
Black and Spanish Olives

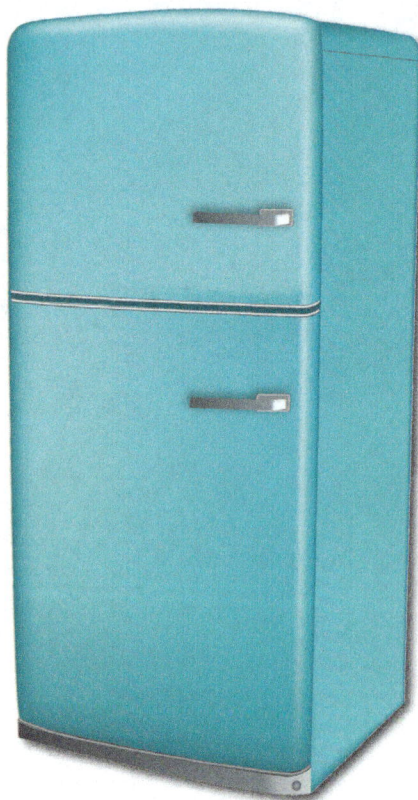

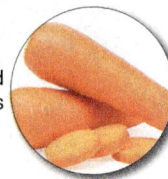
Blanched Carrots

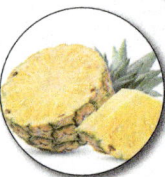
Pineapple

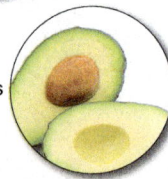
Avocados

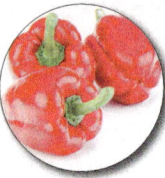
Red Bell Peppers

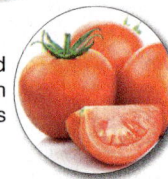
Plum and Common Tomatoes

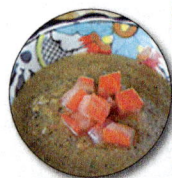
Shredded Chicken

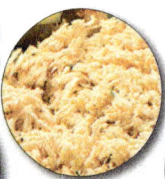
Homemade Salsa

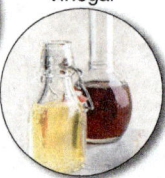
Olive Oil and Red Wine Vinegar

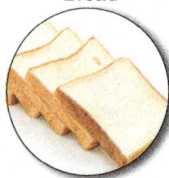
LoFO Gluten-Free Bread

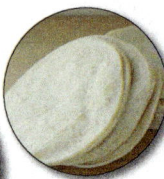
Homemade Chicken Broth

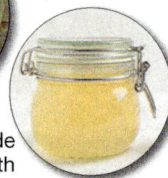
LoFO Gluten-Free Corn Tortillas

Please refer to the Monash University FODMAP Diet Smartphone App for serving size information.

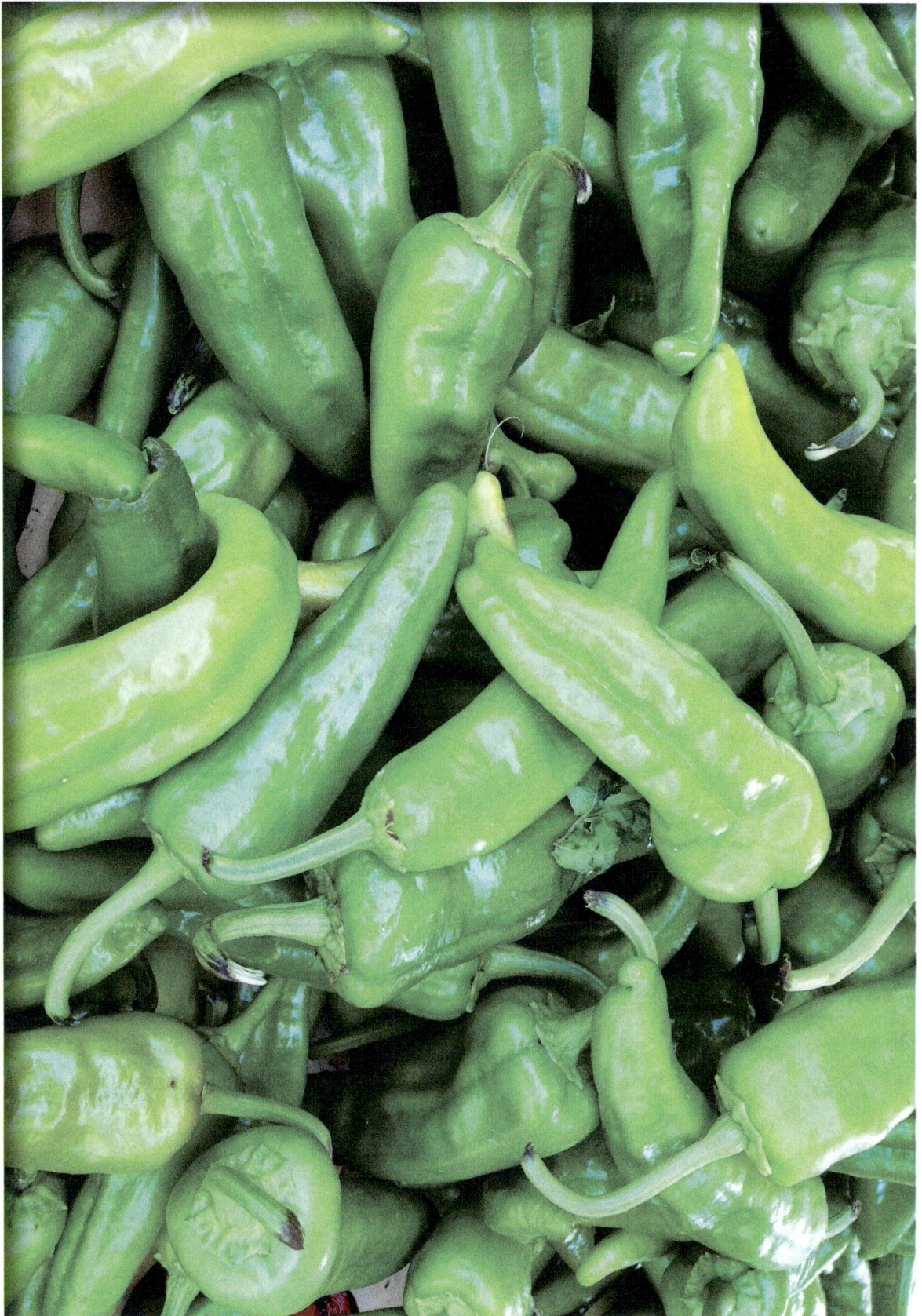

Notes To The Cook

The following notes offer helpful information about measurements, ingredients, kitchen equipment, dairy, gluten-free, soy and tips to help you navigate this cookbook and prepare your pantry and fridge for low FODMAP cooking with great results.

The Low FODMAP Diet is neither dairy-free, nor gluten-free, however this book is based upon how I cook according to my sensitivities. I have included dairy-free and gluten-free notes, with some conventional dairy options (found under Tips at the end of recipes), so that you can make choices depending on your own needs.

When I started the diet and my symptoms began to ease up, I gradually added more LoFO ingredients to my pantry and fridge. Don't feel that you have to give or throw away your HiFO foods. Freeze and keep what you can to serve to family and friends who have no food intolerances, or save them for when you begin the Reintroduction Phase.

MEASUREMENTS
When setting out to convert my recipes into LoFO, I was reminded that the United States is one of only three countries that use the Imperial / U.S. Standard system of weights and measurements. Thanks to my new kitchen scale, Metric measurements are listed beside Imperial. If you are working on a cookbook and live in the United States I would like to offer the suggestion to add Metric measurements to make it easier for everyone else!

CUPS
In many parts of the world, the U.S. cup is smaller. Also, cup Metric amounts vary. 1 cup of granulated sugar weighs 200 g while 1 cup of confectioners' powdered sugar is 100 g. This is why every ingredient listed in this cookbook has been weighed.

TABLESPOONS
All tablespoon measurements in this book are U.S. tablespoons that equal 3 teaspoons. Other countries such as Australia and the UK use 4 teaspoons per tablespoon.

When using the Monash University FODMAP Diet Smartphone App, the tablespoon amount is 4 teaspoons because Monash is located in Australia.

LARGE EGGS
Unless otherwise noted in the recipe, all eggs are size large.

A PINCH
A pinch equals 1/16 teaspoon.

SALT
All salt called for in this book is fine sea salt. This is because when I was in school and began to cook in mom and pop made-from-scratch cafes, I was taught to use fine sea salt because it is not highly processed and contains some minerals. 1 teaspoon = 5 g. Kosher and other salts differ in weights, so you will want to measure the same 5 gram weight, along with increments (1/2 and 1/4 teaspoon) accordingly.

ABOUT DAIRY
Low FODMAP is not a dairy-free plan. Many people who suffer from IBS experience zero to slight digestive issues with lactose or casein in dairy products. Others find that conventional dairy can be a trigger and you will discover your own

sensitivities through your Food + Mood Journal. When starting out, the LoFO plan assumes that you will begin with lactose-free LoFO servings of dairy.

My experience was to remove all dairy during the Elimination Phase and slowly add back cheeses and products that contain only trace amounts of lactose. Still, it didn't settle well with my tummy and took many attempts for me to tolerate small amounts. In time, I discovered that my IBS symptoms are oftentimes fine with proper amounts of lactose-free milk, sour cream, cream cheese and cottage cheese. However, my food program remains primarily dairy-free. That's my comfort zone at the moment. I know people with IBS who are able to eat an entire scoop of cow's milk ice cream and this gives me hope!

All recipes in this book are dairy-free within the body of the recipe. For those who are able to tolerate lactose-free and conventional dairy, suggestions with amounts are given in the TIPS section at the bottom of those recipes.

LOFO DAIRY SWAPS
Following are swaps for conventional dairy products, per your tolerance. Please bear in mind that lactose-free can contain dairy.

Cow's Milk: My go-to combination for cooking is plain unsweetened almond milk mixed with canned full-fat coconut milk for cooking, containing no inulin.

Coconut Milk: Give canned full-fat coconut milk, containing no inulin, a good stir before measuring to combine the milk and cream, which rises to the top.

Butter: Butter contains only trace amounts of lactose. I use vegan butter alternative sticks that are a non-GMO vegan vegetable oil combination with water, salt, natural

flavor, pea protein, sunflower lecithin, lactic acid and annatto extract for color. Ghee, a clarified butter with trace amounts of lactose, is another option.

Sour Cream: Lactose-free sour cream, dairy-free sour cream (although not all plant-based sour cream is LoFO), lactose-free yogurt or plain, dairy-free unsweetened coconut yogurt.

Cream Cheese: Lactose-free cream cheese or LoFO plant-based dairy-free cream cheese, (note: plant-based results in a thinner consistency when making things like cake icing).

Cheeses: The Low FODMAP Diet is not dairy-free, but it is lower in lactose. I was very surprised to learn that many cheeses like Monterey Jack and cheddar are low FODMAP in proper serving amounts. That said, for me personally, I continue to eat mainly dairy-free, but have given dairy options in several recipes. Some plant-based cheeses are LoFO, but not all; you have to be an educated label reader. In addition, plant-based cheeses will bring their own flavors and ability (or not) to melt, so you might have to go through some trial and error. Adding nutritional yeast to sauces such as béchamel (page 65), to eggs and frittatas adds a cheesy flavor.

For brands and products I use, please visit the **fodifyit.com** Foods and Brands We Love on our online shop.

NOT ALL GLUTEN-FREE IS LOW FODMAP
Reading labels is the way to go when searching for gluten-free products that are also LoFO. For example, a gluten-free coffee cake may contain cherries, apple juice and dried fruits that may cause a flare-up.

The Monash FODMAP website and app offer several postings on how to select low FODMAP servings of breads, pastas and gluten-free foods. Gluten-free swaps I use are: low FODMAP rice flour blend breads, corn tortillas, rice flour based pastas, Monash certified breads, and cornbread made with LoFO flours and cornmeal.

Some high FODMAP flours are: wheat, coconut, rye, amaranth, barley and almond meal. LoFO gluten-free swaps are: rice flour, brown rice flour, cornmeal, quinoa flour, potato and tapioca starch, and even small servings of almond meal! The Low FODMAP Diet is very much about serving size. For an extensive explanation see Choosing Low FODMAP Flours (page 55).

If you are gluten-free or have Celiac Disease, more item labels to check are: cornbread mixes, cornstarch, certain vinegars and candy, canned soups and sauces.

If you are Celiac, always check labels for products that may have been processed in a facility where cross-contamination is possible.

ABOUT SOY

Monashfodmap.com posts information describing high and low FODMAP serving sizes of soy products. They have also written articles on Vegan Guides – How To Get Enough Protein and Being Vegan on a Low FODMAP Diet. A few notes on soy to keep in mind are:

Edamame is LoFO in servings of 1/2 cup (90 g) and is appropriate for the Elimination Phase.

Soy Sauce: Generally contains small amounts of wheat and is LoFO in 2 tablespoon servings. Several gluten-free soy sauce brands are available in U.S. markets.

Tofu: In the U.S. Firm and Extra Firm is LoFO while Silken tofu contains higher amounts of FODMAPs. In Australia, both Firm and Plain are LoFO.

Tempeh: is made from fermented whole soy beans and is LoFO as long as it is not made with any HiFO ingredients.

Soy Milk: LoFO if made from soy protein isolate, while soy milk made from whole soy beans is HiFO.

MORE LOFO PANTRY ITEMS

Burrito Wraps: LoFO gluten-free burrito wraps are improving, with more options all the time. I prefer a brown rice flour wrap with tapioca flour, safflower oil, rice bran, xanthan gum and sea salt. Ingredients to avoid; wheat flour or HiFO flours, inulin, honey and any HiFO spices.

Chicken Stock: There is something so comforting about having containers of homemade LoFO Chicken Stock (page 135) in the freezer. Most store-bought stocks (and broths) contain high FODMAP ingredients, onion and garlic in particular, so it's a good idea to have LoFO brands or homemade on hand to thaw as you need it.

One of my favorite recipes is Whole Poached Chicken (page 82) because it yields approx. 2 1/2 – 3 cups (375 - 450 g) of shredded chicken meat and 8 cups (2 L) of stock.

Corn Tortillas and Taco Shells: Store-bought corn tortillas and shells are naturally gluten-free, unless otherwise indicated on the package. Monash has tested those with both added gums and without and both have LoFO servings. For hard shell tacos, I prefer the sturdier flat bottom type.

Cornmeal: When listed in this book means low FODMAP medium grind whole grain yellow cornmeal.

Cornmeal Mix: Mixes vary. The one I use contains: whole grain cornmeal, potato starch, whole grain sorghum flour, cane sugar, whole grain corn flour, tapioca flour, baking powder (baking soda, cornstarch, monocalcium phosphate), fine sea salt and xanthan gum. (For more information on brands we love go to: **fodifyit.com**).

Green Chiles, Fresh and Canned: Canned brands have added salt or none at all, so it's best to taste before adding salt to your recipe. You want mild plain green chiles, chopped or whole, and be sure to check the label for any added onion or garlic. Hot and Medium Hot green chiles have not been tested at the time of this writing.

For information on fresh chiles, please refer to page 44 for identifying them with notes on flavors, and which have inedible skins that require roasting and prepping.

Masa Harina: Masa harina, corn flour and cornmeal are not the same things. Masa is corn that has been cooked with alkaline (nixtamalization) and when ground is smoother and more flavorful for making dough. Corn flour is ground corn that does not offer the same texture for tortillas and tamale dough.

Red Chile Powder: Chile powder and Chili powder look the same but are very different. See page 48 on how to read labels for HiFO seasoning ingredients.

Spices: Commonly used are: cayenne, pure chipotle powder, cinnamon, ground coriander, ground cumin, oregano, paprika, smoked paprika, pure mild red chile powder, and crushed red pepper flakes.

Sugars: White, brown and certain raw sugars are low FODMAP in proper portions. Piloncillo has not yet been tested, however, it is a non-processed brown cane sugar that you may find is not a trigger.

Tomatoes, Canned: My preferences are plain, whole peeled, diced or puréed, and organic when available.

VEGETABLE AND FRUIT SKINS

While sensitivity to the skins of certain vegetables and fruits are not a FODMAP issue, I feel that it's important to mention because I have this sensitivity. This is why you will notice recipe steps calling for blanching and peeling tomatoes, and roasting chiles and red bell peppers to remove the skins.

EQUIPMENT

Blender: Many recipes, particularly sauces, require a blender.

Citrus Squeezer: This is a must for getting the most juice out of your limes, lemons and oranges. If you microwave the citrus for 10 seconds before squeezing they will release even more juice.

Comal: A flat cast-iron griddle used for toasting tortillas. You can also use a stovetop griddle, nonstick or cast-iron skillet.

Dutch Oven: These sturdy, heavy pots are perfect for stocks, stews and braises. I also use mine to make chile hollandaise sauce. You can use the Dutch oven as the bottom of a double-boiler. Simply place a tight fitting bowl on top, fill the Dutch oven with water to below the bottom of the bowl, and use to melt chocolate (in the bowl). You can use this double-boiler for anything that needs gentle heating. A medium-size saucepan and metal mixing bowl that fits snugly into the pan will also work when water is brought to a boil just below the pan level.

Flan Mold: A mold designed for flans delivers a lovely presentation; a metal pie pan will work, as well.

Food Processor: For blending, slicing, and shredding recipes such as fiesta slaw.

Kitchen Scale: My measurements are more accurate when using a digital scale, particularly when weighing out even amounts of tortilla dough.

Mixer, Hand or Stand Mixer: Another kitchen must-have.

Skillet - Ovenproof & Nonstick: For countless recipes and finishing dishes in the oven like frittatas and steaks.

Soup Pot with Steamer Basket: A large soup or stock pot for making LoFO chicken stock and chili, and a steamer basket for cooking tamales.

Spatulas - Silicone & Wooden: For mixing and scraping down the sides of a bowl; a wooden spatula is great for browning and breaking up ground beef.

Tortilla Press: A 6 or 8-inch (15 cm to 20 cm) metal press for making homemade tortillas. You can also roll them with a rolling pin or flatten with the bottom of a saucepan, however they won't be as even.

Tortilla Warmer: For keeping tortillas soft and warm before serving, or for rolling into enchiladas and making tacos.

LoFO / HiFO

In this book you will find references to LoFO meaning Low FODMAP and HiFO meaning High FODMAP.

FOOD BRANDS WE LOVE

Please visit our website **fodifyit.com** for products that contain low FODMAP ingredients and can be found in most U.S. grocery stores or ordered online. Items that have been Monash certified are noted. We only list food and equipment brands that we continually use. Our selections are not based on advertising collaborations. In other words, if we don't love it, we don't recommend it.

Be sure to consult with your dietitian or the Monash University Low FODMAP Smartphone App for proper serving sizes.

NOTES: _____

_____

_____

_____

_____

_____

_____

_____

_____

_____

_____

_____

I love opening up the fridge. It's like a painter's palette of ingredients, and my creation will most likely be some sort of taco.

— Amy Laura

Identifying Chiles

POBLANOS **The chile meat of 1 medium poblano pepper will yield approx. 1/4 cup (45 g) of small chopped chile, after it has been roasted, with stem, skin and seeds removed.**

Dark green, shiny and heart-shaped, poblanos have a mild, deep herbaceous flavor. Their average length is 4.6 inches (11.7 cm). The skins are inedible and need to be peeled off, and the seeds also require removing (see page 46 for instructions). However, some sauce recipes call for leaving the skins on after charring, then puréeing in a blender and cooking in a pan – in which case, skins on are fine. Poblano chile meat is thicker than most chile varieties and hold their shape well for making rellenos (stuffed chile peppers).

GREEN CHILES **The chile meat of 1 medium green chile will yield approx. 2 tablespoons (23 g) of finely chopped chile, after it has been roasted, with stem, skin and seeds removed.**

Medium green in color, banana-shaped, with an earthy, herby buttery flavor, green chiles are known by names such as: Hatch, Anaheim, Colorado Green and Chiles Verde Del Norte, to name a few. Their average length is 5.5 inches (14 cm). At the writing of this cookbook, mild green chiles have been tested. They also come in medium, hot and extra hot heat levels. The skins are inedible (see page 46 for preparation steps).

JALAPEÑOS **A medium-sized jalapeño will yield approx. 1/4 cup (35 g) diced, after the stem, seeds and inner membrane have been removed.**

While known for their heat, some of these small, stout banana-shaped peppers are very mild. Medium green in color, they taste spicy, peppery and bright. Their average length is 3.4-inches (8.6 cm). The skins and seeds are edible, and the heat is mainly found in the seeds and pith (membrane).

SERRANOS **A medium-sized serrano will yield approx. 2 generous tablespoons (20 g) diced, after the stem, seeds and membrane have been removed.**

Shaped like thin Jalapeños, these peppers pack more heat than a Jalapeño and are generally fiery, peppery and snappy in flavor. Depending on the region or country, they average 3 inches (7.6 cm) in length. The skins and seeds are edible. For less heat, remove the seeds and pith (membrane) before cooking.

RED HABANEROS **A medium-sized habanero will yield approx. 1 tablespoon (3 teaspoons) (8 g) diced, after the stem, seeds and inner membrane have been removed.**

Unripe Habaneros are green and turn red and hotter as they mature. They are one of the most scorching peppers in the world with a blazing, fruity flavor. Their average length is 1.5 inches (3.8 cm). The skins and seeds are edible. The heat may be toned down by removing the seeds and inner ribbing, however, you will still feel the burn. Habaneros add delicious flavor and heat to rice, jams, stews, salsas and numerous other dishes.

CANNED GREEN CHILES **1, 4-ounce can of chopped green chiles yields: 1/2 cup (113 g) including the can juices, and 1/3 cup (70 g) when drained.**

Monash Note: Although chiles (chillies) are generally low in FODMAPs, some people with IBS may be sensitive to the capsaicin they contain. Capsaicin is a natural compound that gives chiles their spicy quality. You may need to limit how much chile you eat if your IBS symptoms are triggered by spicy food.

Varieties of Chiles

POBLANO

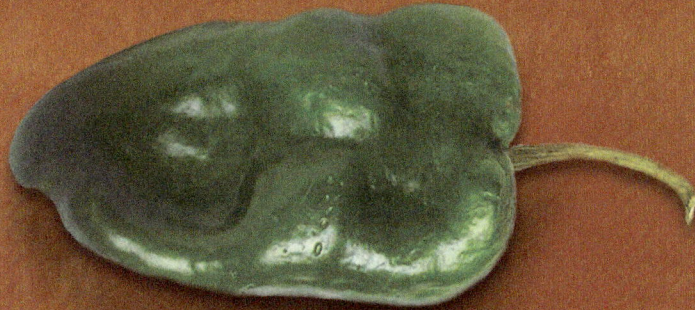

GREEN CHILE

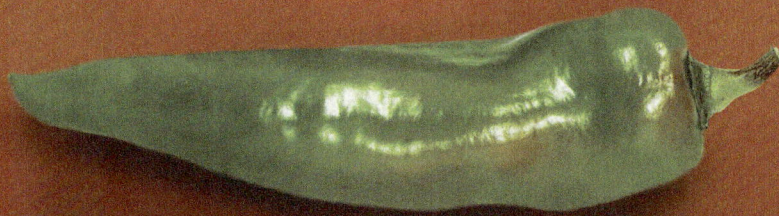

JALAPEÑO

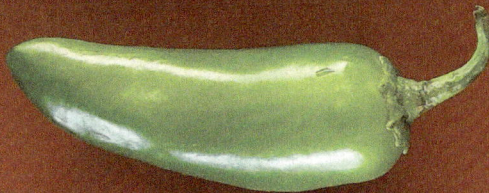

SERRANO

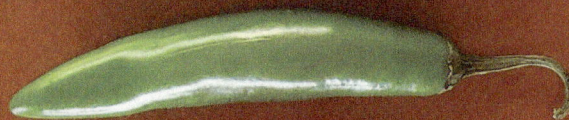

RED HABANERO

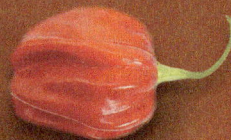

Chile sizes vary per region and country. Check the Monash University FODMAP Diet Smartphone App for proper serving amounts.

How To Roast and Prep Green Chiles

Green chiles go by names like: Hatch, Anaheim, New Mexican, Colorado Green and Chiles Verde Del Norte to name a few. They are about the shape and size of a banana, an average green chile is 5.5 inches long (14 cm), and the flavor is a unique combination of earthy, herbaceous, buttery pepper. The skins are tough and inedible so you'll need to roast and steam them first to peel away the skins from the chile meat. Also, roasting the chiles enhances their delicious flavor. The steps are easy and your kitchen will smell like August-September chile roasting season in the Southwest. This method also works in removing the skins from poblanos, bell peppers and tomatoes.

1. Wash the chiles under cool water.

2. Char roast them over medium high heat using your bbq grill, stovetop gas burner, electric burner using a stovetop grill, or in your oven broiler on a rimmed baking sheet.

3. Turn them with metal tongs until all sides are blistered and charred, but not burnt. A little green should still show through. This step usually takes 7 to 10 minutes.

4. Use tongs to place them in a bowl, then cover with a clean, heavy kitchen towel, plastic wrap or a heavy plate. Allow to steam for at least 30 minutes. This loosens the skins from the chile meat. You can also put them in a sealed plastic baggie.

5. Place them on a cutting board.

6. Peel off the skins with your hands. Always use gloves and don't touch your face or eyes because oils from the chiles can sting. Rub and peel off as much of the loosened skins as possible. Experienced chile cooks discourage running them under water because you lose some of the char flavor. But if you happen to have a stubborn chile, use a paper towel to scrub it a bit and run under cool water if needed.

7. Cut off the stems and discard. (Unless you are making chiles rellenos, in which case leave the stems intact).

8. Slice the chiles in half lengthwise and use a knife to scrape away the seeds.

9. You now have beautiful fillets to chop or slice according to your recipe.

10. For rellenos you want the chiles to hold together for stuffing. Once you've removed the skins, leave the stems on, then make a gentle clean cut lengthwise along the side leaving 1/2-inch intact on the top and bottom of the chile. This creates a pocket for your fillings. Use your hands to gently scoop out the seeds. Photographed is a poblano (left) and green chile (right).

11. Give yourself a round of applause – you are now an official chile roasting expert!

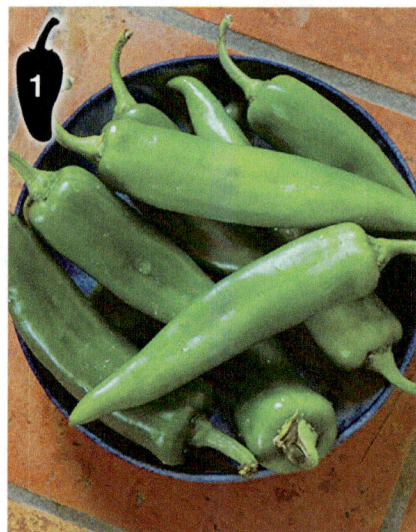

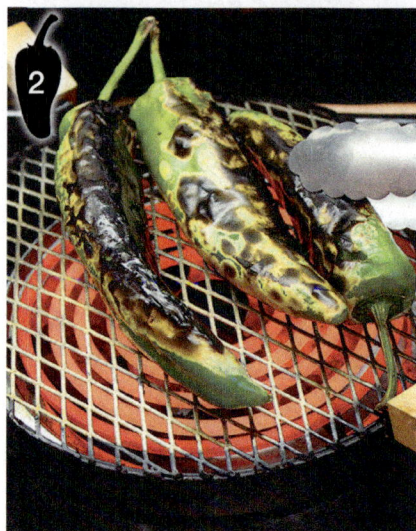

Monash Note: Although chiles (chillies) are generally low in FODMAPs, some people with IBS may be sensitive to the capsaicin they contain. Capsaicin is a natural compound that gives chiles their spicy quality. You may need to limit how much chile you eat if your IBS symptoms are triggered by spicy food.

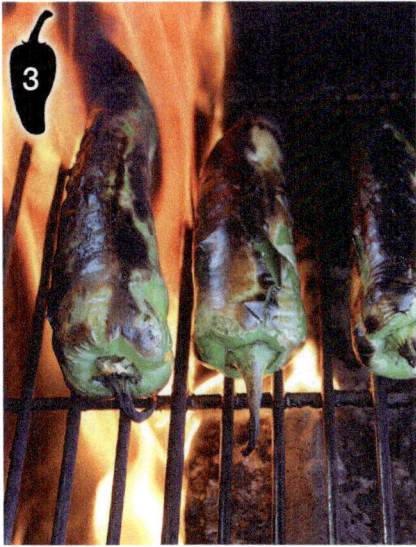

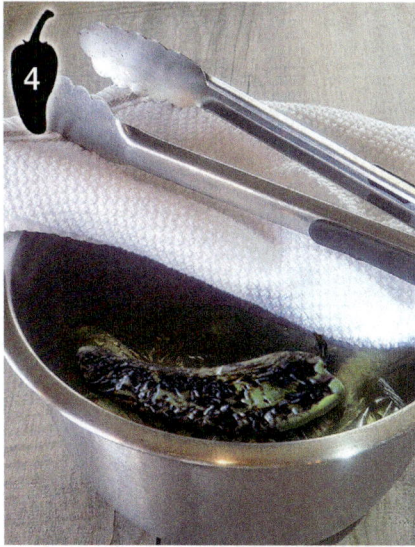

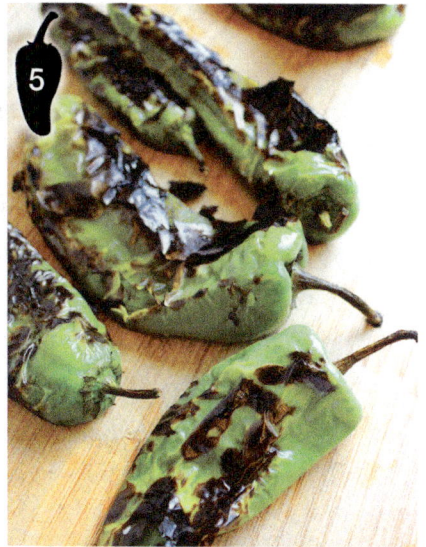

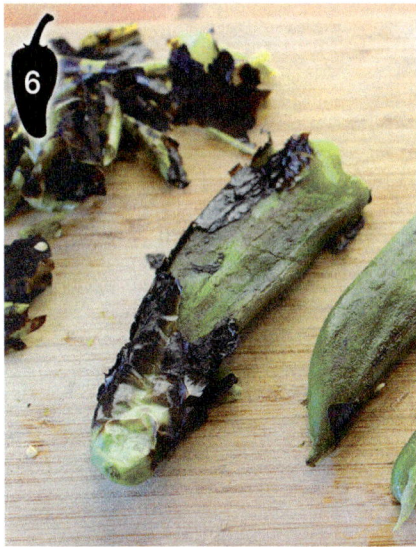

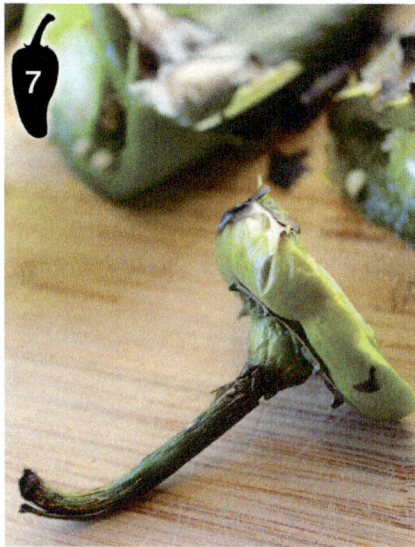

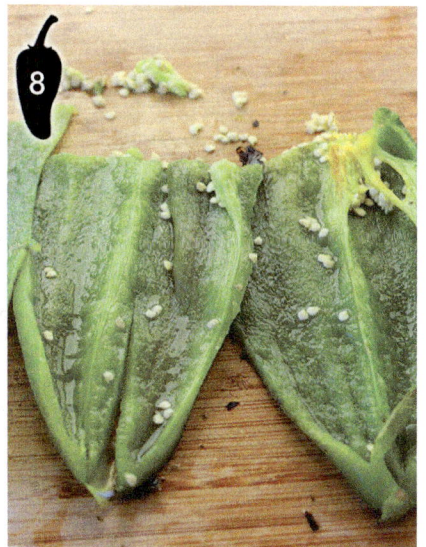

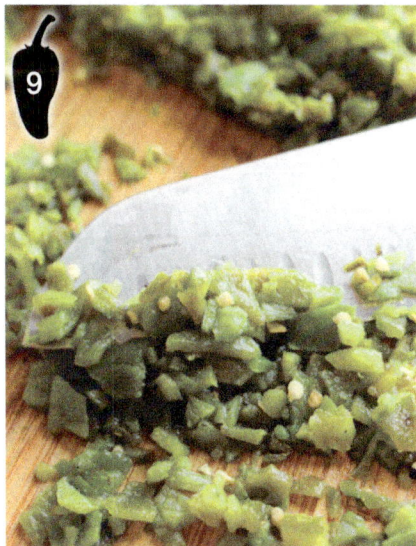

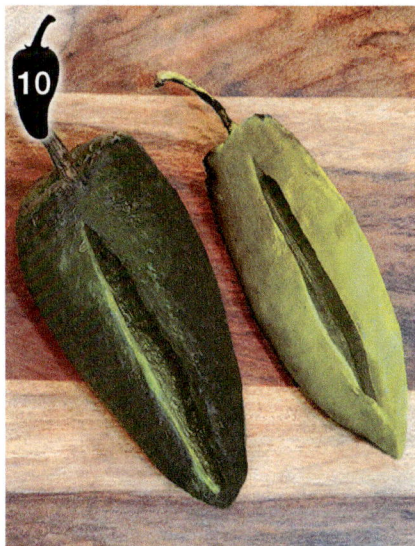

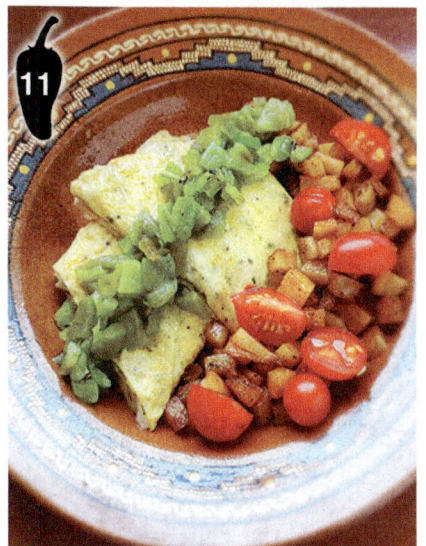

Chile Powder vs Chili Powder

They look the same. The packaging is similar. But there's a big difference for the LoFO cook. They are also not interchangeable in recipes.

CHILE POWDER In the U.S. and particularly in the Southwest, chile powder with an 'e' is ground pure red chiles with no garlic, onion or other HiFO seasonings. The label should read: ground red chile, red chile or chiles rojo enteros. 1 teaspoon (2 g) is a LoFO serving.

CHILI POWDER In the U.S., chili powder with an 'i' is a mixture of pure red chile powder and other seasonings – similar to taco or fajita seasoning. It most likely has onion and garlic powder that can trigger an upset. So read those labels!

That said, I bought Chili Powder with an 'i' at a market in Texas and it was pure red chile powder with no added seasonings. So again, it's always a good idea to read the label for ingredients, as the 'e' vs. 'i' can change from region to region, state to state.

Here is my favorite blended red chile powder mix to use with 1 pound (454 g) ground beef.

LOW FODMAP TACO SEASONING MIX
8 SERVINGS

1 tablespoon (6 g) ground cumin

2 teaspoons (4 g) pure mild red chile powder (containing no onion or garlic, the ingredients should list only: red chile. On the Monash App this is called Chilli (chili) red, powdered)

2 teaspoons (4 g) smoked paprika, or plain paprika

1 teaspoon dried oregano

1/2 teaspoon (2.5 g) fine sea salt

1/2 teaspoon fresh ground black pepper

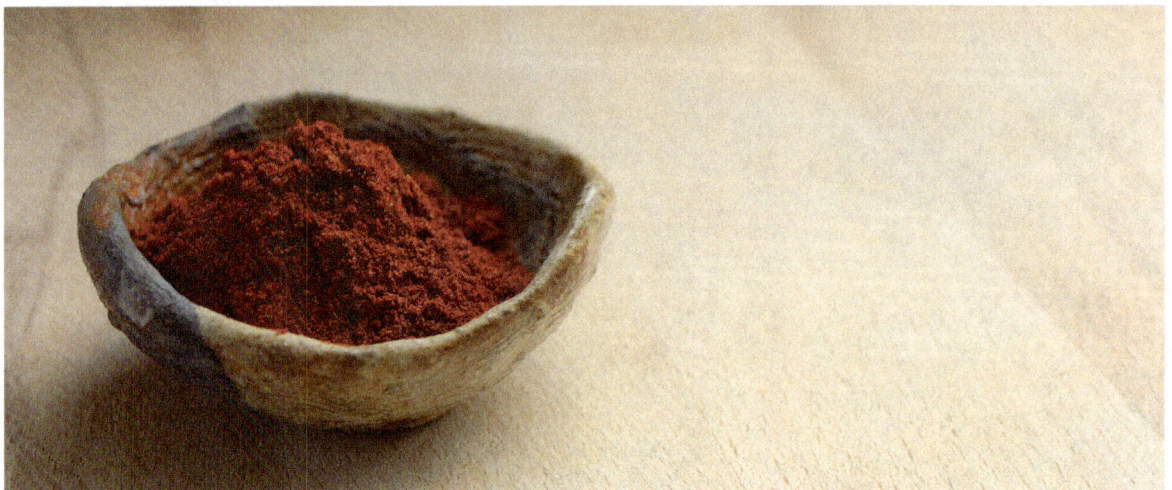

Monash note: Although chiles (chillies) are generally low in FODMAPs, some people with IBS may be sensitive to the capsaicin they contain. Capsaicin is a natural compound that gives chiles their spicy quality. You may need to limit how much chile you eat if your IBS symptoms are triggered by spicy food.

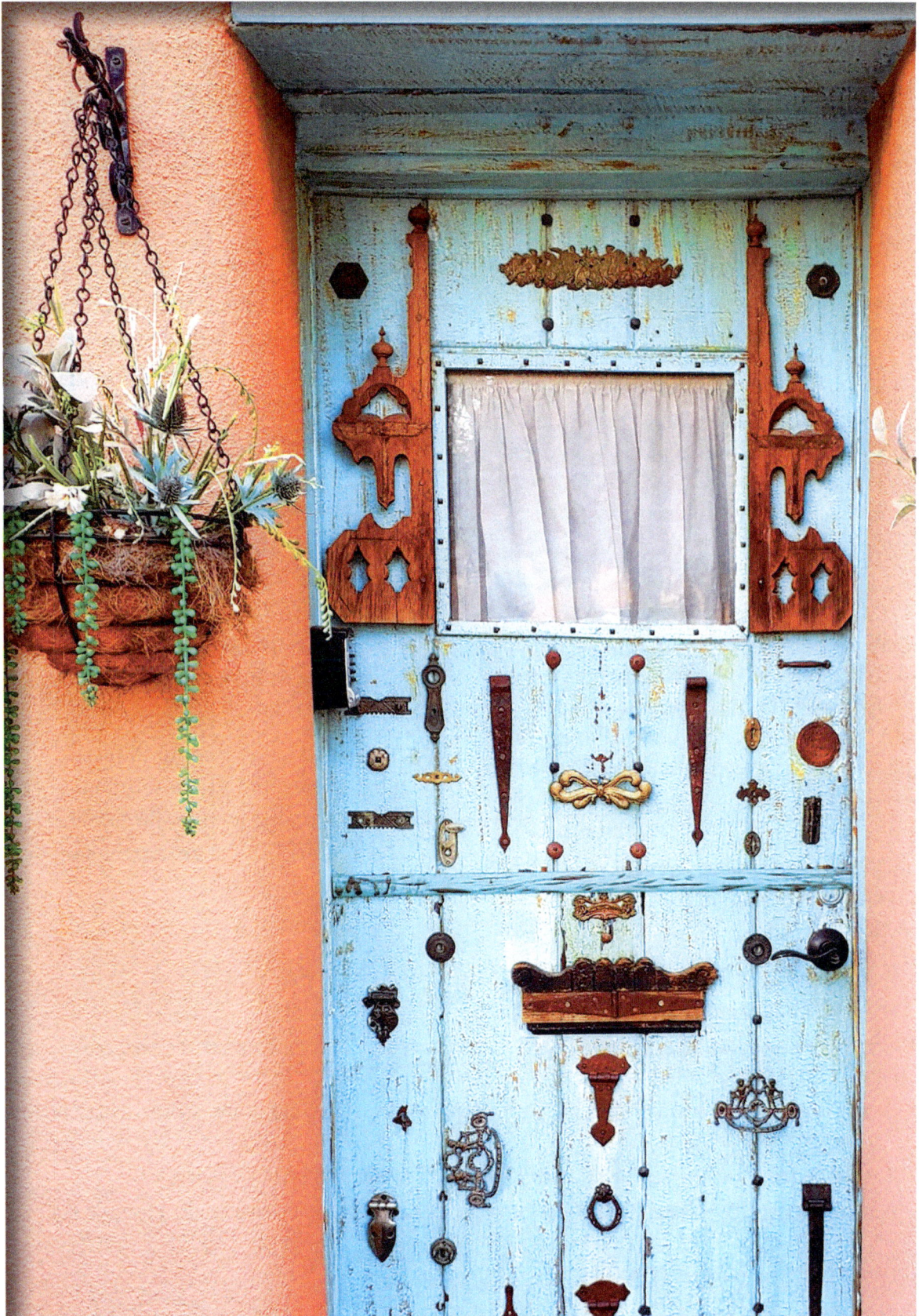

How To Make
Low FODMAP Garlic-Infused Oil
Small and Large Batch Methods

Garlic contains fructans (part of the O for oligosaccharides in FODMAP) that leach into water as you cook. If you make a soup or sauce, add garlic cloves for flavor and then remove them before serving, some of the fructans remain and oftentimes cause a digestive upset. The good news is that fructans are not oil soluble. When garlic pieces are sautéed in oil and then removed, the FODMAPs have not leached into the oil and you are left with flavorful, properly infused garlic oil!

In addition, oil is a fat and contains no FODMAPs, therefore you can choose whatever pure oil you like for the recipe such as canola, olive or vegetable. Therefore, we do not have to be as concerned with serving sizes, however, if you are one of those with IBS who are triggered by fat, watch your portions and eat to your personal tolerance.

The two preparations I use are to; infuse small amounts of oil as I'm cooking, or make a large batch to keep in the fridge and use as needed.

For example, Eggs From Hell (page 164) calls for 2 tablespoons (30 ml) of Low FODMAP Garlic-Infused Oil, so I use the Small Batch Method that takes less than 10 minutes to infuse, discard the garlic pieces and finish up my flavor-packed recipe. Also, while Eggs From Hell requires 2 tablespoons, I prefer to make 3 because some of the oil is lost while draining and transferring back to the pan.

The Large Batch Method is convenient when preparing several recipes for weekly meal prep, for Char Grilled Chimichurri Oysters (page 92) that calls for 1/3 cup (80 ml) of infused oil, or just having on hand ready-made.

Either way, be sure to use your infused oil within 3 days, and pay close attention to storage recommendations for safety as explained in the Large Batch Method on the following page.

SMALL BATCH METHOD: MAKES 3 TABLESPOONS (45 ML):

1. Peel 2 garlic cloves and slice into 4 pieces each.

2. Heat 3 tablespoons (45 ml) extra virgin olive oil, canola, pure olive oil or unseasoned oil of your choice over medium heat in a small saucepan.

3. Reduce heat to simmer and add the garlic. Sauté until they are just light brown. Overcooking to dark brown will result in a bitter flavor.

4. Pour the oil through a fine mesh metal strainer into a small heatproof bowl or measuring cup.

5. Be sure to discard all the garlic pieces from the oil before adding any other ingredients and proceeding with your recipe.

6. Use right away, or cool first as required

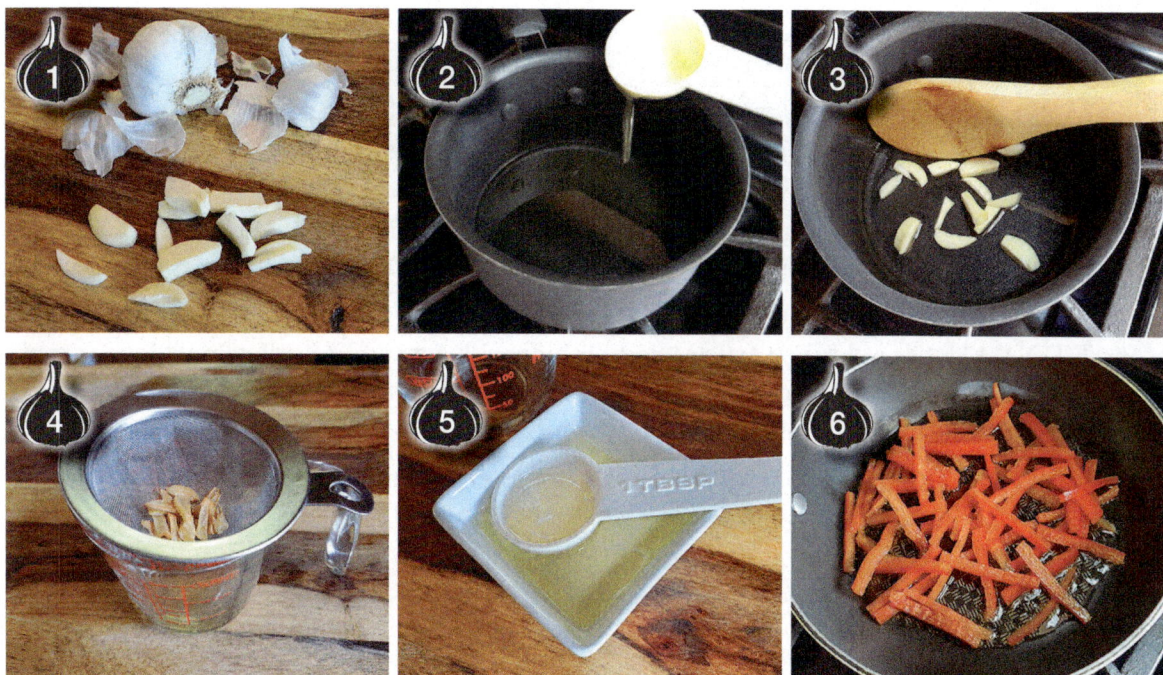

LARGE BATCH METHOD: MAKES 1/2 CUP (120 ML):

1. 1/2 cup (120 ml) unseasoned oil of your choice: canola, olive, vegetable, etc.

2. 5 peeled garlic cloves, sliced into 4 pieces each

3. Rinse an airtight container with a lid with boiling water and allow it to completely dry.

4. Heat the oil over low-medium heat in a small saucepan until it comes to a low simmer, but do not bring to a boil; add the garlic slices. Simmer gently for 10 minutes, stirring occasionally, or until the garlic slices are just turning light golden brown. Take care as overcooking to dark brown will result in a bitter flavor. Remove from heat. Let cool and infuse for 1 hour.

5. Pour the oil through a fine mesh metal strainer into the sterilized container; cool and secure the lid. Discard the garlic pieces. Mark the container with the date of infusion and use within 3 days; keep refrigerated. After 3 days there is a botulism risk. Infused oils can also be frozen in ice cube trays, then flexed into freezer baggies and stored in the freezer for up to 3 months.

Tip: Both methods also work for making LoFO Onion-Infused Oil as well; for 1/2 cup (120 ml) oil use 10 thin slices (approx. 30 g) of onion. For 3 tablespoons (45 ml) oil, use 4 thin slices (approx. 12 g) of onion.

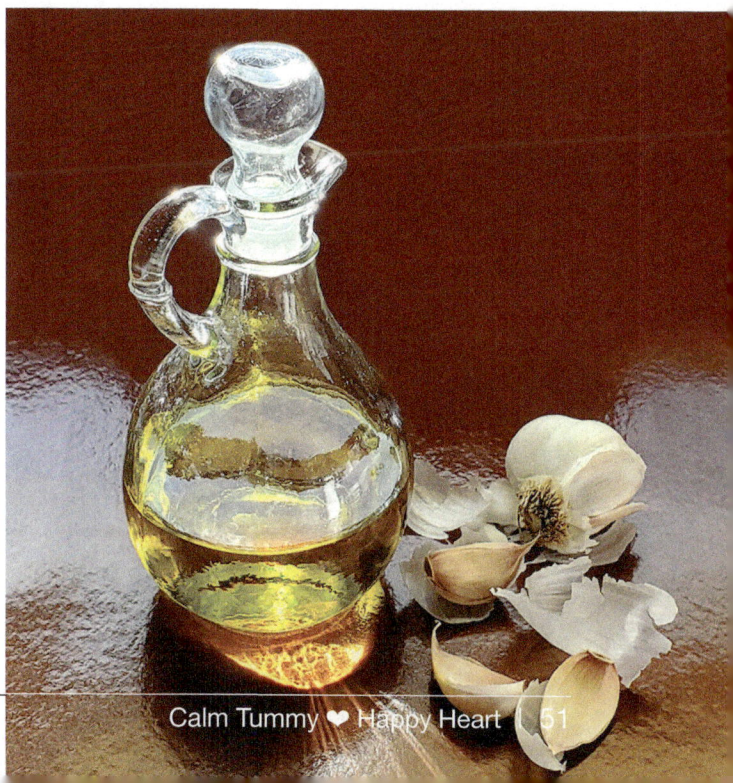

About FODMAP Stacking

Now you know that the acronym FODMAP stands for Fermentable, Oligosaccharides, Disaccharides, Monosaccharides and Polyols. These are the short-chain carbohydrates that Monash University researchers have identified as IBS triggers. Luckily for us, Monash University has tested (and continues to test) raw and prepared foods that you can quickly look up in their smartphone app. There you can easily see which FODMAP(s) certain foods contain, and also if there is a low FODMAP serving size noted by a green traffic light.

Monash FODMAP has published articles to their blog with explanations that "stacking is when multiple "green light servings " of foods are eaten in one sitting, there is an accumulation of FODMAPs in the gut, triggering symptoms."

Further, they explain that "FODMAP amounts are cumulative, and that in one sitting the total amount of FODMAPs consumed influences whether the meal is tolerated or if symptoms are triggered."

Rather than reinterpreting their findings, I find it best to refer you to the following Monash article on stacking.

FODMAP STACKING EXPLAINED
https://www.monashfodmap.com/blog/fodmap-stacking-explained/

We know this can feel daunting, but it gets easier with practice. And always remember, if you have been eating a greater amount of a FODMAP – perhaps without realizing it – and you have not been triggering your IBS, then you might not have to lessen the amount.

Of course, always consult your Registered Dietitian for the best approach and implementation of the diet for your individual situation.

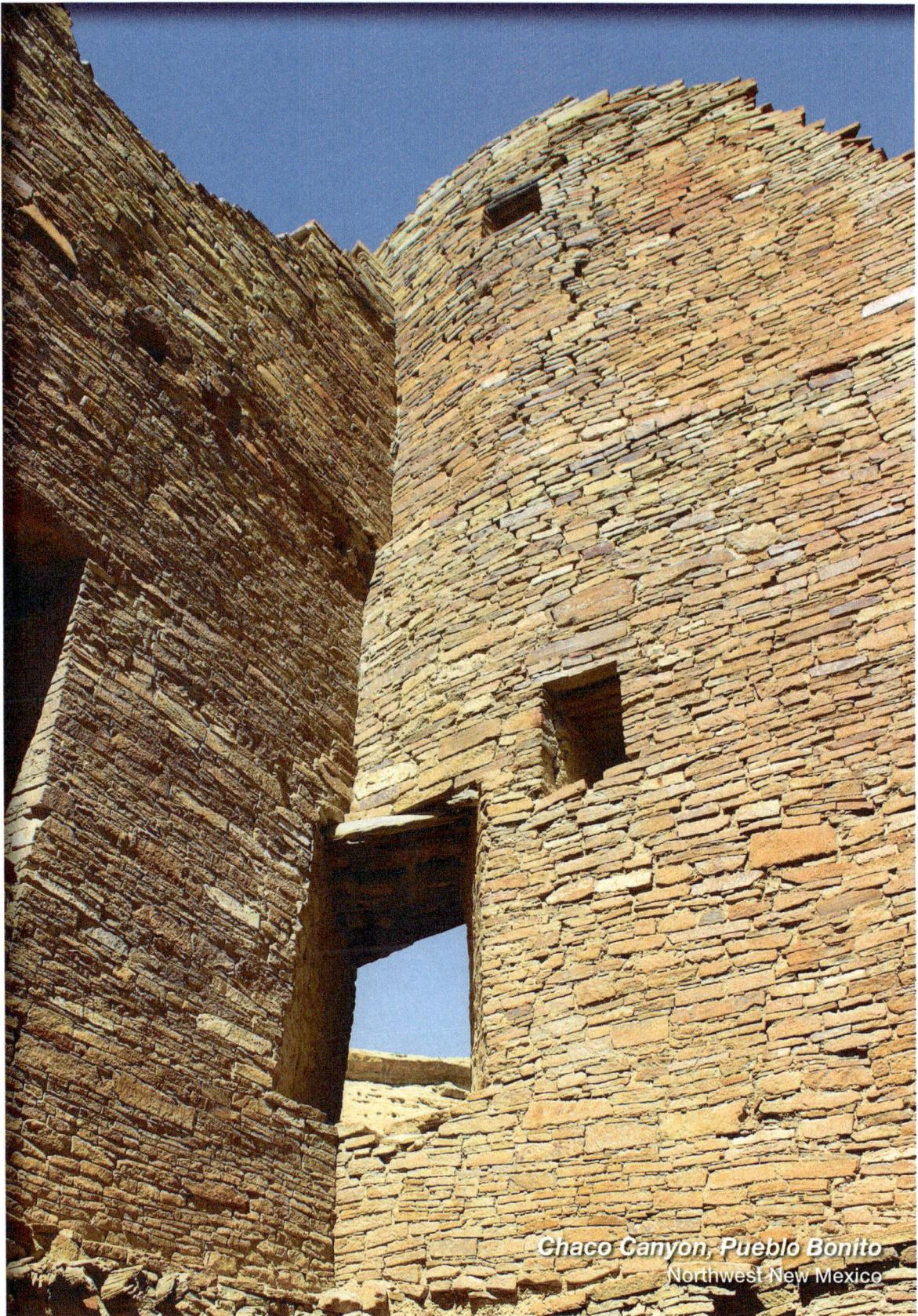
Chaco Canyon, Pueblo Bonito
Northwest New Mexico

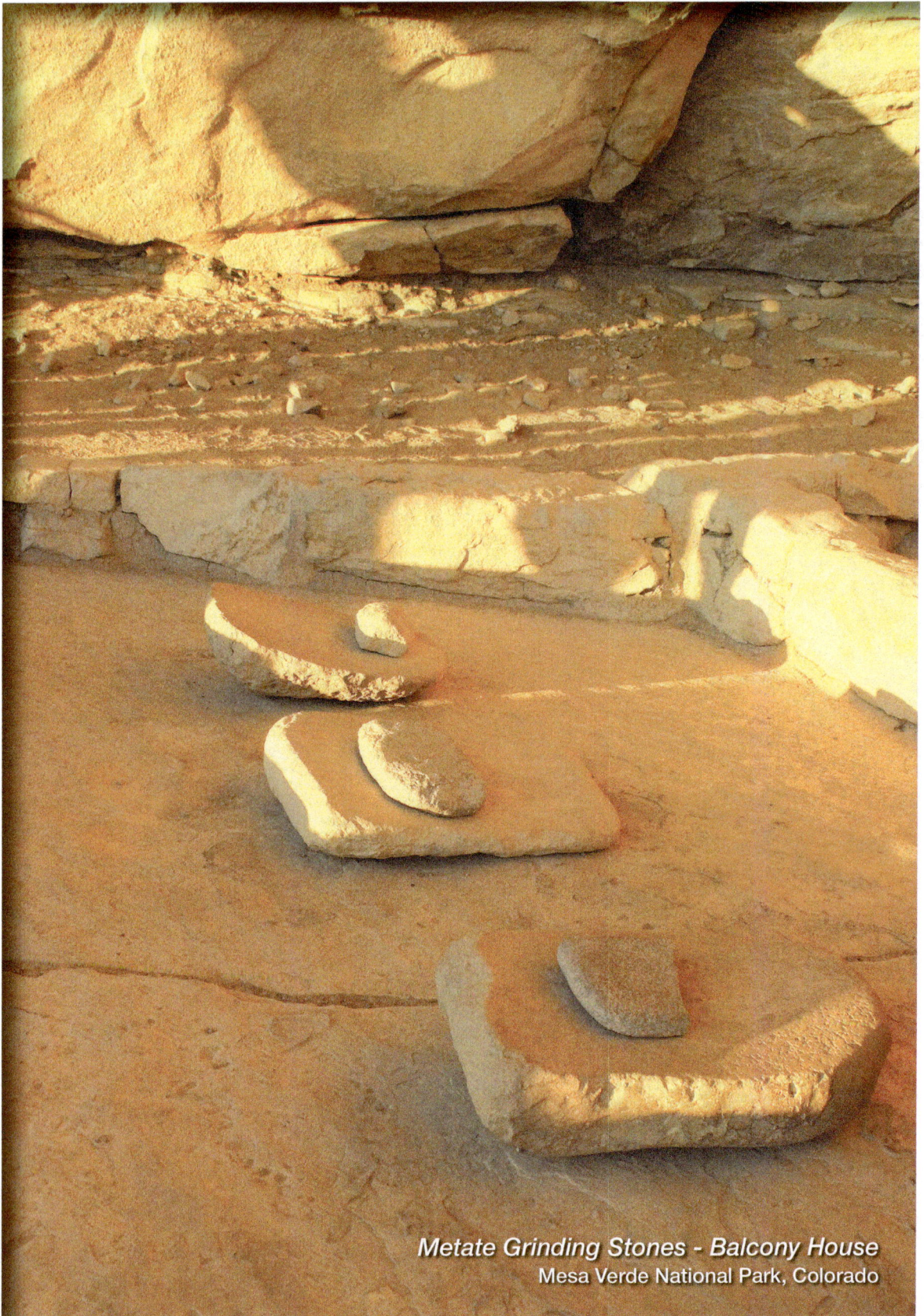

Metate Grinding Stones - Balcony House
Mesa Verde National Park, Colorado

Choosing Low FODMAP Flours

Flour is considered a standard pantry ingredient, and so it is even in the low FODMAP, gluten-free kitchen. We use flour in baking recipes, as well as in cooking, and your choice of flour is important to ensure the best final results.

LOW FODMAP DOES NOT EQUAL GLUTEN-FREE

One thing to point out right away is that not all gluten-free flours, or gluten-free flour blends, are low FODMAP. And of course, not all low FODMAP flours, or flour blends, are gluten-free! I am going to focus on a flour blend that I have used with great success that is both low FODMAP and gluten-free.

In this book, and in my own kitchen, I use the following U.S. produced flour blend for the very best low FODMAP, gluten-free and dairy-free recipes possible.

FLOUR BLEND CALLED FOR IN THIS COOKBOOK

I use gluten-free 1 to 1 baking mix containing: sweet rice flour, whole grain brown rice flour, potato starch, whole grain sorghum flour, tapioca flour and xanthan gum.

It does not contain bean or chickpea flours, baking powder or baking soda.

In this book I will refer this blend as, "low FODMAP gluten-free all-purpose baking flour, containing xanthan gum."

This flour brand has not yet been lab tested for FODMAP levels by Monash, and because this book is a Monash certified cookbook, I am not listing the brand name. However, you can find more information about it, along with other flours and Monash certified brands by visiting our website: **fodifyit.com**.

FLOUR BRANDS DIFFER

Flours from different brands have different formulations. The reason why I like this flour blend, as opposed to using just rice flour, for instance, is because the blends better replicate a final result in your dish that is more similar to conventional baked goods and savory recipes.

And, by the way, xanthan gum is low FODMAP and gluten-free.

Trust that I have kitchen-tested the recipes in this book with various flours, and the one suggested will give you great results. If you use a different flour than what is recommended, I cannot guarantee your results. And, let me tell you, I have tested recipes side-by-side using different flour blends and while the 1 to 1 blend I use made the most heavenly Tres Leches Cake, another brand I tried turned it to mush. It can be that dramatic.

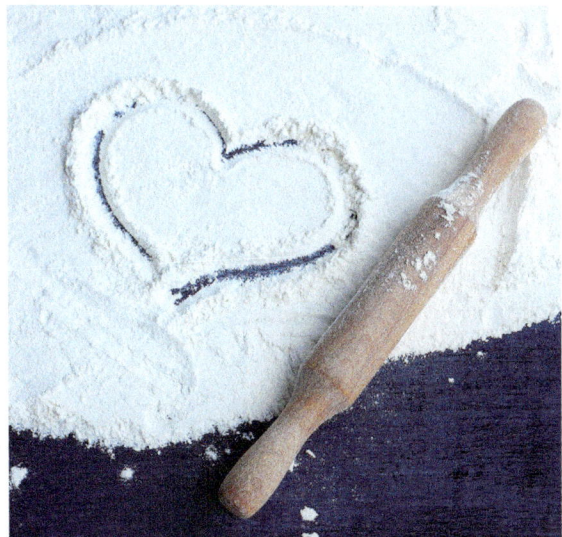

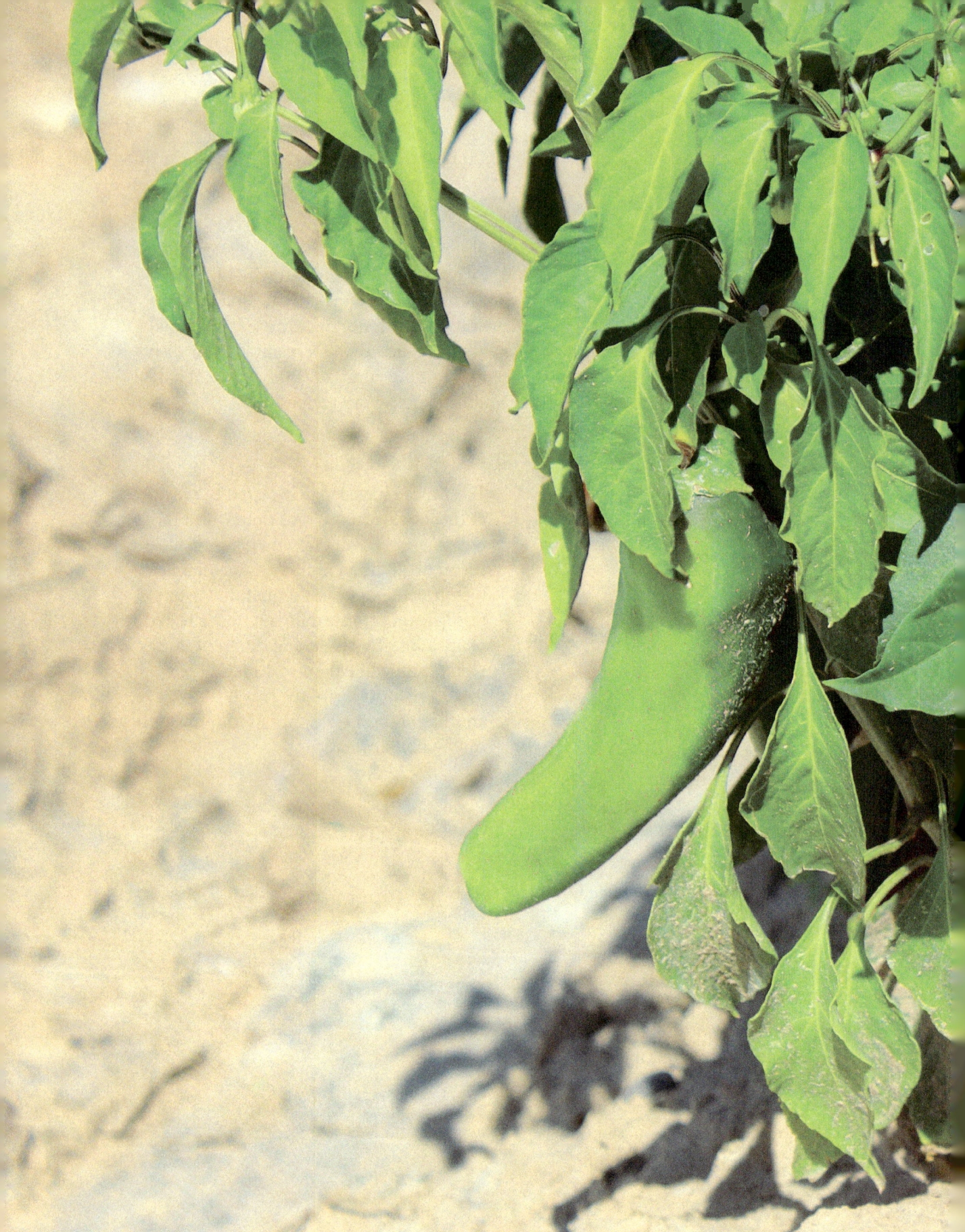

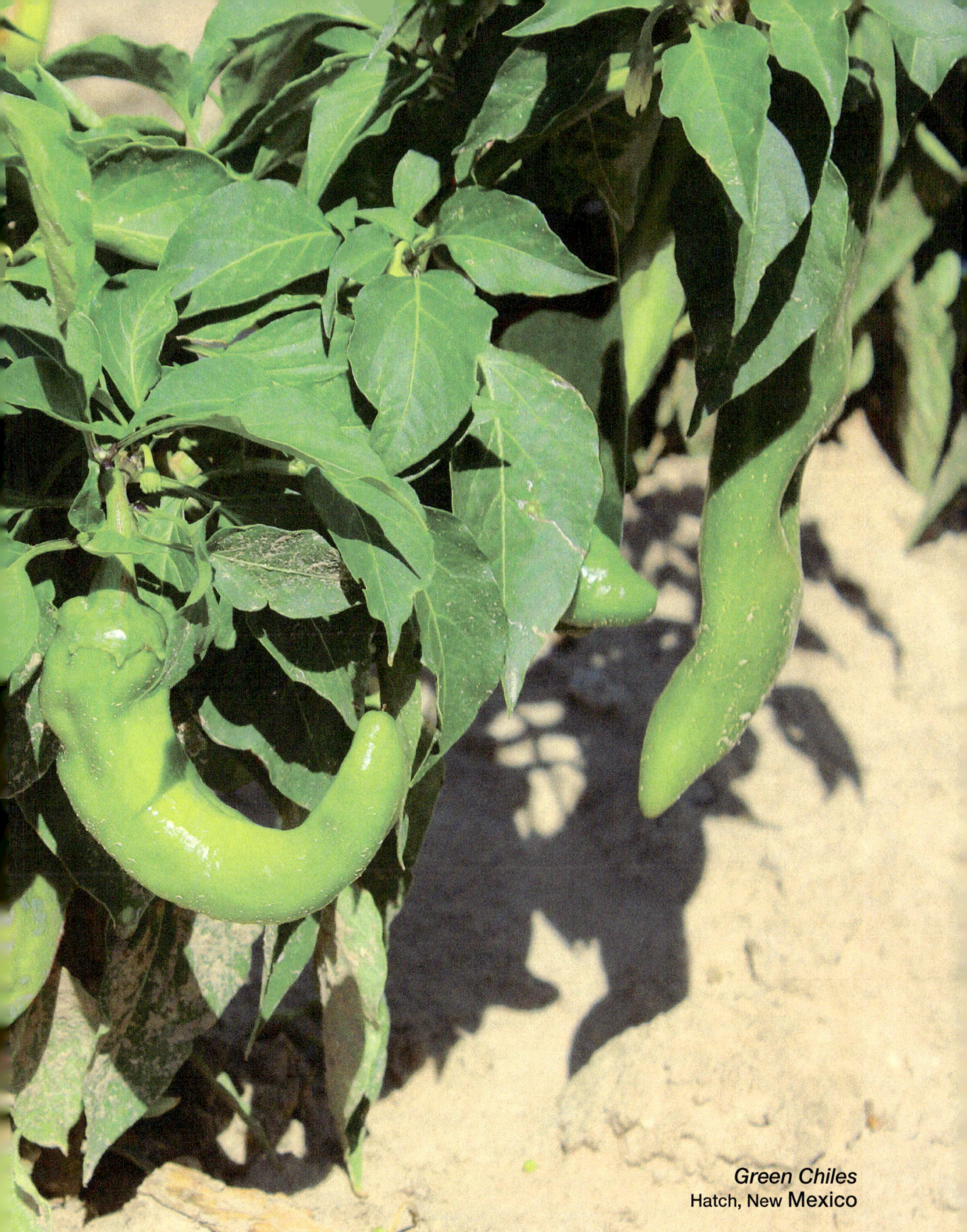

Green Chiles
Hatch, New Mexico

Sauces & Salsas

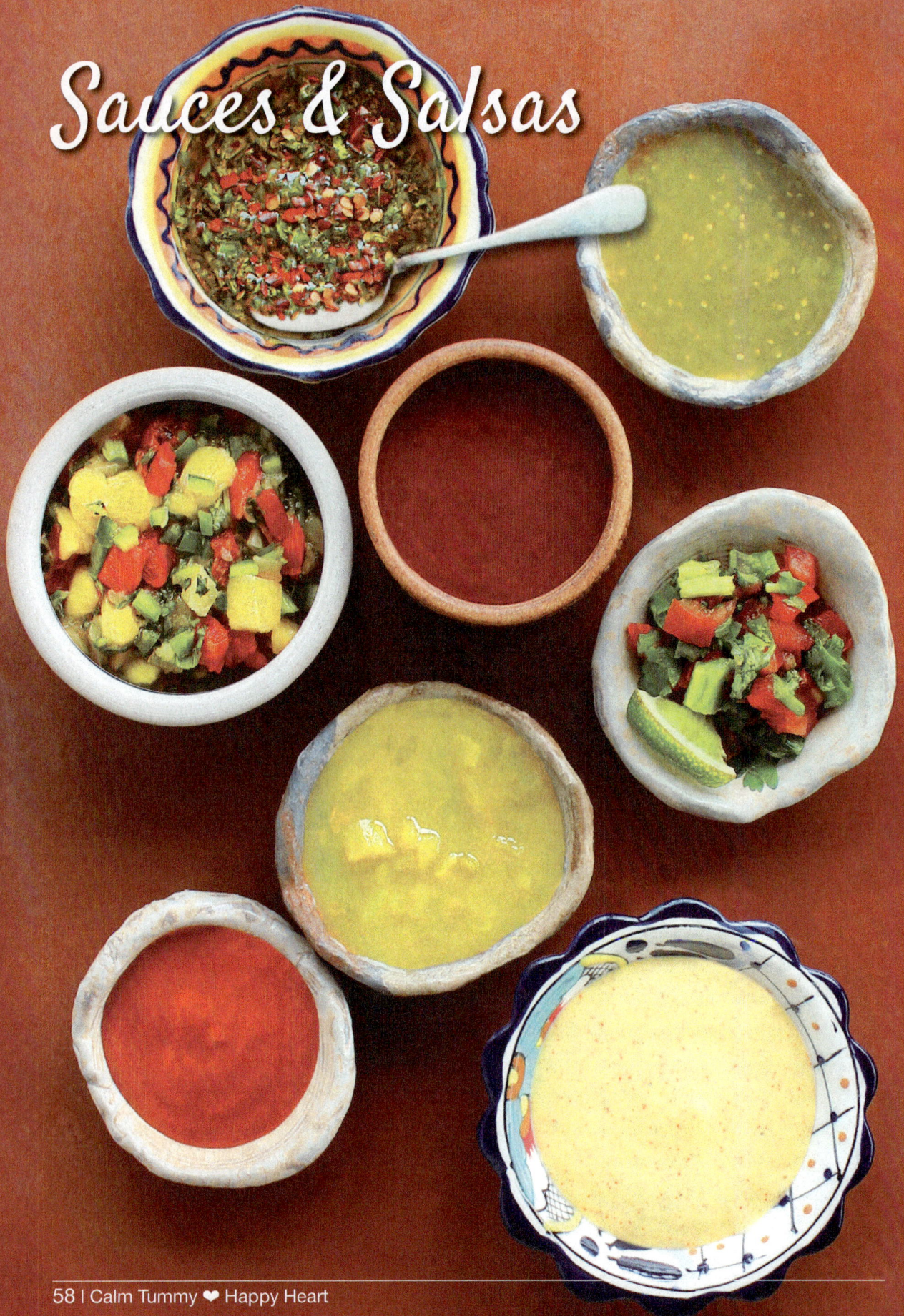

- ♥ **New Mexican Green Chile Sauce**

- ♥ **New Mexican Red Chile Sauce**

- ♥ **Pico de Gallo**

- ♥ **Cheesy Béchamel Sauce with Gluten-Free Roux**

- ♥ **Cilantro Parsley Chimichurri Sauce**

- ♥ **Fresh Grilled Pineapple Salsa**

- ♥ **Extra Tangy Green Chile Hollandaise Sauce**

- ♥ **Spicy Chipotle BBQ Sauce**

- ♥ **Tomato Ketchup / Catsup**

Food brand names are sometimes listed within a recipe, and this means they are Monash Certified. For more brand options we use and love, please visit **Fodifylt.com**

Monash Note: Although chiles (chillies) are generally low in FODMAPs, some people with IBS may be sensitive to the capsaicin they contain. Capsaicin is a natural compound that gives chiles their spicy quality. You may need to limit how much chile you eat if your IBS symptoms are triggered by spicy food.

New Mexican Green Chile Sauce

LOW FODMAP ❤ IBS FRIENDLY ❤ GLUTEN-FREE ❤ DAIRY-FREE

Green chiles (New Mexican, Hatch, Anaheim, Big Jim, Colorado Green) are herby, a little peppery and one chile has as much vitamin C as 5 oranges. I was introduced to them while living in Santa Fe, New Mexico and was told that I would begin to crave them once a week. This was misleading. It's actually more like every day.

While technically it is a sauce, when placing your order at a café you simply ask for "Green Chile." Were you to add "sauce" to that your waiter will ask "so, where are you visiting from?"

There are many recipe variations for Green Chile. Some add diced pork or ground beef, tomatoes, lots of onion, or straight up plain spooned over a burger or taco. This LoFO version is sans meat, uses garlic-infused canola oil in place of chopped garlic, scallion green parts for white onion, and water may be substituted for chicken stock for a vegetarian version.

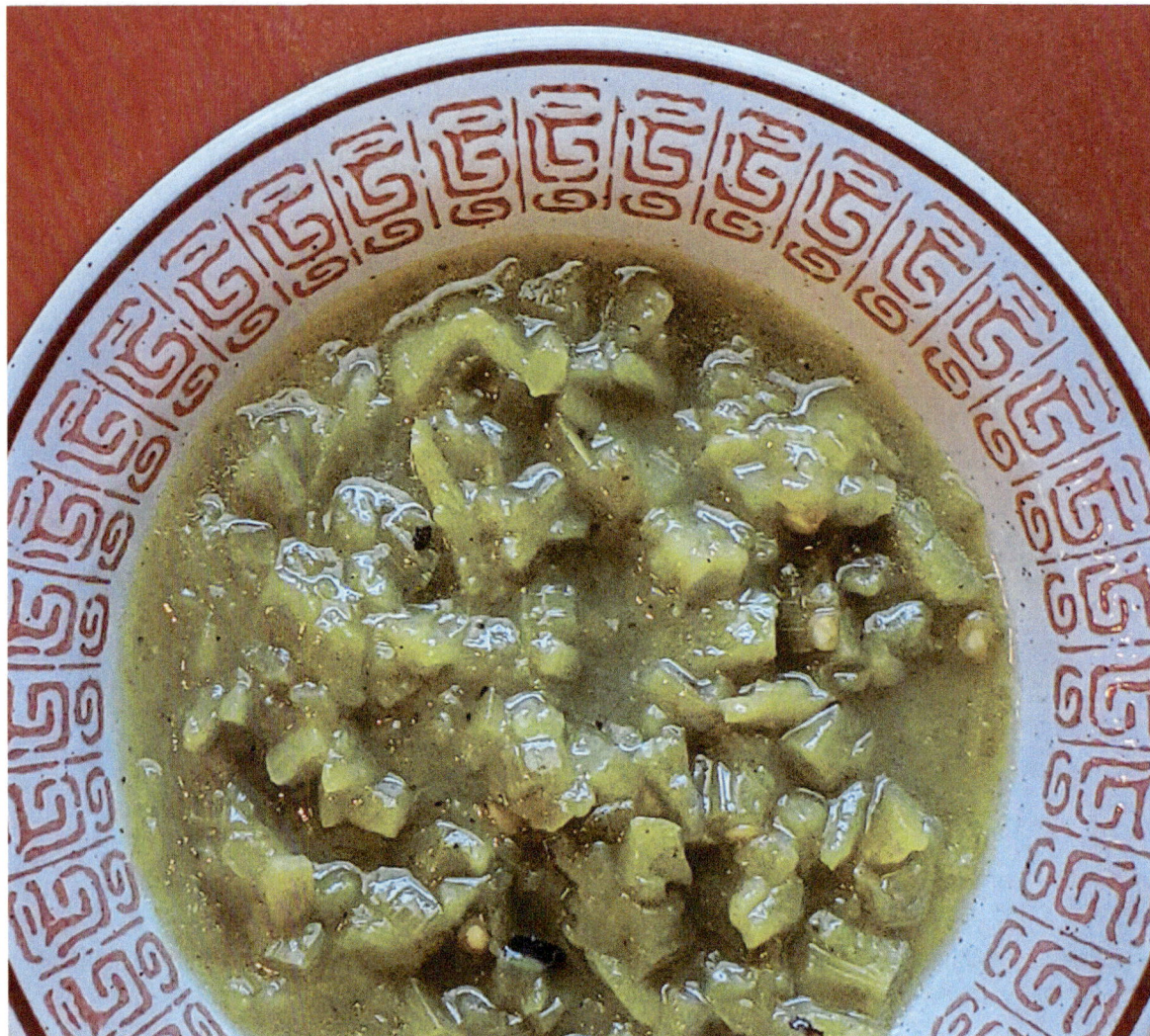

MAKES 1½ CUPS (350 ML) – 4 SERVINGS OF GENEROUS 1/3 CUP (80 ML) EACH
INGREDIENTS

1 tablespoon (15 ml) Low FODMAP Garlic-Infused Oil (page 50), made with canola oil

1/2 cup (25 g) thin sliced scallions, green parts only (or 1/4 cup (13 g) for less onion flavor)

2, 4-oz (226 g total) cans plain chopped green chile (containing no onion, garlic or other high FODMAP ingredients, drained. On the Monash App they are noted as Chilli (chili) green, mild, chopped, canned)
-OR-
8 medium (61 g each) mild fresh green chiles, roasted and prepped (page 46), (on the Monash App they are noted as: Chile, green, peeled, deseeded)

1/2 cup (120 ml) Low FODMAP Chicken Stock (page 135) or water for vegetarian

1/4 teaspoon ground cumin

1/4 teaspoon fresh ground black pepper

Slurry of 1 teaspoon cornstarch and 1 teaspoon cold water, plus another 1:1 teaspoon of slurry if you prefer a thicker consistency

Method: Heat the oil in a medium saucepan over medium high heat until shimmering. Add the scallion greens and chiles. Stir for 1 minute. Add the stock, cumin and black pepper. Bring to a low boil for 5 minutes. Add the cornstarch to the water in a small bowl and stir to create a slurry. Add it to the pan. Briskly whisk and cook for about 30 seconds to 1 minute more until thickened.

Some cooks like to pour the chile into a blender and purée until smooth. I prefer to leave mine chunky for a rustic homemade look and texture. Either way, it's magical.

Tips: Some canned green chile brands are salty. Best to taste before adding salt.

Optional – if you are able to tolerate butter, add 1 teaspoon as you whisk in the slurry to create a silky finish.

Monash Note: Although chiles (chillies) are generally low in FODMAPs, some people with IBS may be sensitive to the capsaicin they contain. Capsaicin is a natural compound that gives chiles their spicy quality. You may need to limit how much chile you eat if your IBS symptoms are triggered by spicy food.

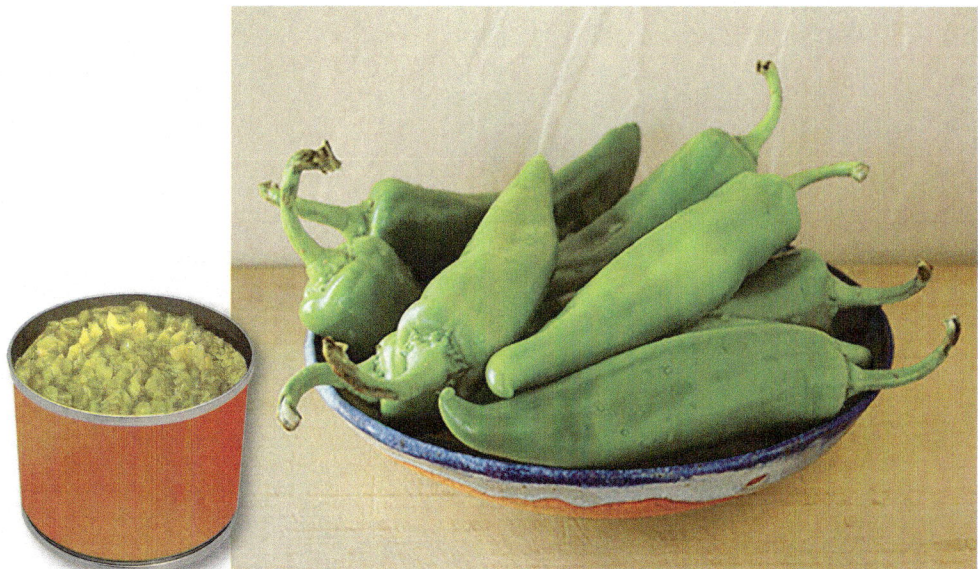

New Mexican Red Chile Sauce

LOW FODMAP ❤ IBS FRIENDLY ❤ GLUTEN-FREE ❤ DAIRY-FREE

Red Chile Sauce has an unmistakable earthy, peppery and fruity flavor. It's right up there on the iconic condiment pedestal with Green Chile and Salsa. And while it is a sauce, the traditional name is simply Red Chile.

The traditional preparation uses dried red chile pods that are re-hydrated in hot water and blended into a purée with spices. At the writing of this cookbook, these pods have not yet been tested. Based on other chile pods that have been evaluated I suspect they will be high FODMAP in the amount needed to make enough for a proper serving. That's my guess, so let's keep an eye on Monash newly tested foods for results from the source.

After countless recipe developments, I found that the closest applicable ingredient to use were red bell peppers roasted over a flame, peeled, seeded (as shown on page 46) and blended with seasonings. Along with garlic-infused canola oil in place of minced garlic, chives in place of white onion, and pure, mild red chile powder, any concerns you may have of feeling Red Chile deprived will be satisfied.

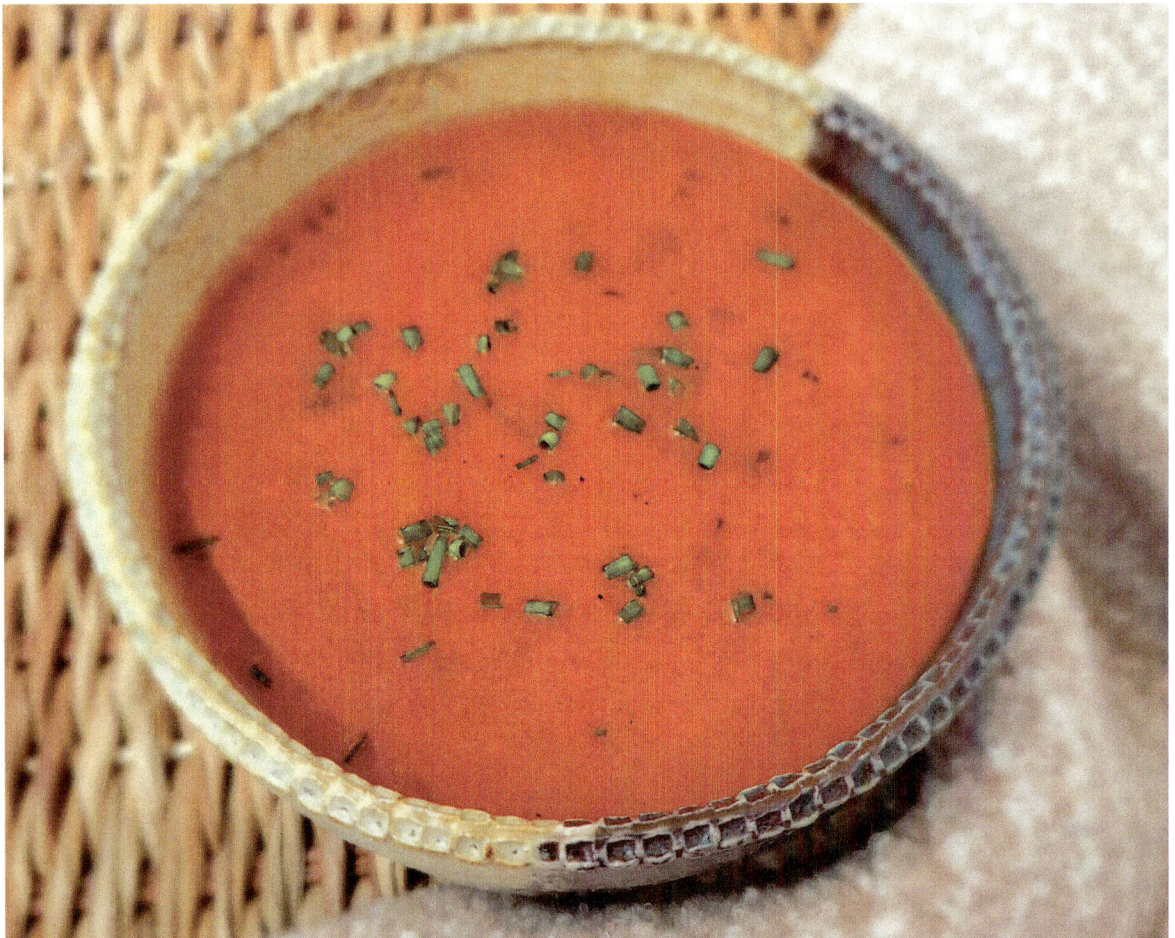

MAKES 16 SERVINGS: APPROX. 4 CUPS (946 ML) TOTAL – 1/4 CUP (59 ML) EACH

INGREDIENTS

4 (28-ounces / 800 g total) fresh red bell peppers, roasted and prepped as shown on page 46, after which you will have 21-ounces (600 g) of pepper meat to work with

3 tablespoons (45 ml) Low FODMAP Garlic-Infused Oil (page 50), made with canola oil, ready to use

2 teaspoons (4 g) pure mild red chile powder (containing no onion or garlic, the ingredients should list only: red chile. On the Monash App this is called Chilli (chili) red, powdered)

2 1/2 cups (590 ml) Low FODMAP Chicken Stock (page 135), or use water for vegetarian

1 tablespoon plus 1 teaspoon (4 g) minced fresh chives

3/4 teaspoon (3.75 g) fine sea salt

1/2 teaspoon (1 g) ground cumin

1/4 teaspoon fresh ground black pepper

Method: Prepare the red bells using the same method shown on page 46 for green chiles. As your kitchen fills with a delicious aroma, picture in your mind the millions of Southwesterners doing this very thing along with you, right at this moment. Roasting some type of chile pepper throughout the week is as familiar to us as breathing.

Give the pepper meat a rough chop.

Heat the oil in a medium saucepan over medium high heat until it shimmers. Add the peppers and cook for 4 minutes, stirring often. Add the remaining ingredients and stir until bubbly hot, about 3 minutes.

Remove from heat and allow to cool for 5 minutes. Carefully spoon into a blender. Cover the top lid with a heavy, clean kitchen towel to avoid splatters. Purée until smooth. If too thick add more stock or water, a little at a time to desired gravy consistency. If too thin, pour back into the pan and simmer to reduce, stirring often.

Tips: For information on red chile powder with an 'e' vs. red chili powder with an 'i', see page 48.

Optional – if you are able to tolerate butter, add 1 teaspoon as you purée the sauce for a silky finish.

Monash Note: Although chiles (chillies) are generally low in FODMAPs, some people with IBS may be sensitive to the capsaicin they contain. Capsaicin is a natural compound that gives chiles their spicy quality. You may need to limit how much chile you eat if your IBS symptoms are triggered by spicy food.

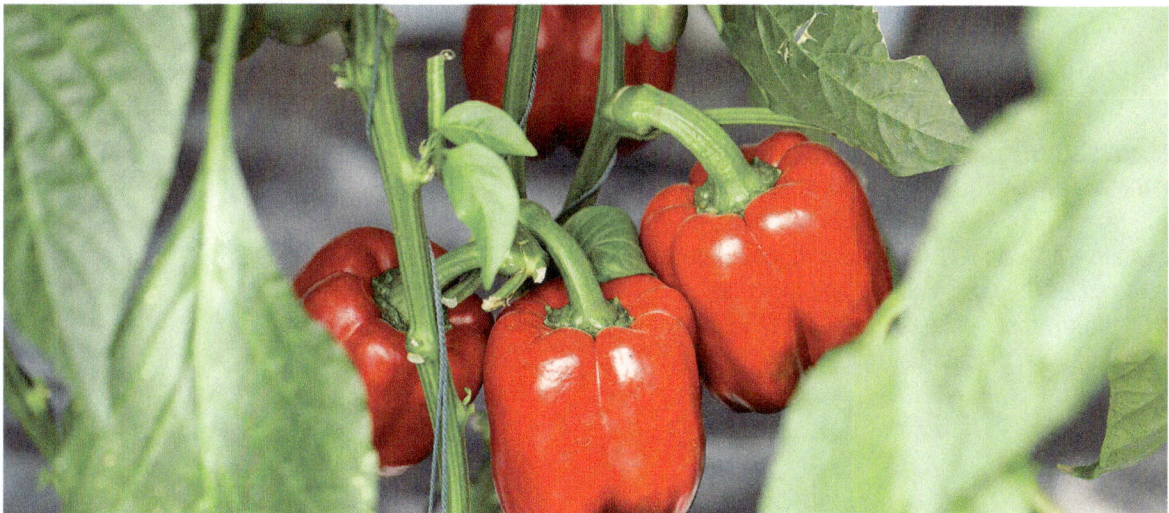

Pico de Gallo

LOW FODMAP ❤ IBS FRIENDLY ❤ GLUTEN-FREE ❤ DAIRY-FREE

Pico de Gallo (meaning: rooster's beak) is a chunky, hand chopped salsa that is very versatile. You can dip it with chips, spoon it over omelets, huevos rancheros, baked potatoes, juicy grilled steaks, salads, fajitas, and layer it in sandwiches and tacos. In our corner of the U.S., this condiment is more popular than ketchup.

MAKES 8 SERVINGS
INGREDIENTS

1 tablespoon (15 ml) Low FODMAP Garlic-Infused Oil (page 50), made with canola oil, cooled

3 large (1.07 kg total) ripe firm common tomatoes, cored and chopped fine

1 medium jalapeño (41 g) stem, seeds and ribs removed, minced, or use only half if it's a really hot one, your preference

3/4 cup (38 g) thin sliced scallions, green parts only

1/2 cup (8 g) fresh medium packed cilantro, mostly leaves, finely chopped

1/2 teaspoon (1 g) ground cumin

1/2 teaspoon (2.5 g) fine sea salt, plus more to your taste

1/4 teaspoon fresh ground black pepper

Juice of 2 limes

Method: Combine all ingredients in a medium bowl. Stir gently to mix. Adjust for salt or lime juice to your taste. Spoon into a serving dish.

Tips: Microwave the limes for 10 seconds before squeezing to release more juices.

Pice de Gallo can be made a day in advance, and will keep in the refrigerator for approximately one week in a tightly sealed container.

Monash Note: Although chiles (chillies) are generally low in FODMAPs, some people with IBS may be sensitive to the capsaicin they contain. Capsaicin is a natural compound that gives chiles their spicy quality. You may need to limit how much chile you eat if your IBS symptoms are triggered by spicy food.

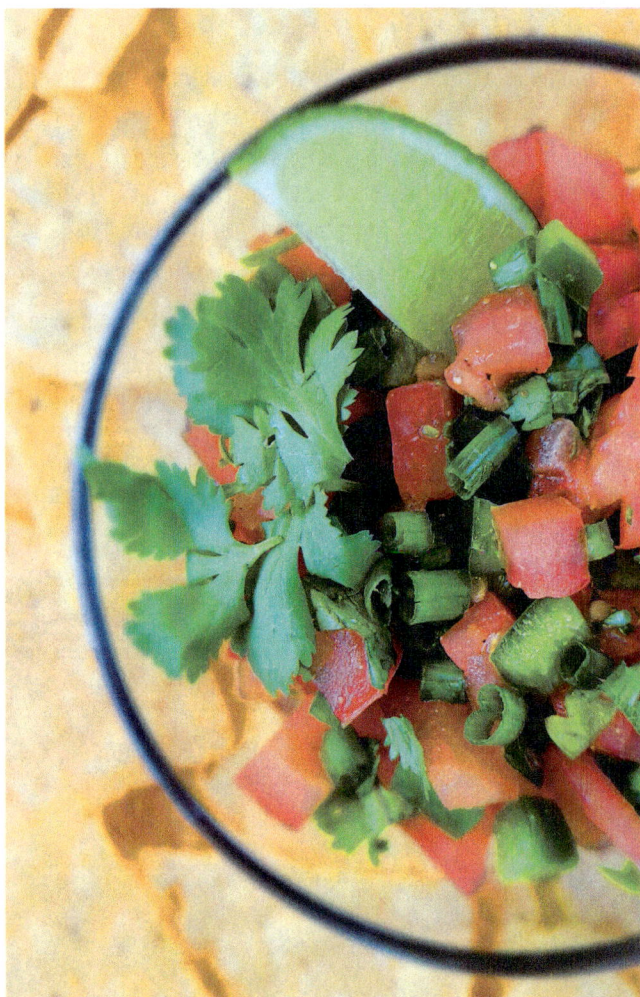

Cheesy Béchamel Sauce with Gluten-Free Roux

LOW FODMAP ❤ IBS FRIENDLY ❤ GLUTEN-FREE ❤ DAIRY-FREE

This silky white sauce is easy to prepare for Mexican Lasagna (page 204) and Seafood Enchiladas (page 206). Classically made with conventional butter, milk and wheat-based flour, this creamy low FODMAP version is a cinch.

In place of cream, my go-to dairy-free combination is plain, unsweetened almond milk combined with canned full-fat coconut milk. The addition of nutritional yeast brings a lovely, earthy cheese flavor. Dairy-free butter alternatives are improving all the time, and the green parts of scallions remain one of LoFO's best onion swap friends.

MAKES APPROX. 2 3/4 CUPS (650 ML) – 6-8 SERVINGS
INGREDIENTS

2 cups (475 ml) plain, unsweetened almond milk

1/2 cup (120 ml) canned full-fat coconut milk for cooking, containing no inulin, well-stirred

6 scallions, green parts only, whole stalks cut in half lengthwise

12 parsley leaves, no stems as they can be bitter

Scant pinch ground nutmeg

1/4 cup (56 g) dairy-free butter alternative

1/4 cup (37 g) low FODMAP gluten-free all-purpose baking flour, containing xanthan gum (page 55)

1 tablespoon plus 1 teaspoon (8 g) large flake nutritional yeast

1/2 teaspoon (2.5 g) fine sea salt

1/4 teaspoon fresh ground black pepper

Method: In a small saucepan, heat the milks, scallion stems, parsley and nutmeg over medium high heat. Bring to a low boil, stirring occasionally. Turn off heat, cover with a lid and let infuse for 15 minutes. Discard the scallions and parsley. Set aside.

In a medium saucepan, create the roux by melting the butter alternative over medium high heat. Add the flour and whisk for 15 seconds. Reduce to medium heat. Add the yeast, salt and pepper. Quickly whisk to combine.

Gradually add the milk infusion, constantly whisking until the sauce is the consistency of heavy thick cream, for about 3 to 4 minutes.

Tips: If too thick, add 1 tablespoon more of the almond milk, and a bit more if needed. If too thin, mix a slurry of 1 teaspoon LoFO gluten-free flour and 2 teaspoons almond milk. Stir well, add to the sauce and whisk to thicken.

Béchamel will keep in the refrigerator for up to 3 days in a tightly sealed container.

Always stir canned full-fat coconut milk well before measuring to combine the milk and cream, which rises to the top.

Cilantro Parsley Chimichurri Sauce

LOW FODMAP ❤ IBS FRIENDLY ❤ GLUTEN-FREE ❤ DAIRY-FREE

This recipe is low in FODMAPS, however, the amount of oil that may be tolerated is highly individualized, in which case I've reduced the ratio of oil for a slightly thicker, less drizzly sauce.

Chimichurri is a garlic-forward, herby, oil and red wine vinegar sauce that is traditionally used as a finishing condiment over grilled steak. The consistency is a coarse sauce with bits of texture from the fine chopped herbs. It is excellent with fish, shrimp, chicken, pork, other meats, tofu and grilled vegetables. We also spoon it over scrambled eggs and tacos, add a dollop to soups, grill it with Oysters on the Half Shell (page 92), whisk it into dips and hollandaise, spoon it over salads or spread it on toasted LoFO gluten-free breads.

Thanks to LoFO Garlic-Infused Oil (page 50), the pungent, aromatic flavor remains robust.

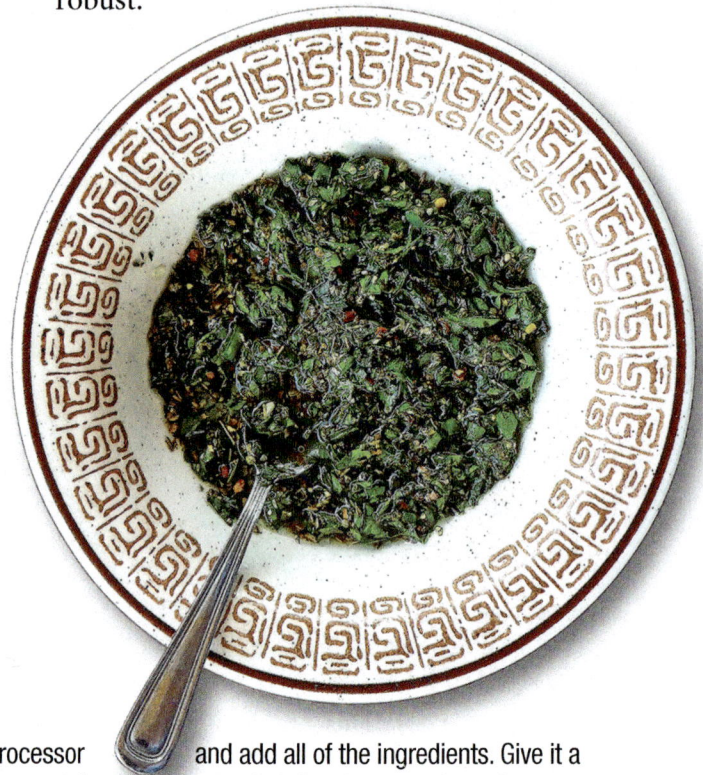

INGREDIENTS

1/2 cup (8 g) fresh medium packed cilantro, mostly leaves, finely chopped

1/2 cup (16 g) finely chopped flat leaf parsley leaves, parsley stems can be bitter

1/4 cup (13 g) thin sliced scallions, green parts only

1/3 cup (80 ml) Low FODMAP Garlic-Infused Oil (page 50), made with canola oil, cooled

1/4 cup (60 ml) red wine vinegar

Juice of 1/2 lime

2 tablespoons dried oregano

1/2 teaspoon (1 g) crushed red pepper flakes, plus 1/2 teaspoon more if you like heat

3/4 teaspoon (4 g) fine sea salt

1/2 teaspoon fresh ground black pepper

Method: Secure the metal chopping blade in a food processor and add all of the ingredients. Give it a few pulses and scrape down the sides of the bowl with a spatula as needed. Continue to pulse a few more times until everything is combined but still has texture – not creamy smooth. Taste for salt and vinegar. Chill in the refrigerator in a airtight container until ready to serve.

Tips: Chimichurri adds excellent flavor to hamburgers. Just mix in 1 tablespoon per patty and grill as normal.

Chimichurri will keep for 3 days in the refrigerator in a tightly sealed container.

Monash Note: Although chiles (chillies) are generally low in FODMAPs, some people with IBS may be sensitive to the capsaicin they contain. Capsaicin is a natural compound that gives chiles their spicy quality. You may need to limit how much chile you eat if your IBS symptoms are triggered by spicy food.

Fresh Grilled Pineapple Salsa

LOW FODMAP ❤ IBS FRIENDLY ❤ GLUTEN-FREE ❤ DAIRY-FREE

Grilling the pineapple is not a crucial step, but that beautiful char truly adds a yummy smoky flavor and lets you know that grilling season has arrived. This is a sweet, tangy salsa that pairs beautifully with grilled fish, pork tacos, or for dipping with corn tortilla chips.

MAKES 4–6 SERVINGS
INGREDIENTS

Canola oil for greasing the grill grates

1 medium (119 g) fresh red bell pepper

6, 1/2-inch (12 mm) thick fresh, cored pineapple rings (to total 350 g)

1/2 cup (8 g) fresh medium packed cilantro, mostly leaves, finely chopped

1/4 cup (13 g) thin sliced scallions, green parts only

Juice and zest of 1 lime

2 teaspoons (10 ml) Low FODMAP Garlic-Infused Oil (page 50), made with canola oil, cooled

1/4 teaspoon (1.25 g) fine sea salt

Method: Heat your grill to medium high heat. Using metal tongs and a paper towel doused with a bit of canola oil, grease the grates.

To prepare the red bell, place it on the grill and turn it every few minutes until most of the skin has charred with nice black markings. Be sure to char the top and bottom, too; char it all over. This should take 7 to 10 minutes. Place it in a sealed plastic baggie or a bowl covered with a clean heavy kitchen towel for 25 minutes to steam.

Arrange the pineapple rings on the grill. Cook 3 minutes per side or until you have distinct grill marks on both sides. Move to a cutting board and let cool for 5 to 10 minutes. Finely chop the pineapple. You should have 2 1/2 cups (350 g).

Back to the red bell, use your hands to remove the charred skin and discard. You may need to run it under cool water to help remove stubborn parts of the skin. Cut off the stem top, remove inner seeds and ribs and discard. Cut the pepper meat to a small dice.

Add all ingredients to a medium bowl. Stir gently with a spoon to fully mix.

Tips: Microwave the lime for 10 seconds before squeezing to release more juices.

Stored in an airtight container, this salsa will keep up to 3 days in the refrigerator.

Monash Note: Although chiles (chillies) are generally low in FODMAPs, some people with IBS may be sensitive to the capsaicin they contain. Capsaicin is a natural compound that gives chiles their spicy quality. You may need to limit how much chile you eat if your IBS symptoms are triggered by spicy food.

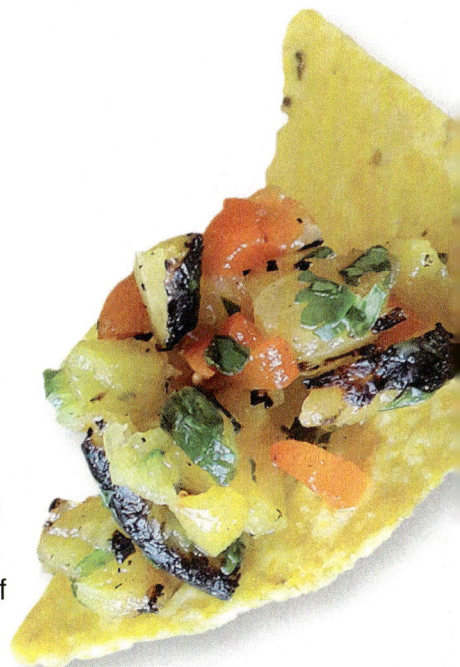

Extra Tangy Green Chile Hollandaise Sauce

LOW FODMAP ❤ IBS FRIENDLY ❤ GLUTEN-FREE ❤ DAIRY-FREE

Lemon and egg yolks whipped with lots of melted butter -- who doesn't love Hollandaise? This version substitutes plain dairy-free, unsweetened coconut yogurt for the butter resulting in a fluffy tanginess. I find that LoFO coconut-based yogurts are creamy and blend nicely with this recipe. Adding green chiles brings an earthy mild pepper flavor and they're also a great source of Vitamin C.

Making Hollandaise goes slowly at first, but once the yolks begin to thicken you'll want to have all of your ingredients nearby and ready to add very quickly before the eggs try to scramble. If you do happen to see small curdles as you're whisking, quickly drop in the green chiles and yogurt and whisk like mad. Oftentimes those little bits are so soft they will blend back in and your sauce is saved.

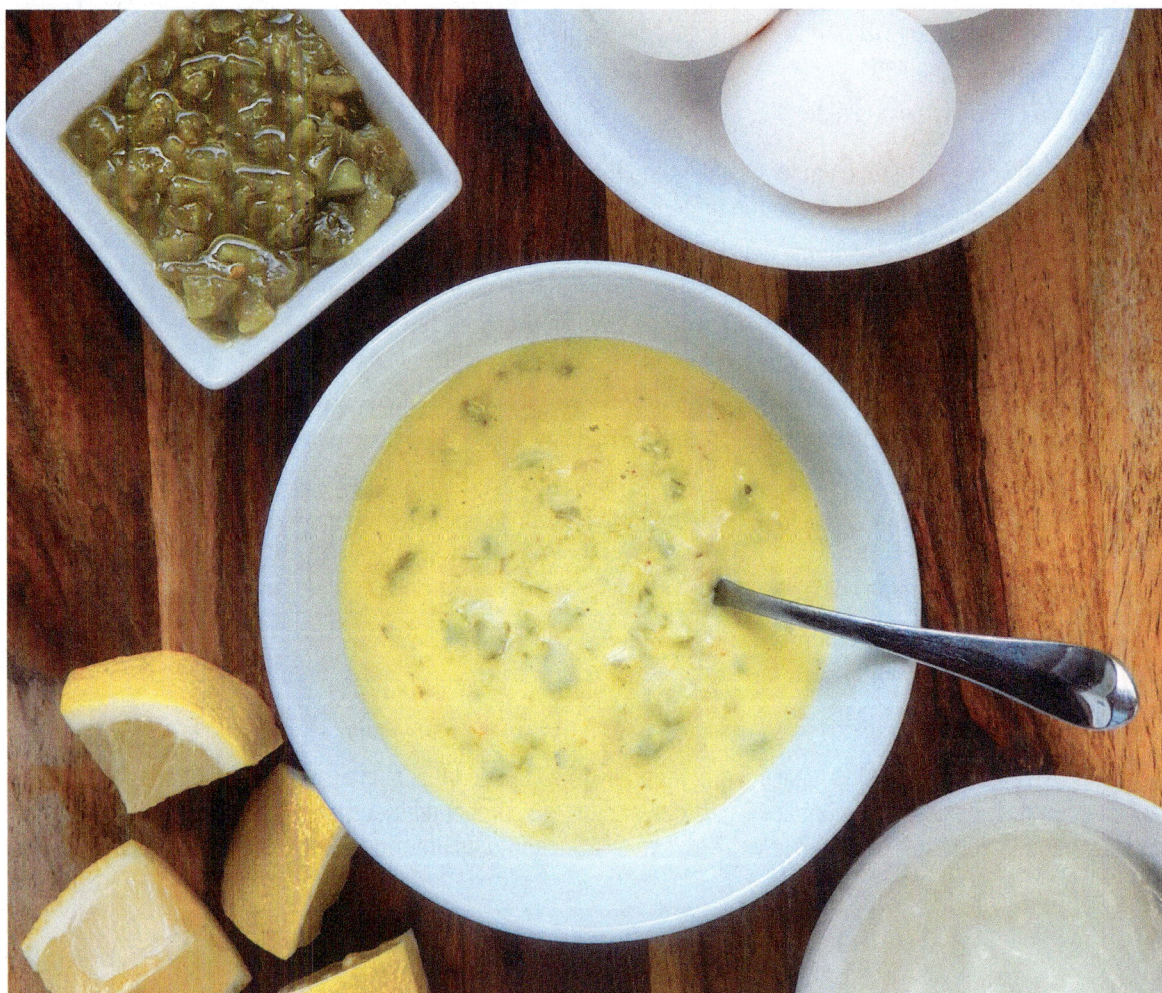

4 SERVINGS – APPROX. 1-11/4 CUPS (300 ML)
INGREDIENTS

1 medium stainless steel mixing bowl that fits snugly into a medium saucepan

4 egg yolks (save the whites for tomorrow's meringue or egg white omelet)

1 tablespoon (15 ml) cold water

1, 4-oz (113 g) can plain mild chopped green chiles, drained (containing no onion, garlic or other high FODMAP ingredients. On the Monash App they are noted as Chilli (chili) green, mild, chopped, canned)
-OR-
2 medium (122 g total) fresh mild green chiles, see page 46 for roasting and prep instructions, chopped fine (on the Monash App they are noted as: Chile, green, peeled, deseeded)

1/4 cup (60-72 g) plain dairy-free, unsweetened coconut yogurt containing no high FODMAP ingredients

Juice of 1 lemon

1/8 teaspoon cayenne

Pinch fine ground black pepper

Slurry of 2 teaspoons cornstarch and 2 teaspoons (10 ml) cold water, mixed in a small bowl, for thickening

Method: Whisk the yolks and 1 tablespoon (15 ml) water in the stainless steel bowl for 1 minute until light and frothy.

Fill the saucepan with 1-inch (2.5 cm) water and bring to a low boil. Place the bowl with yolks over the pan, making sure that the bottom of the bowl does not touch the water. Reduce the heat to low. (You may also use a double boiler).

Vigorously whisk for 3 to 4 minutes until the eggs begin to thicken. Whisk in the chiles, yogurt, lemon juice, cayenne and black pepper. Continue whisking until the sauce is smooth and creamy. You'll need an oven mitt to handle the hot bowl.

If the consistency is too loose, add 1 teaspoon of the cornstarch slurry at a time and whisk for 2 minutes for desired thickness. If too thick, remove it from the heat and whisk in 1 teaspoon hot water.

If you prefer a completely smooth Hollandaise, pour it in a blender or use a hand immersion blender to purée. It will then have a slightly greenish tint from the chiles.

Canned green chiles are oftentimes heavily salted, in which case you most likely won't need to use salt. Add salt to your taste, beginning with a scant 1/4 teaspoon (1.25 g) at a time. Serve immediately.

Tips: I've tried using an additional egg yolk to thicken the sauce but it resulted in an eggy, distinct cackleberry flavor that overpowered the other ingredients.

Use plain, unsweetened lactose-free or conventional cow's milk yogurt, per your tolerance.

Microwave the lemon for 10 seconds to yield more juice before squeezing.

Monash Note: Although chiles (chillies) are generally low in FODMAPs, some people with IBS may be sensitive to the capsaicin they contain. Capsaicin is a natural compound that gives chiles their spicy quality. You may need to limit how much chile you eat if your IBS symptoms are triggered by spicy food.

Spicy Chipotle BBQ Sauce

LOW FODMAP ❤ IBS FRIENDLY ❤ GLUTEN-FREE ❤ DAIRY-FREE

Great flavor with a nice kick of chipotle and cayenne heat, this sauce is perfect for mixing with: plain shredded chicken or shredded pork, glazing hamburgers, steaks and pork chops, blending with mayonnaise for a burger sauce, and marinating tofu and skewered meats.

MAKES 1 CUP (240 ML) – 4, 1/4 CUP (60 ML) SERVINGS
INGREDIENTS

3/4 cup (180 ml) water

1/3 cup (60 g) medium packed light brown sugar, plus 1 tablespoon (10 g) more to your taste

3/8 cup (90 g) tomato paste, containing no high fructose corn syrup or other high FODMAP ingredients

2 tablespoons (30 ml) white or apple cider vinegar

2 teaspoons (10 ml) soy sauce; gluten-free if you are following a gluten-free diet

2 teaspoons (2 g) minced fresh chives

1 teaspoon (5 g) prepared Dijon or yellow mustard, containing no onion or garlic

1/2 teaspoon (1 g) pure chipotle powder

1/2 teaspoon (1 g) cayenne

1/2 teaspoon (2.5 g) fine sea salt

1/4 teaspoon (.5 g) fresh ground black pepper

Method: Place all ingredients in a medium saucepan, using 1/3 cup (60 g) brown sugar. Bring to a low boil. Reduce to simmer for 5 minutes, stirring occasionally. If too thick, add 1 tablespoon more water, more if needed. Taste and add remaining 1 tablespoon (10 g) brown sugar, if desired.

Monash Note: Although chiles (chillies) are generally low in FODMAPs, some people with IBS may be sensitive to the capsaicin they contain. Capsaicin is a natural compound that gives chiles their spicy quality. You may need to limit how much chile you eat if your IBS symptoms are triggered by spicy food.

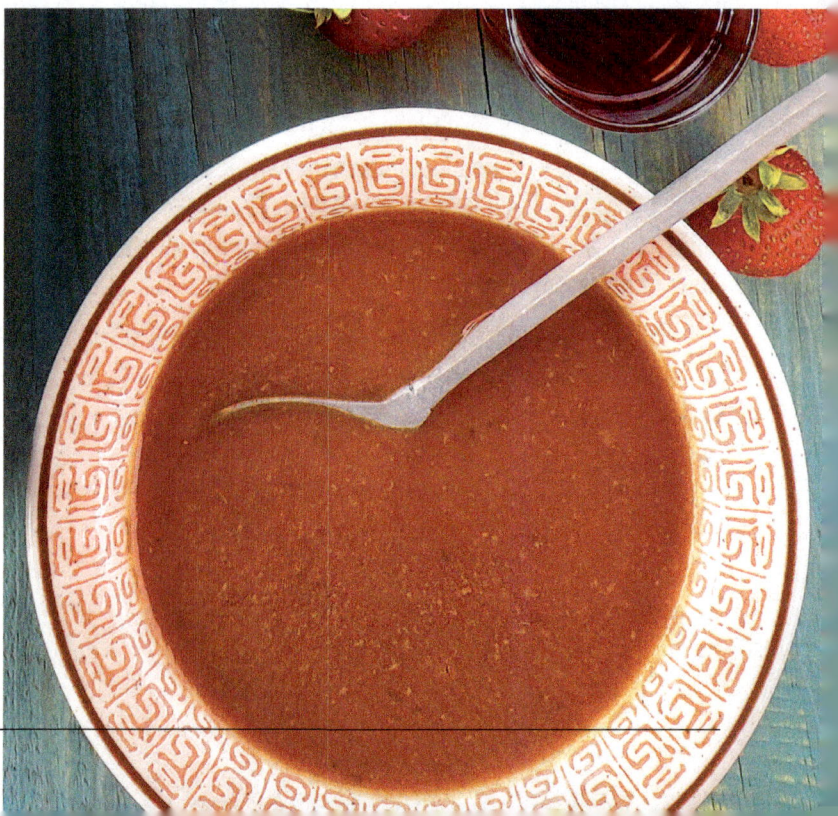

Tomato Ketchup / Catsup

LOW FODMAP ❤ IBS FRIENDLY ❤ GLUTEN-FREE ❤ DAIRY-FREE

Based on the fresh tomato-based ketchup with vinegar, sugar and spices, it's never a bother to make because it tastes so much better than store-bought. Stored in a jar with a tightly sealed lid, it will keep in the fridge for 1 week.

MAKES 1 CUP (240 ML) – 8, 2 TABLESPOONS (30 ML) SERVINGS
INGREDIENTS

2 medium (476 g total) common tomatoes

1/4 cup (60 ml) apple cider vinegar

2 tablespoons (20 g) medium packed light brown sugar

2 tablespoons (25 g) sugar

1/4 cup (60 g) tomato paste, containing no high fructose corn syrup or other high FODMAP ingredients

1 teaspoon (1 g) fine minced fresh chives

1 teaspoon (2 g) paprika

1 teaspoon (5 g) fine sea salt

1/2 teaspoon (2.5 g) plain, prepared yellow mustard, containing no onion or garlic

1/8 teaspoon ground nutmeg

1/8 teaspoon ground cinnamon

Pinch ground cloves

Method: To blanch the tomatoes: Fill a medium saucepan three-quarter full with water and bring to a full boil. Use a sharp knife to cut a shallow X on the bottom and top of the tomatoes and add them to the water. Pour in more hot water if needed to completely submerge them. Set a timer for 2 minutes. The skins will begin to loosen and peel. (There are recipes calling for 30 second blanching but, for me, this never seems long enough for the skins to pull away for easy removal).

Use a fork to turn the tomatoes over. Check to see if the skins are pulling away from the tomato meat. If not, boil for another minute. Using a slotted spoon, place the tomatoes on a cutting board. Use a fork and sharp paring knife to peel the skins off. Cut the meat from the core.

Scoop the tomato meat with seeds and juices into a blender. Add the remaining ingredients and purée 2 minutes.

Discard the blanching water and pour the ketchup into the saucepan. Cook over low-medium heat, bringing to a low boil. Cover with lid and cook for 10 minutes, stirring occasionally until bubbly and thickened to ketchup consistency. For a thicker ketchup, remove the lid and cook a bit longer to reduce, stirring often.

Taste for additional seasoning. You may prefer an additional pinch each of nutmeg, cinnamon, and clove – a tiny pinch at a time, tasting as you add. Allow to cool.

Homemade ketchup will keep in the fridge for 2 weeks when stored in a sterilized airtight container.

Tip: I like to see the seeds and a bit of pulp in my ketchup for that rustic homemade look. If you prefer a more smooth texture, press the warm ketchup through a fine mesh metal strainer and then cool.

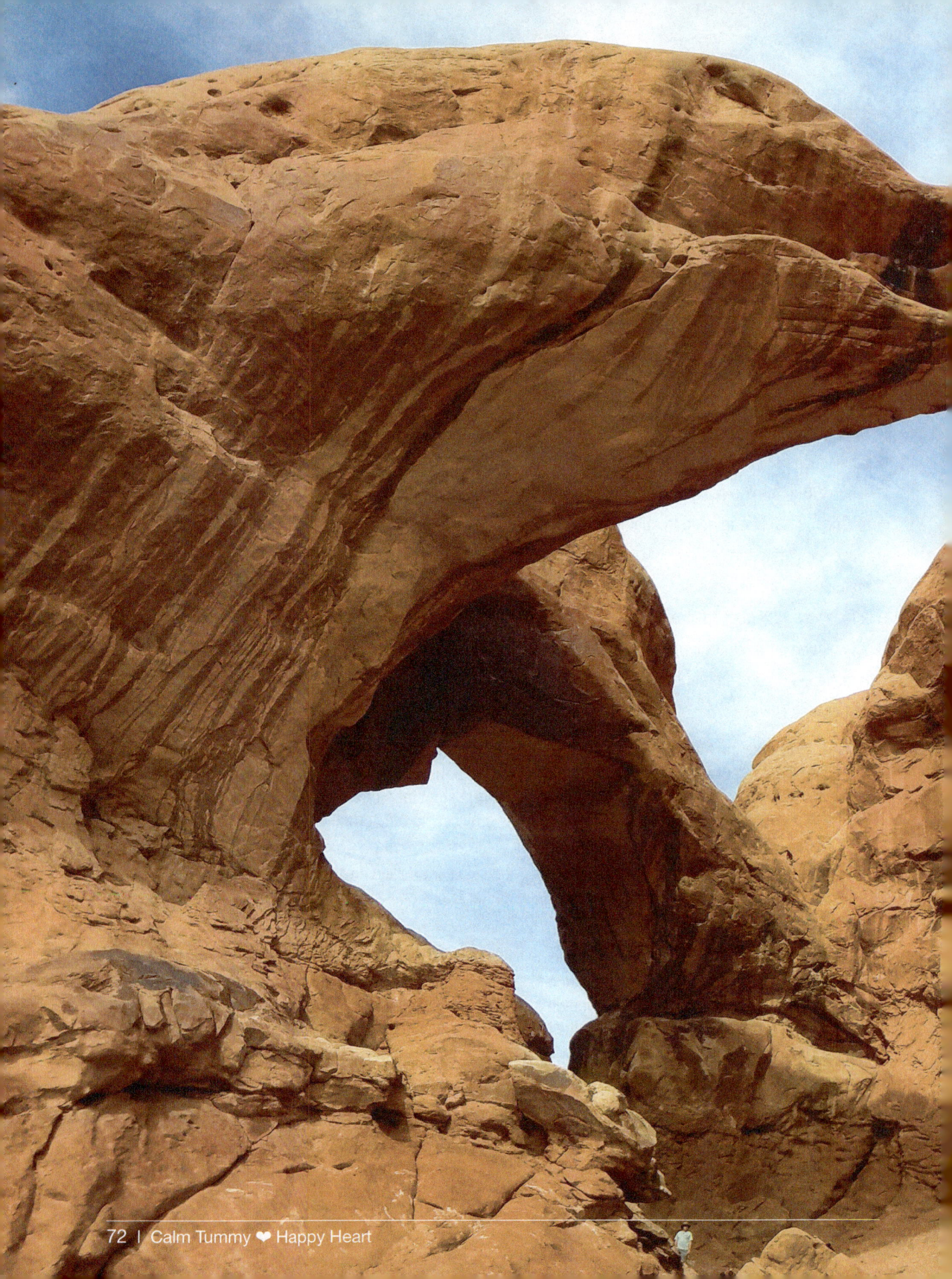

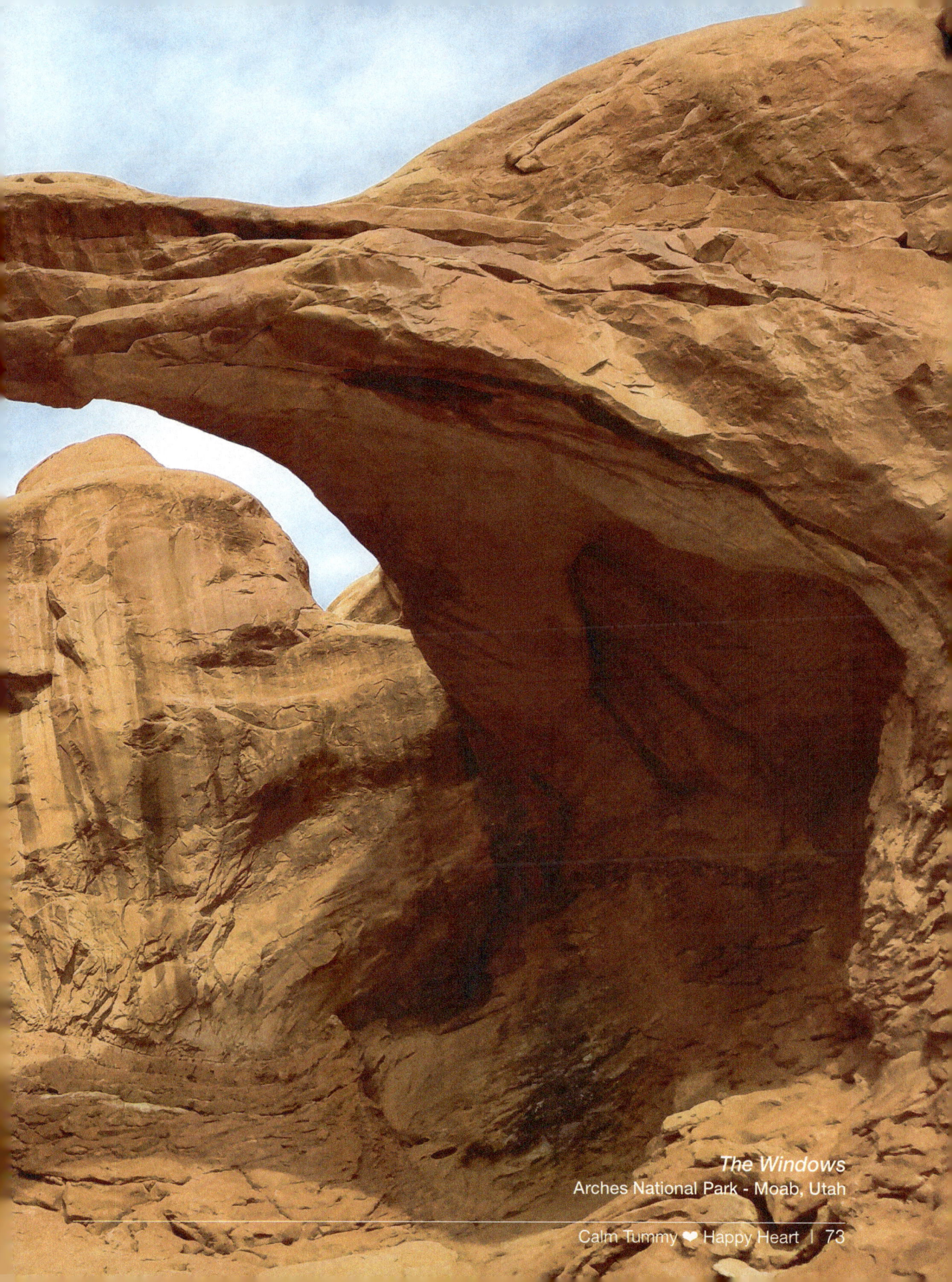

The Windows
Arches National Park - Moab, Utah

Preparing Meats

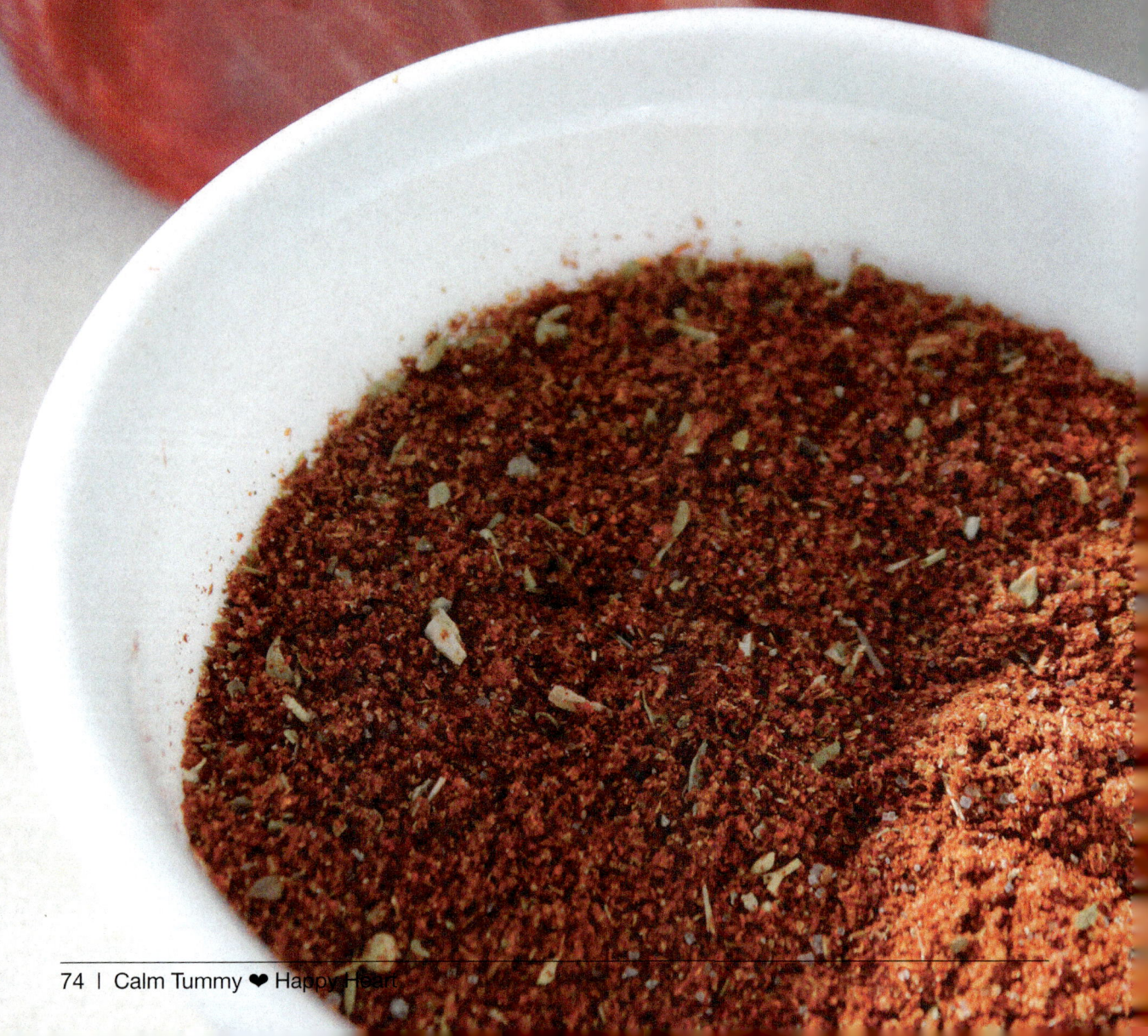

- ❤ **Pa's Slow Cooker Shredded Chicken Breasts**

- ❤ **Pork or Turkey Chorizo (not encased)**

- ❤ **Shredded Beef Barbacoa Style**

- ❤ **Slow Oven-Roasted Pulled Pork**

- ❤ **Whole Poached Chicken for Shredding & Stock**

- ❤ **Poached Chicken Breasts for Shredding & Broth**

Food brand names are sometimes listed within a recipe, and this means they are Monash Certified. For more brand options we use and love, please visit **FodifyIt.com**

Monash Note: Although chiles (chillies) are generally low in FODMAPs, some people with IBS may be sensitive to the capsaicin they contain. Capsaicin is a natural compound that gives chiles their spicy quality. You may need to limit how much chile you eat if your IBS symptoms are triggered by spicy food.

Pa's Slow Cooker Shredded Chicken Breasts

LOW FODMAP ❤ IBS FRIENDLY ❤ GLUTEN-FREE ❤ DAIRY-FREE

A freezer stocked with shredded chicken is a great convenience, particularly if you use it several times a week.

I am forever grateful to my Pa for giving me this recipe that results in a big batch of delicious, juicy chicken that is subtly infused with citrus and scallion greens. The shred is seasoned perfectly and ready for soups, stews, salads, tacos, pizzas, burritos, nachos, you name it. Freeze 1 to 2 portions each, with the pot liquid, in air-tight containers or tightly wrapped freezer baggies and thaw as you need them.

MAKES 10-12 SERVINGS
INGREDIENTS

3 tablespoons (45 ml) Low FODMAP Garlic-Infused Oil (page 50), made with extra virgin olive oil

4-pounds (1.8 kg) boneless, skinless chicken breasts, trimmed of any fat

1 teaspoon (5 g) fine sea salt

1/2 teaspoon fresh ground black pepper

1/2 cup (120 ml) fresh squeezed orange juice

Juice of 1 lime

1/4 cup (13 g) thin sliced scallions, green parts only

water for partially submerging the chicken

Method: Pour the oil in the bottom of 6 quart slow cooker and set cooker to high. Season the chicken breasts on both sides with a light dusting of salt and pepper. Place in the pot. Pour in the citrus juices. Sprinkle the scallion greens on top. If needed, add enough water to the submerge the breasts half-way, but not completely covered. Cover with the lid and cook for 3 1/2 hours.

Check for shredability by using tongs to move 1 breast to a cutting board. Using two forks, it should pull apart and shred easily. If not, place it back in the pot and cook 30 minutes longer.

Place the chicken on a cutting board and allow to cool for 5 minutes. Use two forks to shred.

Chicken will last in the refrigerator for 2 days when stored in an airtight container, and will freeze for 2 to 3 months in an airtight freezer-safe container or heavy zip top bags.

Tip: Microwave the lime on high for 10 seconds before squeezing to release more juices.

Pork or Turkey Chorizo
(not encased)

LOW FODMAP ❤ IBS FRIENDLY ❤ GLUTEN-FREE ❤ DAIRY-FREE

Chorizo is a spicy pork sausage with chiles, garlic, red wine vinegar and spices. You can buy pre-ground pork or ask your butcher to grind 1-pound (454 g) of boneless pork shoulder or pork chops for you. Ground turkey also works well, and the addition of garlic-infused oil keeps it juicy.

Pan cooked chorizo patties add a flavor blast to breakfast sandwiches, and there are countless uses for cooked crumbled chorizo such as mixing into Frittatas (page 166), folding into scrambled eggs, and as a topping for pizzas and gluten-free pasta.

This recipe requires 4 hours of refrigeration and overnight is even better, so plan accordingly. The flavors and texture will improve with this step. When short on time, let it sit for 30 minutes to infuse, then cook.

MAKES 6 SERVINGS
INGREDIENTS

2 tablespoons (30 ml) Low FODMAP Garlic-Infused Oil (page 50), made with canola oil, cooled

1-pound (454 g) ground pork or ground turkey, crumbled

3 tablespoons (45 ml) red wine vinegar

2 teaspoons (4 g) smoked paprika

2 teaspoons (4 g) pure mild red chile powder (containing no onion or garlic, the ingredients should list only: red chile. On the Monash App this is called Chilli (chili) red, powdered)

2 teaspoons dried oregano

1 teaspoon (5 g) fine sea salt

1/2 teaspoon ground cinnamon

1/2 teaspoon fresh ground black pepper

1/4 – 1/2 teaspoon cayenne powder

2 tablespoons (30 ml) canola oil for pan cooking

Method: Mix the garlic oil, pork, vinegar, paprika, red chile powder, oregano, salt, cinnamon, black pepper and cayenne until fully incorporated in a medium bowl. Cover with a lid or plastic wrap and refrigerate for at least 4 hours; overnight is even better to allow the flavors to infuse.

Patties: Divide the meat mixture into 6 even amounts and form into balls. Flatten into patties with your hands.

Pour 2 tablespoons canola oil in a nonstick skillet over medium high heat. Add the patties and cook for 4 minutes. Flip and cook 4 to 5 minutes or until cooked completely through.

Cooked Crumbled Chorizo: Pour 2 tablespoons canola into a nonstick skillet over medium high heat. Add the loose chorizo meat and brown for 4 minutes using a flat wooden spatula to really break up the meat. Turn and stir. Cook 4 to 5 minutes longer or until cooked completely through.

Monash Note: Although chiles (chillies) are generally low in FODMAPs, some people with IBS may be sensitive to the capsaicin they contain. Capsaicin is a natural compound that gives chiles their spicy quality. You may need to limit how much chile you eat if your IBS symptoms are triggered by spicy food.

Shredded Beef Barbacoa Style

LOW FODMAP ❤ IBS FRIENDLY ❤ GLUTEN-FREE ❤ DAIRY-FREE

Barbacoa is a slow cooked beef roast marinated with rehydrated dried red chile and ancho chile pods, spices, vinegar, garlic, and fresh lime juice. Dried chiles that have been Monash tested contain high FODMAP levels, so I've calculated spices and ground chiles in LoFO amounts for a robust Barbacoa. The vinegar, chipotle powder, cumin, oregano, cinnamon and scallion greens infuse flavor into the meat for a sublime, tender shredded beef.

This recipe requires 6+ hours roasting time.

MAKES APPROX. 2 1/2 – 3 1/4-POUNDS (1.134 KG – 1.475 KG) AFTER DISCARDING THE FAT

Depending on your recipe and appetite, 1-pound of barbacoa will serve 3 to 4 people. 1-pound (454 g) yields enough for 8 to 9 tacos. This will vary according to the overall fat content of the roast and how much you prefer to discard when shredding.

INGREDIENTS

1, 4-pound (1.8 kg) boneless beef chuck roast with medium marbling, not too fatty

2 teaspoons (10 g) fine sea salt, divided

2 teaspoons fresh ground black pepper, divided

3 tablespoons (45 ml) canola oil

Juice of 2 limes

1 cup (240 ml) Low FODMAP Chicken Stock (page 135), or water

1/3 cup (80 ml) red or white wine vinegar

1/4 cup (60 g) tomato paste, containing no high fructose corn syrup or other high FODMAP ingredients

1 teaspoon (2 g) pure chipotle powder

1 teaspoon (2 g) ground cumin

1 teaspoon dried oregano

1 teaspoon fresh ground black pepper

1/2 (1 g) teaspoon ground cinnamon

3/4 cup (38 g) thin sliced scallions, green parts only

Method: Place the oven rack to center position. Heat oven to 425 F / 220 C

Coat the roast all over with 1 teaspoon salt and 1 teaspoon pepper. In a large nonstick skillet heat the oil over medium high heat until shimmering and brown the roast on all sides, turning the meat with two large forks as needed. Place the beef in a roasting pan that is lightly coated with oil or cooking spray oil.

In a medium mixing bowl, whisk together the lime juice, stock, vinegar, tomato paste, chipotle powder, cumin, oregano, 1 teaspoon pepper and cinnamon. Pour over the meat and into the pan. Cover with foil being sure to tightly seal around the edges with your fingers.

Place in the oven and roast for 40 minutes.

Reduce the heat to 300 F / 150 C and roast for 5 hours.

When a meat thermometer inserted into the center of the roast reads 200 F / 93 C it is ready to shred. If not yet ready, return to the oven, covered tightly and roast for 30 minutes to 1 hour longer.

Move the beef to a large bowl or casserole dish, tent with foil and let rest for 30 minutes or until cooled enough to handle. Reserve the pan juices.

Using two forks, pull the beef to shred, removing any fatty bits. Pour the reserved pan liquid through a fine mesh metal strainer back over the meat to keep it nice and juicy. Mix in the sliced scallion greens and the result is a flavorful, tender shredded beef with many uses.

Stored in an airtight container, it will keep for 3 days in the refrigerator.

For freezing, divide the shred into 1 to 2 serving size portions and place in freezer baggies or tightly sealed freezer containers. It will keep 2 to 3 months in the freezer.

FOR PLAIN SHREDDED BEEF

Coat the roast with salt and pepper. Brown in oil as instructed. Omit all braising ingredients but the LoFO chicken stock and finishing touch of scallion green parts.

Barbacoa is perfect for tacos, enchilada filling, beef sandwiches, burritos, nachos, on loaded baked potatoes, in stews – the list is long.

Brisket is also great for shredded beef.

Be sure to shred the beef once it's rested and cooled enough to handle. Putting it in the fridge to shred later doesn't work as well because when cold and hardened it's difficult to pull the beef from bits of fat. Best to shred while still warm and then refrigerate.

A favorite preparation is beef barbacoa tacos topped with sliced green parts of scallions, fresh squeezed lime, thin sliced radishes, and shredded cheddar (if tolerated).

Monash Note: Although chiles (chillies) are generally low in FODMAPs, some people with IBS may be sensitive to the capsaicin they contain. Capsaicin is a natural compound that gives chiles their spicy quality. You may need to limit how much chile you eat if your IBS symptoms are triggered by spicy food.

Slow Oven-Roasted Pulled Pork

LOW FODMAP ❤ IBS FRIENDLY ❤ GLUTEN-FREE ❤ DAIRY-FREE

Slow-cooker pulled pork is delicious but this oven roasted method delivers much more flavor, and takes about the same time to cook. Start your roast in the morning to allow for ample cooking time and an all-day fandango of wonderful aromas dancing around your home.

There are countless seasoning combinations for pork rub, but I prefer a simple coating of salt and pepper. This way the pork is seasoned, I've eliminated onion and garlic powder, and later I can select the sauce or preparation to use without worrying about stacking FODMAPs and calculating additional chile powder and other ingredients. Basically, I think of this recipe as a tasty clean slate to work from.

FAVORITE PULLED PORK DISHES

Pulled Pork Sandwich (page 186)

Pulled Pork Caesar Salad (page 126)

Cornmeal Pancakes with Pulled Pork, Tangy Sauce, Strawberries and Cinnamon Maple Syrup (page 158)

If you are a fan of pineapple, pulled pork tacos topped with Grilled Pineapple Salsa (page 67) is divine.

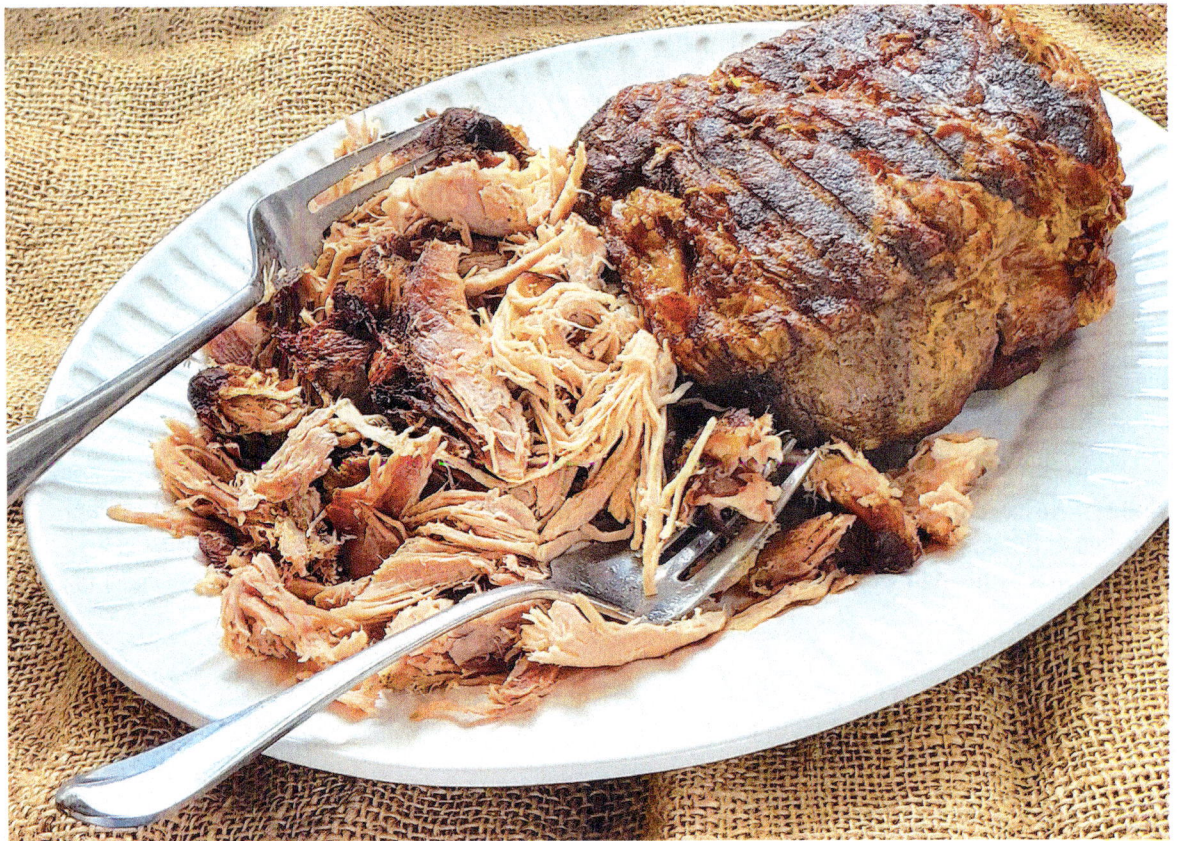

MAKES APPROX. 2 1/2 – 3-POUNDS (1.1 KG – 1.4 KG) AFTER REMOVING AND DISCARDING THE BONE AND FAT

The amount will vary according to the overall fat content and also how much you prefer to discard when shredding the roast. Depending on your recipe and appetite, 1-pound of pulled pork will serve 3 to 4 people, and will yield 8 to 9 tacos.

INGREDIENTS

1, 8-pound (3.6 kg) pork shoulder (Boston Butt) bone-in for better flavor, set out for 30 minutes to room temperature and no longer than 1 hour

3 teaspoons (15 g) fine sea salt mixed with 3 teaspoons (6 g) fresh ground black pepper

Method: Set oven rack to center position. Preheat oven to 350 F / 177 C. Line a roasting pan with foil.

Wash the pork under cool water and pat dry with paper towels. On the fatty side, cut off any large fat pockets, leaving about 1/2–inch (1.25 cm) of fat layer for good roasting flavors to infuse into the meat. Place the pork in the pan and coat both sides with the salt and pepper mix. With the fat side up, cover the pan with foil being sure to tightly seal around the edges with your fingers.

Roast for 5 1/2 hours.

Uncover and carefully, using two big forks, move the roast to a large plate. Using oven mitts, pour the pan juices into a medium-sized bowl or measuring cup. Cover the juices with plastic wrap and place in the fridge for later when you drench the finished shred.

Add 2 cups hot water to the pan and place the roast with the fat side down.

Roast uncovered for 1 to 1 1/2 hours or until a meat thermometer inserted into the center reads 195 F / 90 C. If the internal temperature reaches 200 F / 94 C, that's perfectly fine. It will shred just as well for you.

Move to a cutting board or counter top and tent the pan with foil. Let rest for 30 minutes. Pull the bone out and discard, if present. Using two forks, pull the pork to shred and place in a large bowl as you go. Remove and discard any fatty bits. Pour the reserved pan juices through a fine mesh metal strainer back over the shred to drench. By following this step you will never make a dry pulled pork!

Pulled Pork will keep in the refrigerator for 3 days, and in the freezer for 4 to 5 months. I like to freeze 2 to 4 portion sizes per tightly rolled and sealed freezer baggie, or in a freezer-safe container.

Tip: Be sure to shred the pork once it's rested and cooled enough to handle. Putting it in the fridge to shred later doesn't work as well because when cold and hardened it is difficult to pull the pork from bits of fat. Best to shred while still warm and then refrigerate or freeze.

SLOW COOKER PULLED PORK METHOD

Select a pork shoulder (Boston Butt) that will fit into your slow cooker. Coat it on all sides with a light dusting of salt and pepper. Heat 2 tablespoons (30 ml) canola oil in a large nonstick skillet over medium high heat. Brown the pork on all sides for nice sear. Place it in the slow cooker with 1-inch (2.5 cm) of water in the bottom. Cook on low for 8 to 8 1/2 hours, or the recommended time per pound according to your cooker manual. When the internal temperature reaches 195 F / 90 C it is tender enough to shred. Move the roast to a large casserole dish and let it rest for 30 minutes tented with foil. Use two forks to pull the meat apart. Remove any fatty bits. Pour the pot liquor through a fine mesh metal strainer back onto the pulled pork to keep it juicy. Dig in!

Whole Poached Chicken for Shredding & Stock

LOW FODMAP ❤ IBS FRIENDLY ❤ GLUTEN-FREE ❤ DAIRY-FREE

While Pa's Slow Cooker Shredded Chicken Breasts (page 76) are delicious and easy to make, they take 3 1/2 hours to cook and do not yield enough pan juices for stock. If you're pressed for time, poaching a whole chicken takes a little over an hour to cook, cool and shred. You will also have a delicious stock for freezing in portions and thaw as needed.

MAKES APPROX. 2 1/2 CUPS (375 G) SHRED AND 8 CUPS (2 L) STOCK

This will vary according to how much of the meat you prefer to shred while discarding the bone and fat.

INGREDIENTS

1, 3-pound (1.4 kg) chicken

6 scallions, green parts only, rough chopped

1 carrot (75 g) peeled and cut into 1-inch (2.5 cm) pieces

2 tablespoons (2 g) fresh parsley leaves, without stems as they can be bitter

1 teaspoon whole black peppercorns

Fine sea salt for dusting the shredded meat

Method: Place the chicken in a large stockpot and fill with water to completely submerge the bird. Add the scallion greens, carrot, parsley and peppercorns. Bring to a boil for 10 minutes, covered. Reduce to a simmer for 20 minutes. Use a slotted spoon to skim any foam from the surface. Turn the chicken over, place the lid back on and simmer for another 20 minutes. Add more hot water to cover the bird if the stock has significantly reduced. Turn the bird over and simmer 20 minutes longer, covered. The chicken should be cooked through, with no pink showing. Remove from heat and place on a wire rack or trivet to cool for 10 minutes.

Move the chicken from the pot to a clean work surface and reserve the stock. Let the chicken cool until you are able to handle it. Pull the meat from the bones as best you can. Discard the skins and carcass. Use your hands or two forks to shred the meat. Lightly dust with salt if desired. You now have a beautiful shred for enchiladas, tacos, salads and any number of dishes.

Pour the stock through a fine mesh metal strainer into a large bowl. Discard the solids. Skim off any foam or fat from the surface. Depending on the size of your stockpot and how much the stock reduces while cooking, this method will yield about 8 cups (2 L).

Refrigerate or freeze immediately. Cooked chicken and stock will last in the refrigerator for up to 2 days and can be frozen in airtight freezer containers for 2 to 3 months.

Tip: Those yummy cooked carrot pieces are for the chef!

Poached Chicken Breasts
for Shredding & Broth

LOW FODMAP ❤ IBS FRIENDLY ❤ GLUTEN-FREE ❤ DAIRY-FREE

Pa's Slow Cooker Shredded Chicken Breasts (page 76) are flavorful, easy to make, and take 3 1/2 hours to cook. Whole Poached Chicken (page 82) requires a little over an hour to cook, cool and shred. You will also have a delicious stock for freezing in portions and thaw as needed.

This poaching recipe takes only 40 minutes to boil, poach, cool and shred. It will yield a good amount of broth, however, I find that the stock from a Whole Poached Chicken has a deeper, more robust flavor. That said, this recipe is a time saver and one to have in your repertoire.

MAKES APPROX. 2-POUNDS (907 G) SHRED – 4-5 CUPS (150 G EACH) AND 8 CUPS (2 L) BROTH
INGREDIENTS

8 cups (2 L) water

2-pounds (907 g) boneless, skinless chicken breasts

6 scallions, green parts only, rough chopped

1 carrot (75 g) peeled and diced

2 tablespoons (2 g) fresh parsley leaves, without stems as they can be bitter

1 teaspoon whole black peppercorns

Method: Fill a large stockpot with water and bring to a rolling boil. Add the chicken, scallion greens, carrot, parsley and peppercorns. Cover with lid and reduce heat to medium for a steady, medium boil for 5 minutes. Stir, turn the chicken over. Boil 5 minutes longer. Remove from heat and let poach for 15 minutes, covered and undisturbed. Use a slotted spoon to remove any foam from the surface.

Transfer the chicken to a cutting board. If the breasts are at all pink in the center, return to the pot to boil 5 to 10 minutes longer until they are cooked through. Allow to cool on the cutting board for 10 minutes, or until cool enough to handle. Use your hands to pull the chicken into a fine shred.

Pour the stock through a fine mesh metal strainer into a large bowl.

Refrigerate or freeze immediately. Cooked chicken and broth will last in the refrigerator for up to 2 days and can be frozen in airtight freezer containers for 2 – 3 months.

Tip: Those yummy cooked carrot pieces are for you!

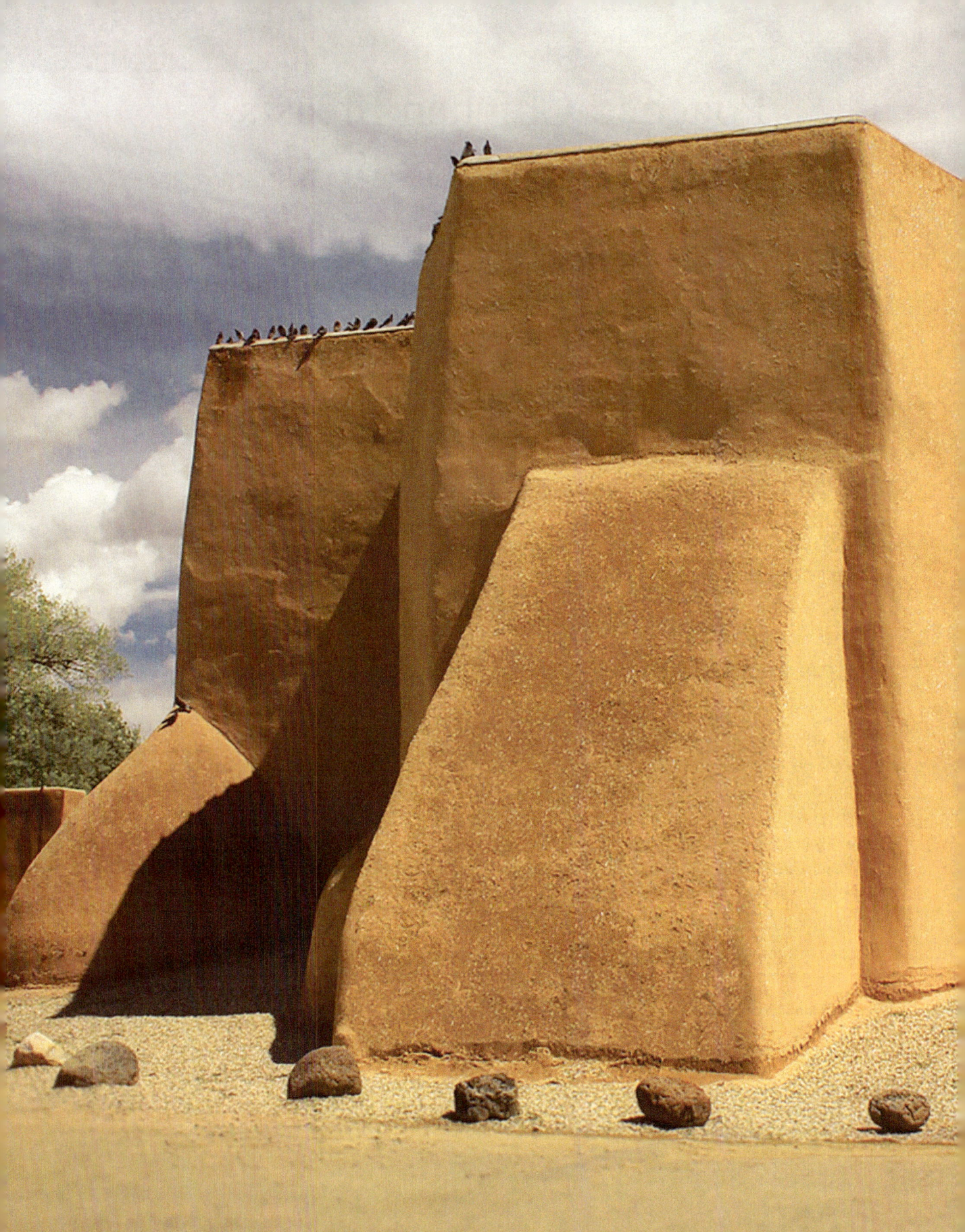

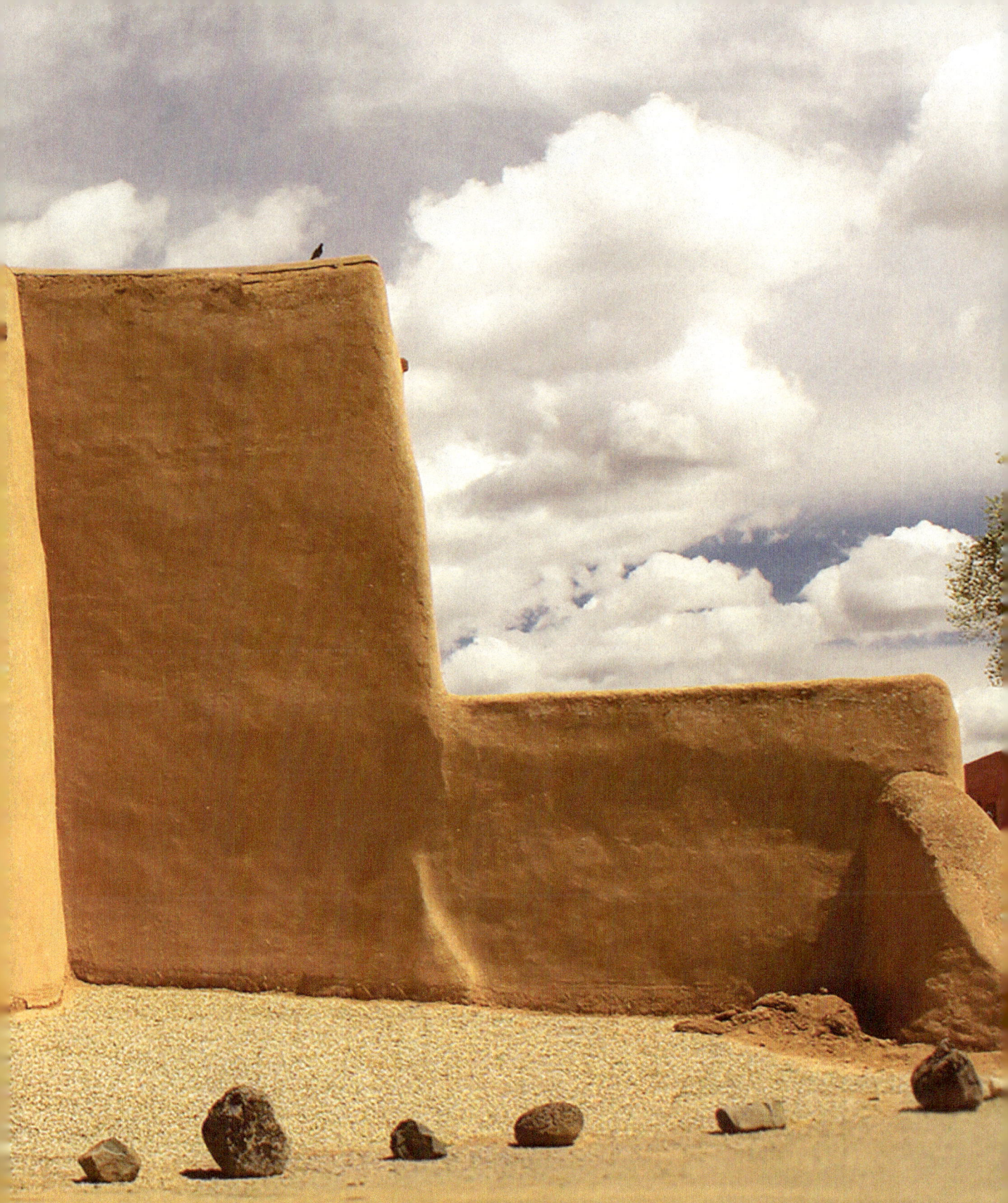

San Francisco de Asis Church
Taos, New Mexico

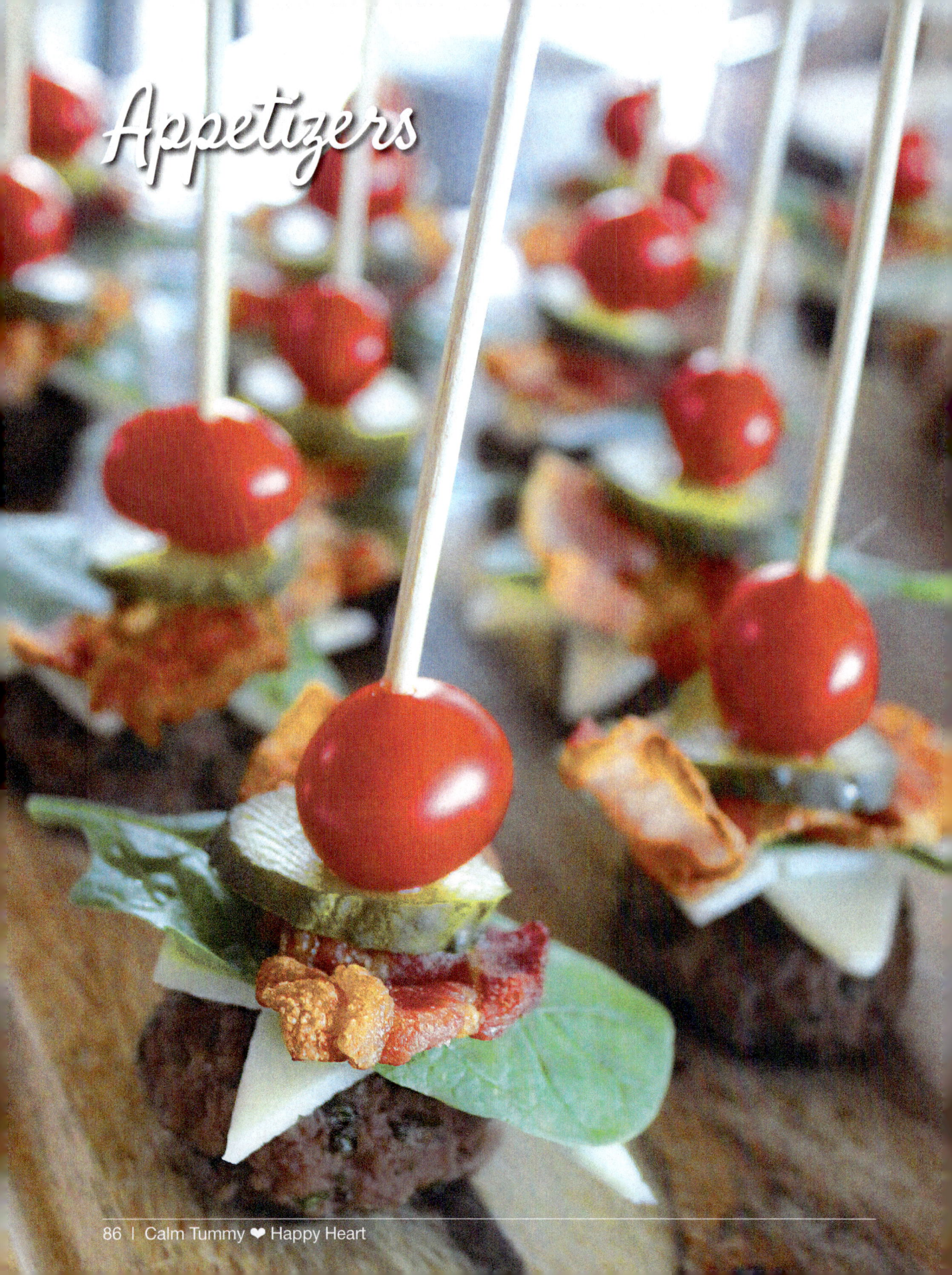

Appetizers

- ❤ **Mexican Restaurant Style Chips & Salsa**

- ❤ **Cilantro Lime Olive Tapenade**

- ❤ **East Meets Southwest Salmon Nachos with Chile Mayo Soy Sauce**

- ❤ **Char Grilled Chimichurri Oysters**

- ❤ **Green Chile Crab Cakes**

- ❤ **Guacamole Mockamole Love**

- ❤ **Chipotle Chive Turkey Burger Bites with Yellow Cornmeal & Pickles**

Food brand names are sometimes listed within a recipe, and this means they are Monash Certified. For more brand options we use and love, please visit **FodifyIt.com**

Monash Note: Although chiles (chillies) are generally low in FODMAPs, some people with IBS may be sensitive to the capsaicin they contain. Capsaicin is a natural compound that gives chiles their spicy quality. You may need to limit how much chile you eat if your IBS symptoms are triggered by spicy food.

Mexican Restaurant Style Chips & Salsa

LOW FODMAP ❤ IBS FRIENDLY ❤ GLUTEN-FREE ❤ DAIRY-FREE

As sure as the sun will rise tomorrow, the moment you're seated at a Mexican restaurant someone will bring a basket of warm corn tortilla chips with a bowl of salsa and place them in the center of your table. Is that a delightful constant in life or what?

The salsa is typically not chunky, but rather a salty tomato purée with small bits of cilantro and lots of onion and garlic. This LoFO version swaps in scallion greens for white onion and garlic-infused oil (page 50) for garlic cloves or powder. Lime juice and cilantro add a spritz of dazzle and herby freshness.

Monash notes that while this is low FODMAP and in proper portions, it is on the higher side of the cut-off. Considering it is an appetizer and will be consumed with other foods, they recommend to spread out the other dishes and eat them over several hours. Or, this recipe may be consumed as a standalone snack.

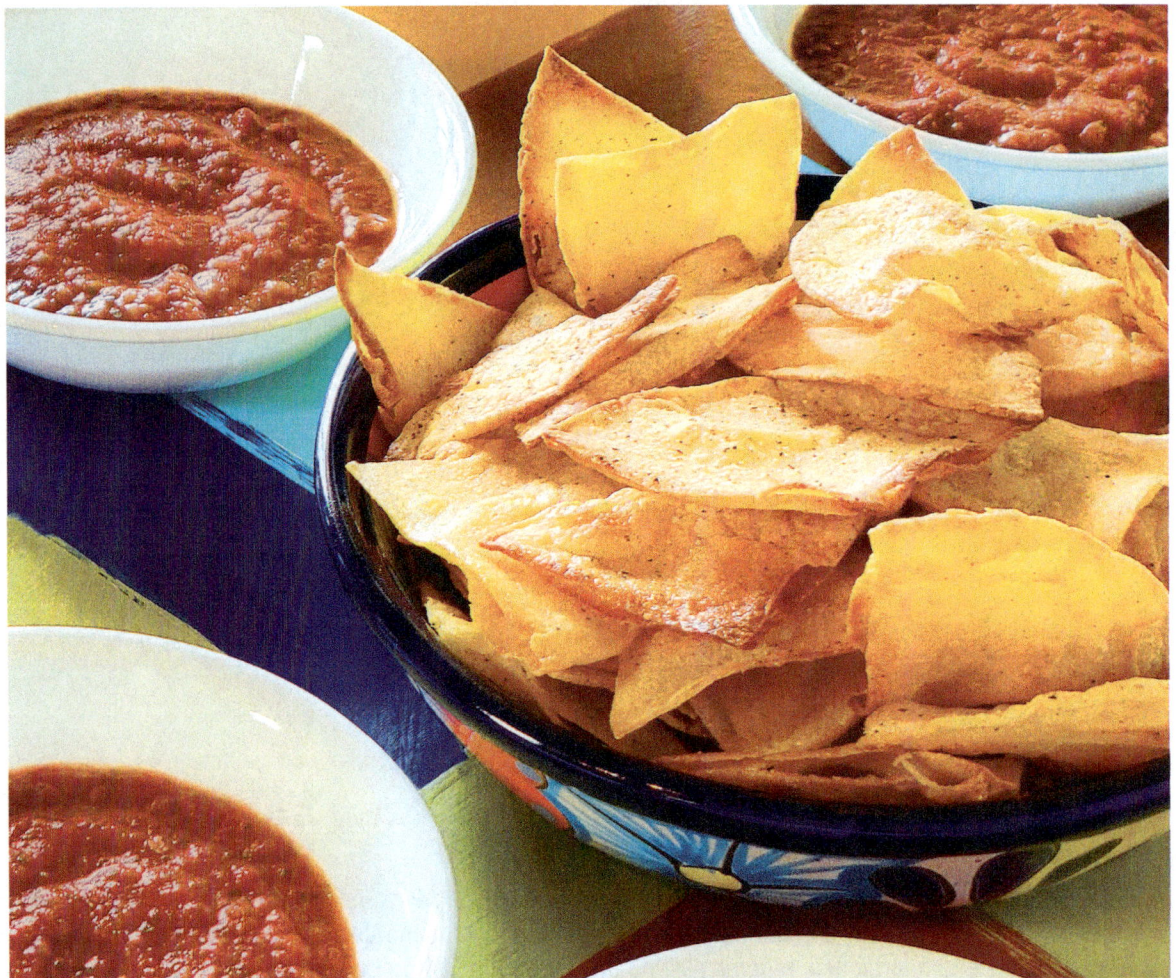

MAKES 8 SERVINGS
SALSA INGREDIENTS

21-ounces (600 g) canned, plain peeled Roma tomatoes, drained

1/4 cup (4 g) fresh medium packed cilantro, mostly leaves

1/2 teaspoon (1 g) ground cumin

1/2 teaspoon (2.5 g) fine sea salt, plus more to your taste

2 tablespoons (30 ml) Low FODMAP Garlic-Infused Oil (page 50), made with canola oil

1/4 cup (13 g) thin sliced scallions, green parts only

Juice of 1 lime

CHIP INGREDIENTS – 9 PER SERVING

14 (6-inch/16 cm) low FODMAP gluten-free white corn tortillas; yellow corn tortillas are fine though you may prefer the lighter white corn texture

Spray cooking oil

Fine sea salt

Fresh ground black pepper (optional)

Method: Preheat oven to 400 F / 200 C

Salsa: Place the metal blade in a food processor. Add the tomatoes, cilantro, cumin, and salt. Pulse a few times to mix, scrape down the sides with a spatula, then purée until you have a smooth consistency with a bit of texture. If you do not have a food processor, the same rustic consistency can be achieved by hand chopping and mincing with a large, sharp knife on a cutting board with a grooved rim to catch the juices.

Pour the oil into a medium nonstick skillet over medium high heat and bring to a shimmer. Add the salsa and scallion greens and cook the mixture for 4 minutes, stirring often. Reduce the heat to low and simmer for 5 minutes or until the consistency is thick enough to scoop with a chip. Remove from heat, stir in the lime juice and taste to adjust for salt. Cool for 10 minutes, then refrigerate in an airtight container until chilled.

Chips: Using a pizza cutter, quarter each tortilla like a pie.

Coat a rimmed baking sheet with cooking spray oil. Place as many tortilla triangles on the tray that will fit without overlapping. Spray them lightly with oil. Coat evenly with a very light dusting of salt, and an even lighter sprinkling of pepper. Bake for 4 minutes. Use a spatula to flip them over and bake for an additional 4 minutes or until they are just browned on the edges. Keep a close watch, they will burn quickly. Place the chips on paper towels to cool. Repeat in batches until all chips are baked.

Traditionally, the chips are served in a bowl, or basket lined with parchment paper. The salsa is served in a chilled serving bowl or divided into smaller bowls and placed in the center of the table.

Stored in an airtight container, salsa will keep up to 3 days in the refrigerator

Tip: Microwave the lime on high for 10 seconds before squeezing to release more juices.

Monash Note: Although chiles (chillies) are generally low in FODMAPs, some people with IBS may be sensitive to the capsaicin they contain. Capsaicin is a natural compound that gives chiles their spicy quality. You may need to limit how much chile you eat if your IBS symptoms are triggered by spicy food.

Cilantro Lime Olive Tapenade

LOW FODMAP ❤ IBS FRIENDLY ❤ GLUTEN-FREE ❤ DAIRY-FREE

Spanish and canned pitted ripe black olives blended, but not too smooth, with fresh herbs and a few more goodies create a delicious, salty olive spread with an enticing, coarse texture. Served with corn tortilla chips, this is a quick and easy recipe for your happy hour.

MAKES 4-6 SERVINGS
INGREDIENTS

1/2 cup (60 g) canned, pitted ripe black olives

1/2 cup (60 g) Spanish plain pitted green olives, not stuffed with pimento, garlic or other ingredients, nor brined in onion, garlic or other high FODMAP ingredients

1/4 cup (4 g) fresh medium packed cilantro, mostly leaves, minced

1/4 cup (13 g) flat leaf parsley leaves, stems can be bitter

1/4 cup (60 ml) Low FODMAP Garlic-Infused Oil (page 50), made with extra virgin olive oil, or plain olive oil is also fine

2 tablespoons (20 g) fresh red bell pepper, rough chopped

2 tablespoons (12 g) capers, drained

Juice of 1 lime, or more if desired

1 1/2 teaspoons dried oregano

1 teaspoon (2 g) ground cumin

Garnish with a round slice of lime

Method: Using the metal blade of a food processor, place all of the ingredients into the bowl. Pulse a few times to mix. Scrape down the sides of the bowl with a spatula as needed. Continue to pulse rather than blend, as you do not want a smooth puréed texture. When the olives and herbs are fully incorporated and the texture is still a bit coarse, spoon into a serving bowl. Place the lime slice on the center top of the tapenade. Chill until ready to serve. Serve with corn tortilla chips at a suggested serving of 10 chips (30 g) per serving.

Stored in an airtight container, tapenade will keep for up to 7 days in the refrigerator.

Tip: As of this writing pimentos, that are oftentimes stuffed into olives, have not yet been tested for FODMAPs by Monash. Be sure to check the Monash App for new testing updates.

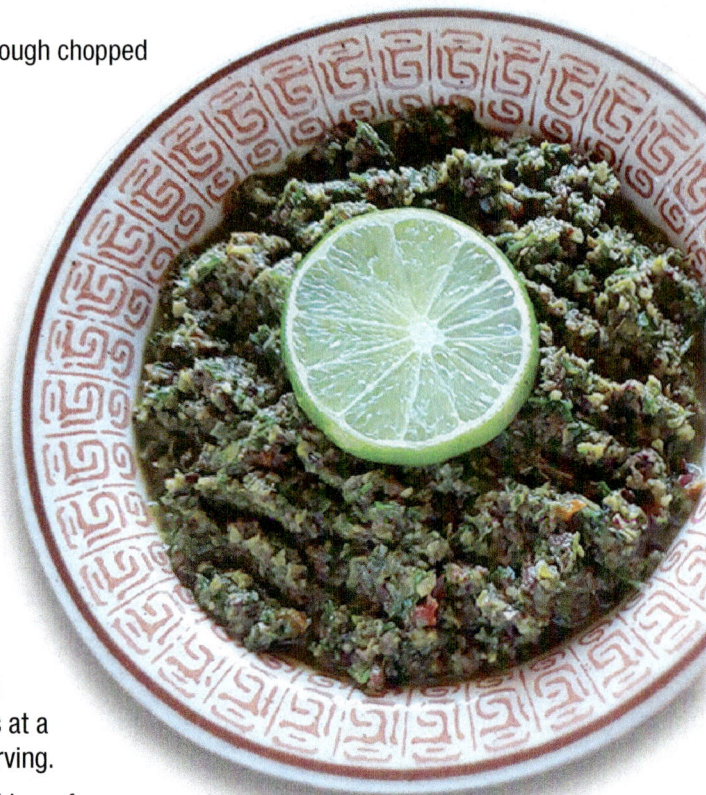

East Meets Southwest Salmon Nachos with Chile Sesame Mayo Soy Sauce

LOW FODMAP ❤ IBS FRIENDLY ❤ GLUTEN-FREE ❤ DAIRY-FREE

If you don't like tacos this is 'nacho' type of dish! Nachos are basically a big plate of corn tortilla chips piled into a mound with taco ingredients, all joined together with melted cheese. And just like tacos, they can be made with all sorts of leftovers from your fridge. This cold dish version is a mix of delicate flaked salmon and toasted sesame oil mayo, topped with bold pickled jalapenos. Nacho average gluten-free dairy-free appetizer platter!

MAKES 8 SERVINGS
CHIP INGREDIENTS

60, (6 1/2-ounces / 180 g) low FODMAP store-bought corn tortilla chips

8-ounces (227 g) salmon, pan cooked in extra virgin olive oil or steamed, flaked with a fork and cooled

1/3 cup (64 g) jarred pickled jalapeños, containing no onion, garlic or other high FODMAPs, drained well

2 tablespoons (7 g) thin sliced scallions, green parts only

8 large (160 g total) red radishes, sliced thin

2 limes, sliced into wedges

SAUCE INGREDIENTS

1/3 cup (77 g) mayonnaise, containing no onion or garlic

2 tablespoons (30 ml) soy sauce; gluten-free if you are following a gluten-free diet

1/2 teaspoon (2.5 ml) toasted sesame oil

Juice of 1 lime

1/2 teaspoon (1 g) pure mild red chile powder (containing no onion or garlic, the ingredients should list only: red chile. On the Monash App this is called Chilli (chili) red, powdered)

Pinch of fine sea salt

Pinch of fresh ground black pepper

Method: Place the chips on a large serving platter, evenly distributed. Place the salmon, jalapeños, scallion greens and radishes evenly over the chips. Arrange lime wedges around the rim of the platter.

Mix the sauce ingredients in a small bowl. Spoon the sauce into a small plastic baggie towards one end. Use scissors to snip a small opening on the end. With swift back and forth motions, squeeze the baggie and drizzle the sauce over the nachos in a "striped" direction. Serve immediately.

Tips: Plain shredded chicken seasoned with a dusting of salt and fresh ground black pepper is a great substitute for salmon.

If pure red chile powder is not available, use smoked paprika.

Monash Note: Although chiles (chillies) are generally low in FODMAPs, some people with IBS may be sensitive to the capsaicin they contain. Capsaicin is a natural compound that gives chiles their spicy quality. You may need to limit how much chile you eat if your IBS symptoms are triggered by spicy food.

Char Grilled Chimichurri Oysters

LOW FODMAP ❤ IBS FRIENDLY ❤ GLUTEN-FREE ❤ DAIRY-FREE

This recipe is low in FODMAPS, however, the amount of oil in the chimichurri that may be tolerated is highly individualized, in which case Monash recommends keeping your portion size to 1 to 2 tablespoons if you are concerned about fat intake.

When you think of Southwest U.S. cuisine, oysters might not immediately come to mind. In the 19th century, mining towns of landlocked Southwestern Colorado considered them to be a delicacy and families would pool their money to have oysters delivered to them via rail. They became so popular that restaurant owners opened oyster houses that were a huge hit with customers, and these mollusks remain on the menus of most historic mining town restaurants today, namely Durango and Telluride, Colorado.

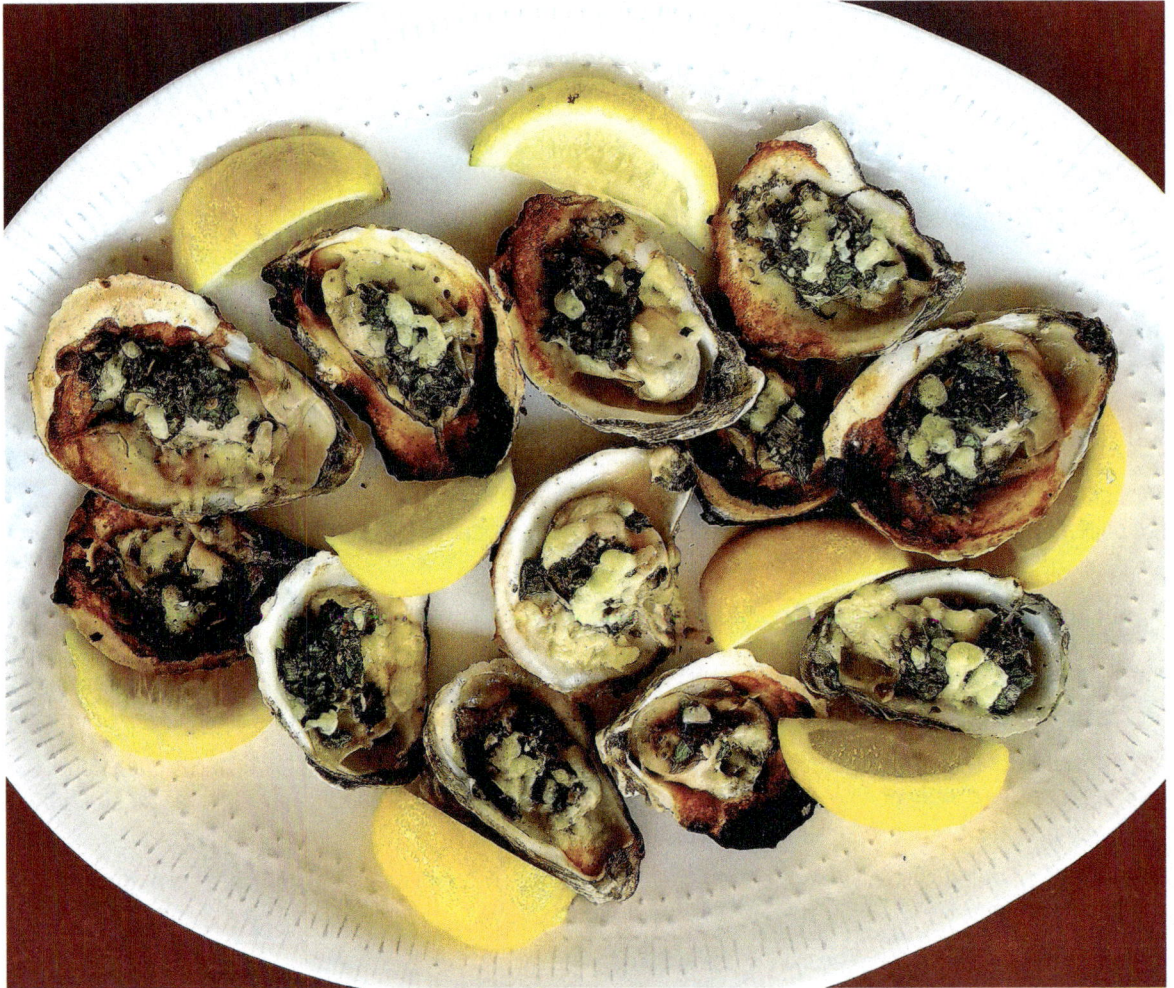

MAKES 4-6 SERVINGS
INGREDIENTS

1/2 cup (8 g) fresh medium packed cilantro, mostly leaves

1/2 cup (8 g) fresh medium packed flat leaf parsley leaves, stems can be bitter

6 scallions, green parts only, rough chopped

1/3 cup (80 ml) Low FODMAP Garlic-Infused Oil (page 50), made with extra virgin olive oil

1/4 cup (60 ml) red wine vinegar

Juice of 1/2 lime

2 tablespoons (4 g) dried oregano

1 teaspoon (2 g) crushed red pepper flakes, more if you like heat

1/2 teaspoon (2.5 g) fine sea salt

1/2 teaspoon fresh ground black pepper

24 fresh large oysters, shucked, with oyster placed in the more cup-shaped shell half, attaching muscle severed

Sliced lemon wedges, optional for garnish

Method: Preheat your grill to high.

Secure the metal blade in a food processor and add the cilantro, parsley, scallion greens, oil, vinegar, lime juice, oregano, pepper flakes, salt and pepper. Give it a couple pulses and scrape down the sides of the bowl with a spatula. Continue to pulse a few more times until everything is combined and the herbs are mixed well but still have a coarse texture – not creamy smooth. Taste for salt and vinegar and adjust as desired.

Place 1 heaping teaspoon of chimichurri onto each oyster. Using metal tongs, place the oysters on the grill grates, close the lid and cook for 3 to 4 minutes. They will bubble and the shells will char a bit around the edges. Use tongs to place on a serving platter with sliced lemon. Allow the oysters to cool a bit until safe to pick up with your hands. Serve immediately.

Tips: Shucking oysters can be tricky. Ask your fishmonger or grocery seafood department for shucked, prepared oysters if you'd like to skip this step.

If you are able to tolerate, 1 teaspoon of fresh grated parmesan or Manchego cheese per oyster adds a salty umami flavor.

Leftover chimichurri is delicious when spooned over eggs and tacos, or used as a spread for sandwiches. It's wonderfully versatile.

Monash Note: Although chiles (chillies) are generally low in FODMAPs, some people with IBS may be sensitive to the capsaicin they contain. Capsaicin is a natural compound that gives chiles their spicy quality. You may need to limit how much chile you eat if your IBS symptoms are triggered by spicy food.

Green Chile Crab Cakes

LOW FODMAP ❤ IBS FRIENDLY ❤ GLUTEN-FREE ❤ DAIRY-FREE

Mild, buttery green chiles do not overpower the delicate crab making them a splendid match. Therefore I now pronounce these chile crab cakes the perfect pair for an appetizer course, main course salad, Eggs Benedict patty, served with breakfast salsa eggs, or for toasted LoFO gluten-free sandwiches with crisp chilled lettuce.

You have the option of using canned drained mild green chiles, or roasting and prepping fresh ones (page 46). On the Monash App they may be displayed as chillis, and there is a green chilli that is a thinner, smaller Serrano. If you are not familiar with the larger banana shaped green chile, please see page 44 for shape and taste descriptions.

Low FODMAP swaps are simply chives instead of white or red onion and gluten-free panko breadcrumbs in place of regular. Now toss the bouquet and let the festivities begin!

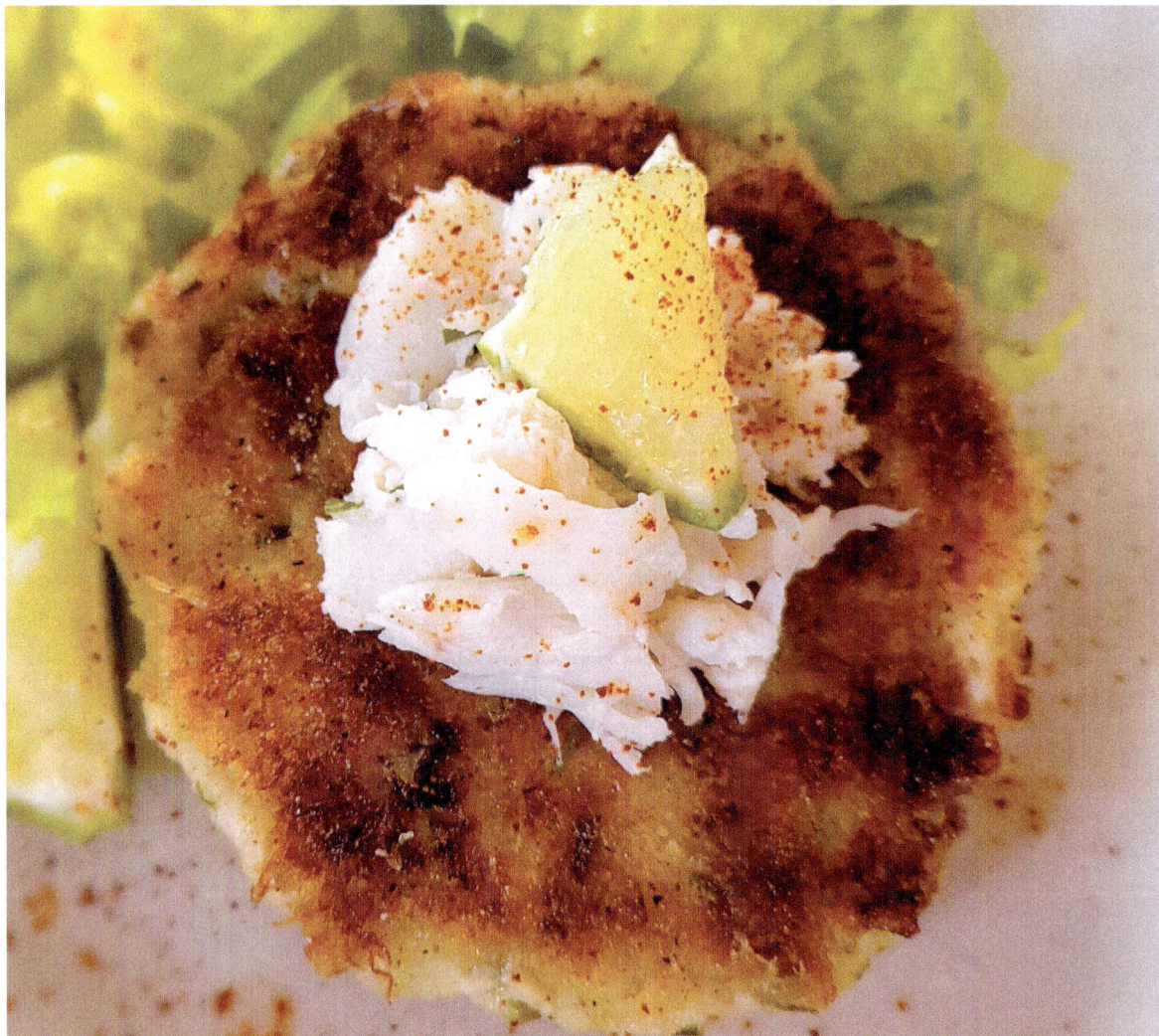

MAKES 4 CAKES – 2 ENTRÉE SERVINGS OR 4 APPETIZERS
CRAB CAKE INGREDIENTS

12-ounces (340 g) lump crab meat, fresh or canned and drained, cleaned and divided

1, 4-ounce can (113 g) mild chopped green chiles, drained (containing no onion, garlic or other high FODMAP ingredients. On the Monash App they are noted as Chilli (chili) green, mild, chopped, canned)
- OR -
5 medium (61 g each) mild fresh green chiles, roasted and prepped (page 46) will yield approx. 5/8 cup (115 g) diced chile meat (on the Monash App they are noted as: Chile, green, peeled, deseeded)

1/3 cup (46 g) plain low FODMAP gluten-free panko breadcrumbs

2 tablespoons (29 g) mayonnaise, containing no onion, garlic or other high FODMAP ingredients

1 egg white, whisked

Juice of 1/2 lime, plus 1 more lime for finishing spritz and garnish

2 teaspoons (2 g) minced chives

1/2 teaspoon fresh ground black pepper

TO COAT AND PLATE THE CAKES

1/4 cup (35 g) low FODMAP gluten-free all-purpose baking flour, containing xanthan gum (page 55)

1/4 teaspoon (1.25 g) fine sea salt

1/4 teaspoon fresh ground black pepper

2 tablespoons (30 ml) canola oil for pan cooking

1 cup (75 g) thinly sliced Romaine lettuce, chilled

1/4 teaspoon smoked paprika for dusting garnish

Method: Place 3/4 of the crab meat in a medium mixing bowl. Chill the remaining crab in the fridge, covered. Add the chiles, breadcrumbs, mayo, egg white, lime juice, chives and pepper. Mix gently to combine. Form 4 patties, pressing into 1/2-inch (1.25 cm) thick rounds. Place on a plate and chill in the fridge for 30 minutes to set.

Whisk the coating flour, salt and pepper in a small wide bowl. Lightly dip both sides of each patty in the flour.

Add oil to a large nonstick skillet; heat over medium-high heat until shimmering, then add the patties. Cook covered for 3 to 4 minutes without disturbing. When the bottom is golden brown, gently flip with a spatula. Reduce the heat to medium low, cover and cook undisturbed for 4 minutes. Check for golden brown color. They should be crispy on the outside and tender inside. If they feel too soft, cover and cook 2 minutes longer. If needed, add 2 teaspoons (10 ml) more oil to the pan. Move to a plate and tent with foil to rest 3 minutes.

To plate as an appetizer: place a handful of shredded Romaine on 4 plates, then place one patty each topped with a dollop of the remaining crab meat. Spritz the cakes and lettuce with lime juice. Garnish with a lime wedge and a pinch of smoked paprika. Serve immediately.

Tips: If you are able to tolerate butter, add 2 teaspoons (10 g) to the pan as you heat the oil for browning the cakes.

Canned chiles and crab are oftentimes plenty salted. Taste before adding salt to the coating flour.

Monash Note: Although chiles (chillies) are generally low in FODMAPs, some people with IBS may be sensitive to the capsaicin they contain. Capsaicin is a natural compound that gives chiles their spicy quality. You may need to limit how much chile you eat if your IBS symptoms are triggered by spicy food.

Guacamole Mockamole Love

LOW FODMAP ❤ IBS FRIENDLY ❤ GLUTEN-FREE ❤ DAIRY-FREE

If you have issues with sorbitol, avocados are limited to 1-ounce (30 g) per serving. This is not nearly close to the portion size for guacamole we're accustomed to. The good news is that there is a way to work around this and it has to do with Mockamole.

Many people in the Southwest prefer this more affordable Mock Guac. The secret to my LoFO version is to sauté poblano chiles, cucumber and a little zucchini, purée and let it cool for an hour, then gently fold in the freshly diced avocado. Also, amping up the spices, cilantro and citrus creates a Mock Guac that's oh so satisfying for sensitive tummies to love.

This recipe requires 1 hour of chilling in the fridge before final assembly.

MAKES 8 SERVINGS
INGREDIENTS

6 medium (97 g each / 582 g total) fresh poblano peppers, roasted and prepped (page 46) will yield 1 1/2 cups (270 g total) of chile meat

1 tablespoon (15 ml) Low FODMAP Garlic-Infused Oil (page 50), made with canola oil

2 cups (10.5-ounces / 300 g) peeled, diced English cucumber (English cucumbers hold less liquid; when using a regular cucumber be sure to remove the seeds)

1/2 cup (98 g) peeled, 1/2-inch (1.25 cm) cubed zucchini

1/2 cup (25 g) thin sliced scallions, green parts only

1/2 cup (118 ml) water

1 (160 g) ripe avocado, small diced

2 small (150 g total) fresh Roma tomatoes, cored and small diced (reserve 2 teaspoons for garnish)

3/4 cup (12 g) fresh medium packed cilantro, mostly leaves, fine chopped, plus more leaves for garnish

Juice of 2 limes

2 teaspoons (4 g) ground cumin

3/4 teaspoon (3.75 g) fine sea salt

80 corn tortilla chips; 10 chips (30 g) per serving

Method: Roast and prep the poblanos as shown on page 46. Chop the chile meat into a small dice.

Make the garlic infused oil as instructed on page 50, using a large nonstick skillet with a lid. Stir in the poblanos, cucumber, zucchini, scallion greens and water over medium high heat. Cover with a lid and let steam and cook for 10 minutes, stirring often. When the zucchini pieces are easily mushed with a fork, it's ready. Scoop the sauté into a blender and purée for 1 minute. Pour it into a large bowl and let cool for 10 minutes. Cover with plastic wrap and place in the fridge for 1 hour or until completely chilled.

Gently fold in the avocado, tomato, cilantro, lime juice, cumin and salt. Taste and adjust for salt. Garnish with cilantro leaves and diced tomato.

Serve with corn tortilla chips.

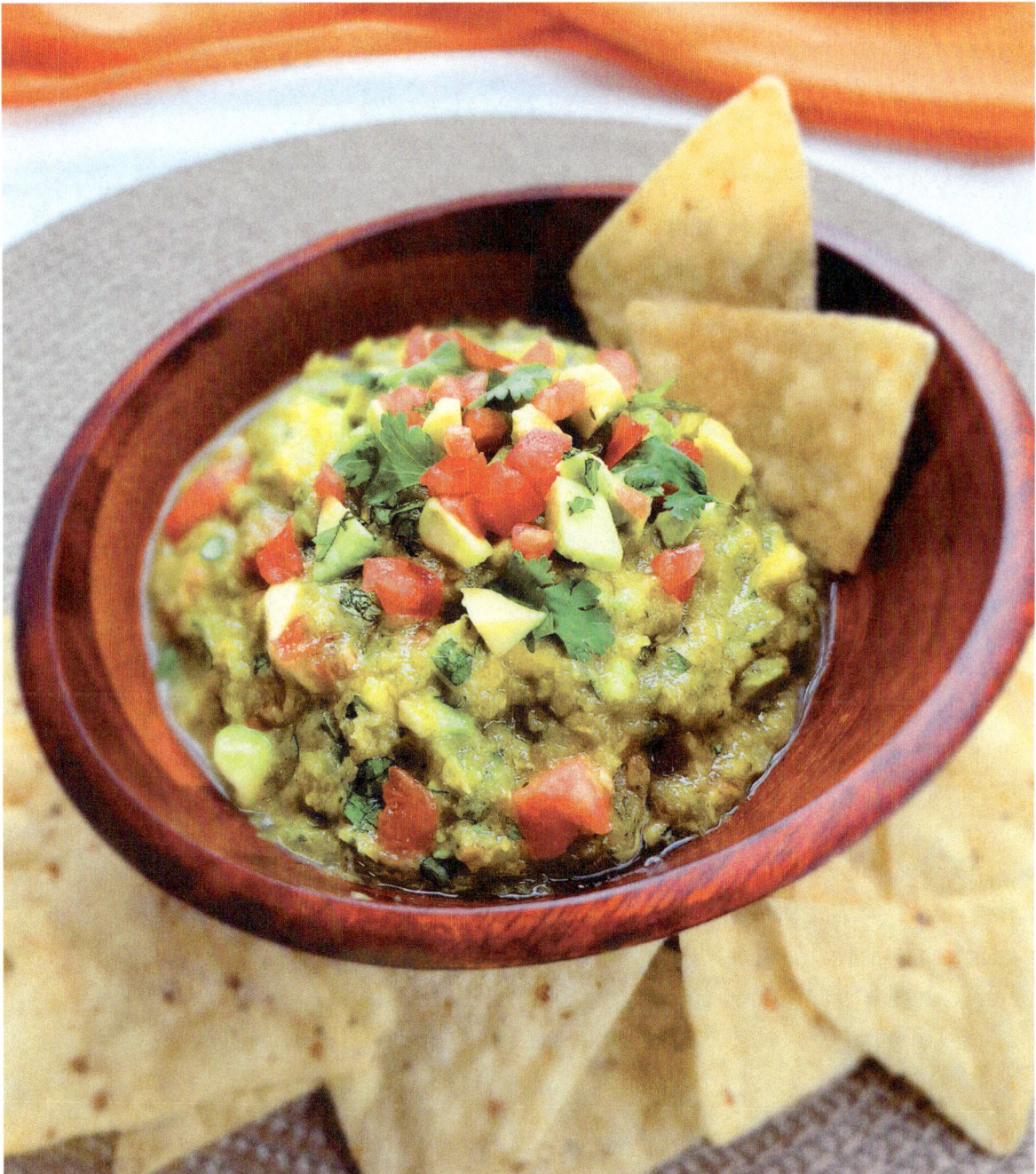

Tips: Guacamole is best eaten the same day you make it, as it tends to turn brown very quickly. To keep in the fridge, scoop the guac into an airtight container. Pour 1/2-inch (1.27 cm) cold water over to completely cover, secure the lid and refrigerate for up to 3 days. Discard and replace the cool water each time you go in for a dip.

Microwave the limes for 10 seconds on high to release more juices before squeezing.

If your pan does not have a lid, cover it with foil.

Monash Note: Although chiles (chillies) are generally low in FODMAPs, some people with IBS may be sensitive to the capsaicin they contain. Capsaicin is a natural compound that gives chiles their spicy quality. You may need to limit how much chile you eat if your IBS symptoms are triggered by spicy food.

Chipotle Chive Turkey Burger Bites with Yellow Cornmeal & Quick Pickles

LOW FODMAP ❤ IBS FRIENDLY ❤ GLUTEN-FREE ❤ DAIRY-FREE

These casual, delicious mini burger skewers are tenderized with cornmeal and almond milk, with easy prep and assembly. A feast for the eyes and taste buds with each little bite!

MAKES 16 BURGER SKEWERS = 8 SERVINGS

QUICK PICKLE CHIPS INGREDIENTS

1 large (410 g) thin English cucumber sliced into rounds a bit over 1/4-inch (.625 cm) thick. (English cucumbers contain less seeds and water content, perfect for pickles)

1/3 cup (66 g) sugar

1/4 cup (13 g) thin sliced scallions, green parts only

3/4 cup (180 ml) apple cider vinegar

3/4 cup (180 ml) water

2 teaspoons (6 g) mustard seeds

BURGER INGREDIENTS

1-pound (454 g) ground turkey

2 tablespoons (22 g) low FODMAP medium grind whole grain yellow cornmeal

2 tablespoons (30 ml) plain, unsweetened almond milk

1 tablespoon plus 1 teaspoon (4 g) minced fresh chives

3/4 teaspoon (1.5 g) pure chipotle powder, if you like heat add 1/2 teaspoon (1 g) more

3/4 teaspoon (4 g) fine sea salt

1/2 teaspoon fresh ground black pepper

2 tablespoons (30 ml) Low FODMAP Garlic-Infused Oil (page 50), made with extra virgin olive oil, or plain olive oil is fine

2 tablespoons (29 g) mayonnaise containing no onion or garlic

16 baby spinach leaves, or arugula for a peppery flavor

5 pieces thick cut bacon, cooked to crisp, drained and broken into 4 pieces each (you will have a few extra pieces to select the best for assembling, and the leftovers are of course for the cook!)

16 small cherry tomatoes

16 long wooden skewers

Method

Pickles: Place all pickle ingredients in a medium saucepan and boil for 5 minutes. Spoon the pickles into a large Mason jar or heatproof bowl and pour in the pickling liquid. Let cool. This makes about 35 chips, twice the amount needed. But if you're going to make these tangy, sweet homemade pickles that are far tastier than store-bought, you'll definitely want extras to snack on for days.

Burgers: Use your hands to thoroughly mix the turkey, cornmeal, milk, chives, chipotle powder, salt and pepper in a medium bowl. Shape into 16 mini burgers approx. 32 grams each. Use your thumb to press an indentation into the center of each so they will cook evenly.

Add the oil to a large nonstick skillet over medium high heat until it shimmers. Cook the burgers 2 minutes, covered with a lid. Flip and cook 1 to 2 minutes longer, covered, until the centers are no longer pink. Place them on paper towels to drain for 1 minute, then arrange on a serving platter to assemble.

Place a small dollop of mayo on each patty. Stack with a spinach leaf or arugula, piece of bacon, and 1 pickle chip. Hold the tomatoes on top and pierce through the layers with a skewer to keep in place. Serve immediately.

Tips: Store-bought mayonnaise often contains onion and garlic in small amounts. I look for the no onion no garlic brands, and LoFO brands are offered online. In the Reintroduction Phase 2 of the diet, many people find that they are able to tolerate mayo that contains onion and garlic.

If tolerated, add 16 (4 g each) thin slices of Monterey Jack or provolone cheese.

Pictured are turkey burger bites skewered with store-bought pickles. They were bought in a pinch when friends were coming over for a get-together and I was out of English cucumbers. Many people find that, as with mayo, they are able to reintroduce and tolerate pickles that contain small amounts of onion and garlic. That said, homemade quick pickles are much fresher and tastier!

The pickles will keep in the refrigerator for 2 weeks, stored in a jar with a tight lid.

Monash Note: Although chiles (chillies) are generally low in FODMAPs, some people with IBS may be sensitive to the capsaicin they contain. Capsaicin is a natural compound that gives chiles their spicy quality. You may need to limit how much chile you eat if your IBS symptoms are triggered by spicy food.

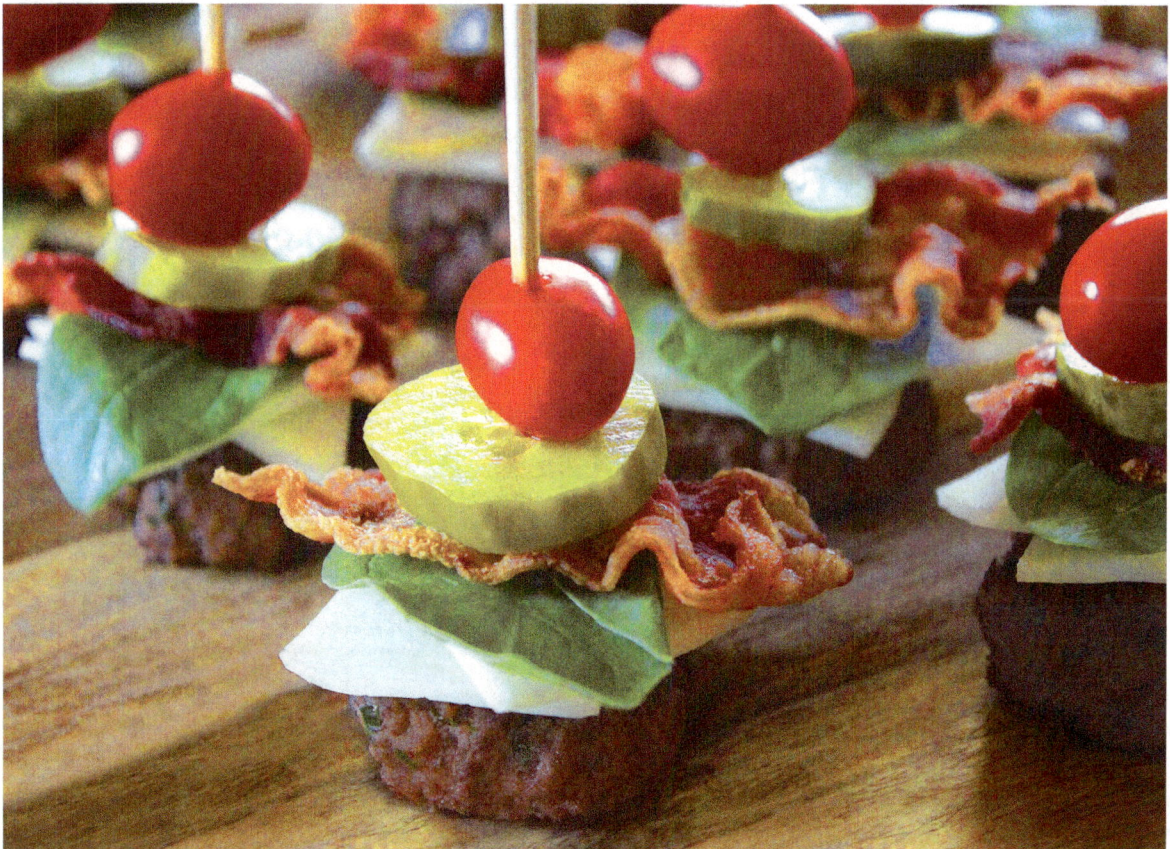

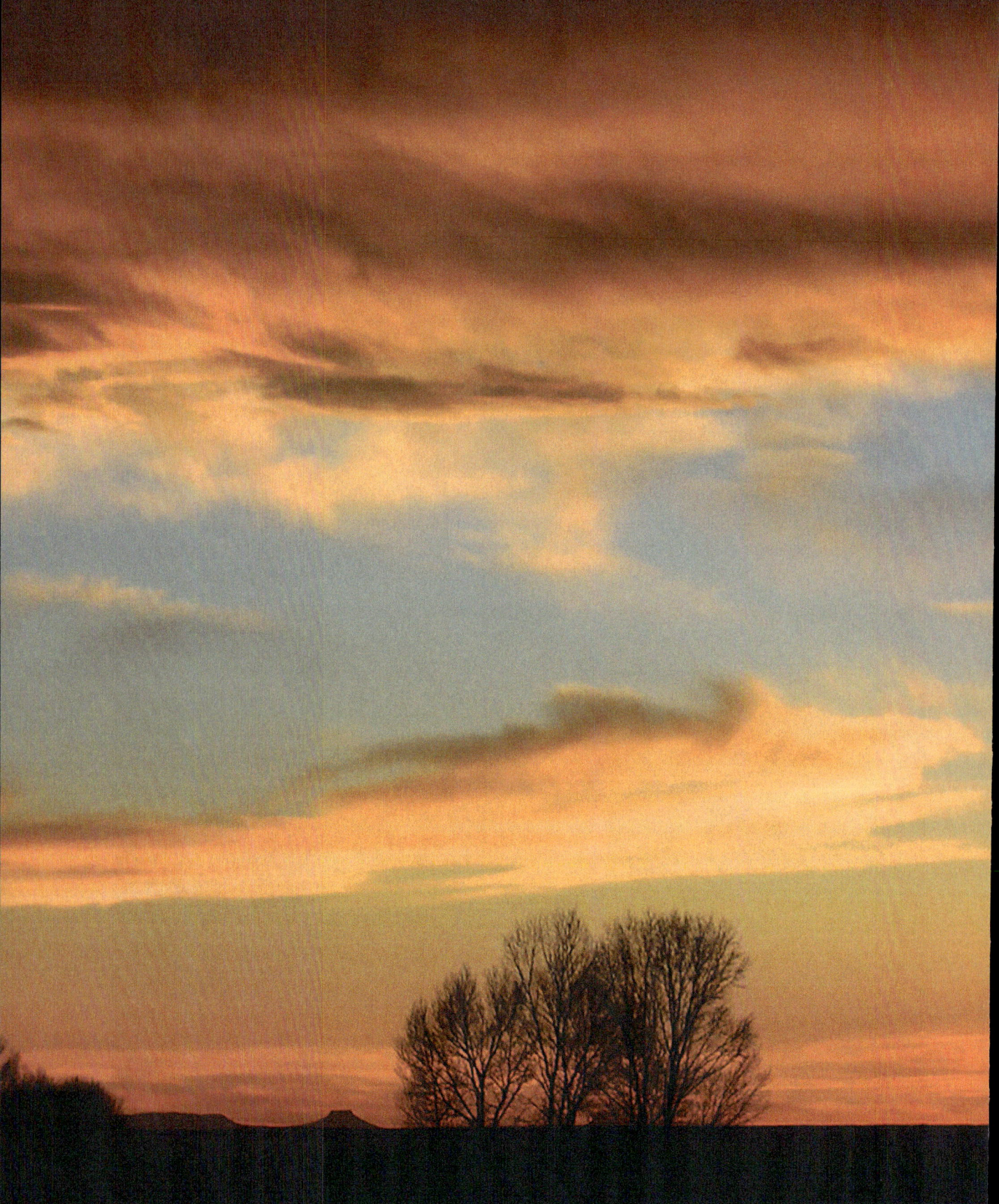

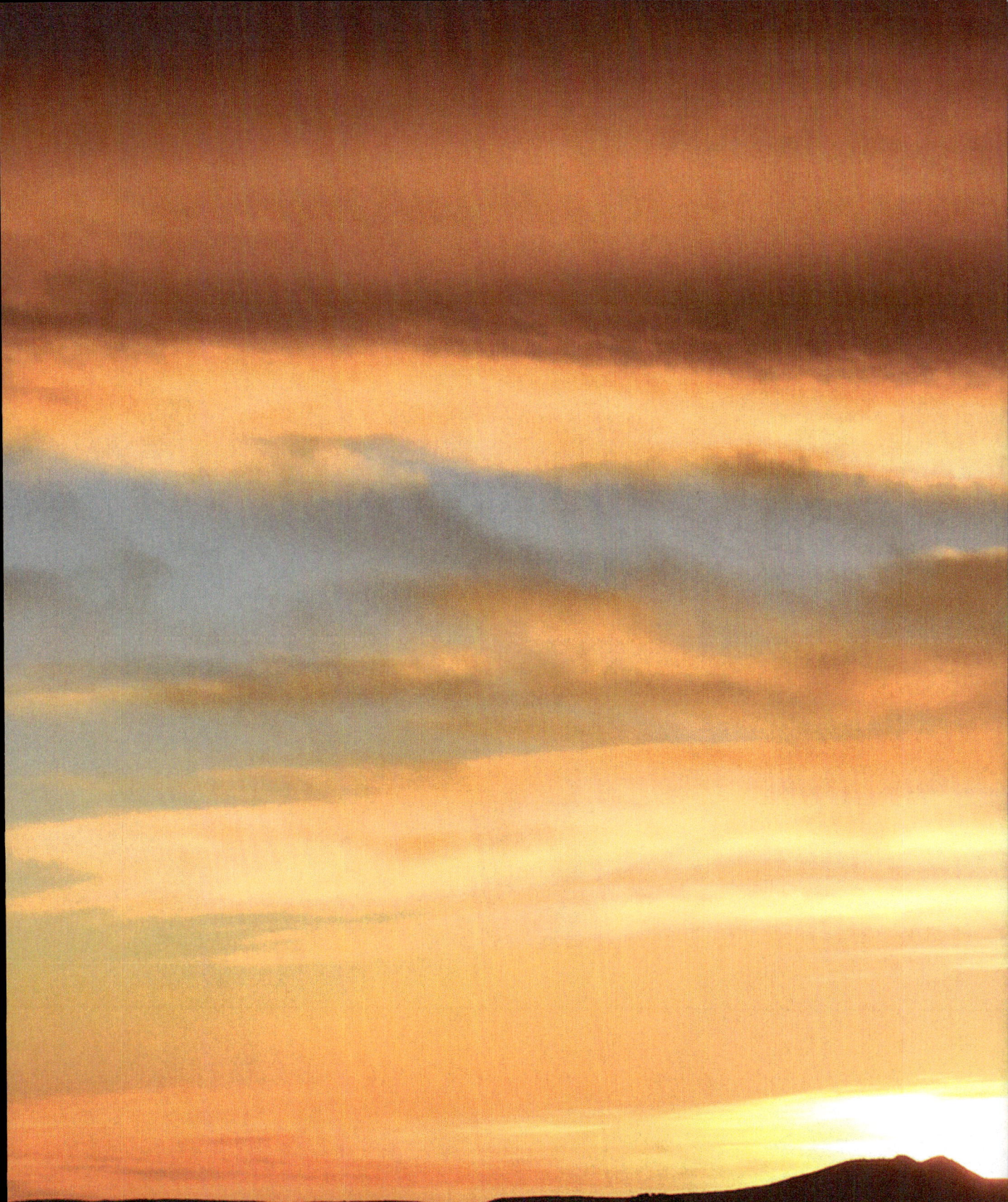

Southwest Sunset, Looking Toward Abiquiu
New Mexico

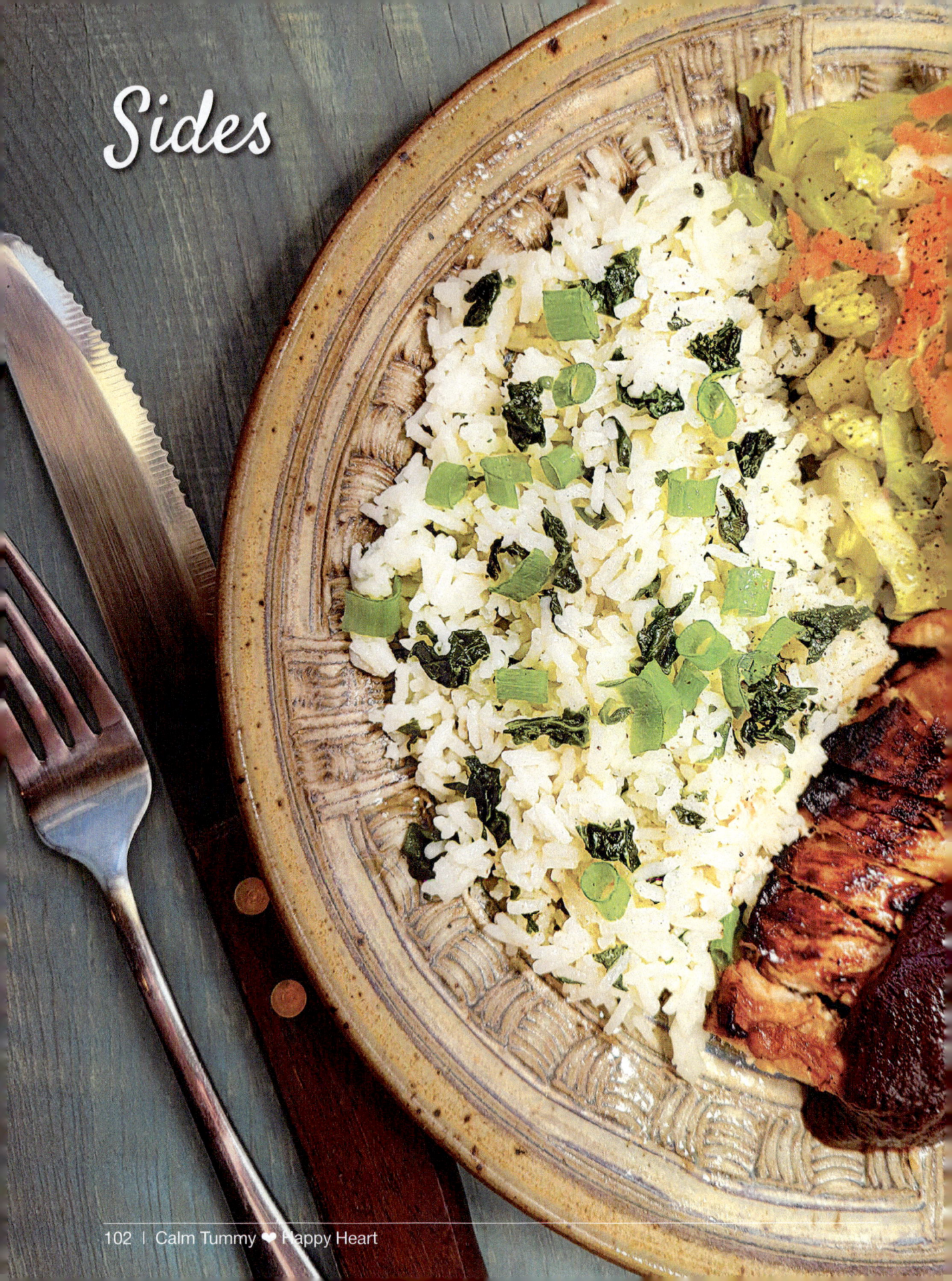

Sides

- ❤ **Homemade Classic Corn & Cilantro Pressed Tortillas**
- ❤ **Lemony Chopped Bok Choy**
- ❤ **Cilantro Green Rice with Spinach & Lime**
- ❤ **Mexican Restaurant Style Rice**
- ❤ **Green Chile Thanksgiving Dressing**
- ❤ **No Beans Refried "Beans"**
- ❤ **Garlic Olive Oil & Chive Mashed Potatoes**
- ❤ **Fiesta Slaw**
- ❤ **Fresh Green Chiles Rellenos with Mashed Potatoes**

Food brand names are sometimes listed within a recipe, and this means they are Monash Certified. For more brand options we use and love, please visit **FodifyIt.com**

Monash Note: Although chiles (chillies) are generally low in FODMAPs, some people with IBS may be sensitive to the capsaicin they contain. Capsaicin is a natural compound that gives chiles their spicy quality. You may need to limit how much chile you eat if your IBS symptoms are triggered by spicy food.

Homemade Classic Corn & Cilantro Pressed Tortillas

LOW FODMAP ♥ IBS FRIENDLY ♥ GLUTEN-FREE ♥ DAIRY-FREE

Many friends from New Mexico, where I first learned to make tortillas, mix their dough without measuring cups or scales. After years of making thousands of tortillas, they can feel the dough with their hands and know when it's just right with a soft cookie dough consistency. They assure me there is no shame in using a timer or measuring out ingredients, and that one day I will feel and "know." It just takes practice. I believe this because each time I make these fresh masa harina tortillas, they just get better and better.

Masa harina is corn that has been cooked with alkaline (nixtamalization) and when ground is smoother and more flavorful for making tortilla (and tamale) dough. You will also need a tortilla press, plastic to cover the press surfaces for easy removal of the pressed dough, a comal (smooth, flat griddle) or large nonstick skillet, and a tortilla warmer.

MAKES ABOUT 12 TORTILLAS – 3 PER SERVING
CLASSIC CORN 4 1/2-INCH (11.25 CM) ROUND
INGREDIENTS

2 cups (250 g) masa harina

1/2 teaspoon (2.5 g) fine sea salt

1 1/2 to 2 cups (350-475 ml) warm water, plus more if needed depending on the humidity of the day
(I typically use 1 1/2 cups (350 ml) plus 2 tablespoons (30 ml)

Tortilla press

1 plastic ziplock baggie that is larger than the tortilla press surfaces, or tortilla parchment circles

Canola oil for lightly greasing the nonstick skillet or comal (traditional tortillas are cooked on a hot comal)

Method: Whisk the masa and salt in a medium mixing bowl. Add 1 cup (240 ml) water and mix lightly with your hand. The dough will begin to combine but will still feel crumbly dry to the touch. Add 1/2 cup (120 ml) more water, knead to mix and assess the texture. The dough will begin to pull away and clean the sides of the bowl. Add 1 tablespoon (15 ml) more water at a time if needed for a very soft but not mushy or sticky texture. Knead with your hands for 4 minutes, in the bowl. Cover with a clean damp kitchen towel. Let rest for 30 minutes.

Cut the baggie into two circles that are larger than the tortilla press surfaces. Open the press, sprinkle water on both plates and stick a plastic circle to each plate.

Heat a large nonstick skillet or comal to high heat. Just before pressing the tortillas, bring the heat down to medium. Using a paper towel, lightly grease the pan with canola oil.

As you work, keep the dough in the bowl covered with the damp towel so it won't dry out. Pull a piece of golf ball sized dough (45 g) and roll it loosely into a 1 1/2-inch (3.8 cm) ball. Push a well into the center with your thumb. Lightly wet your fingers with water and work the moisture into the well as you roll and form a nice round ball. This will help keep the tortillas from cracking and drying out as they toast.

(continued on next page)

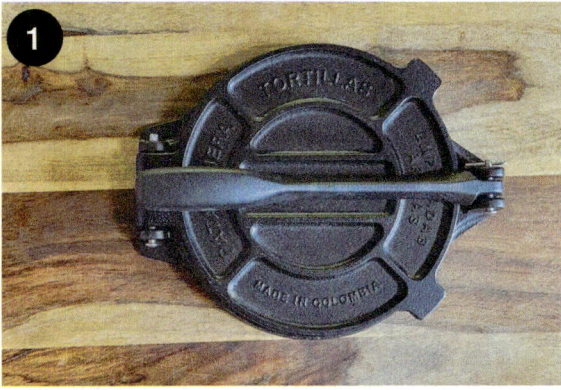

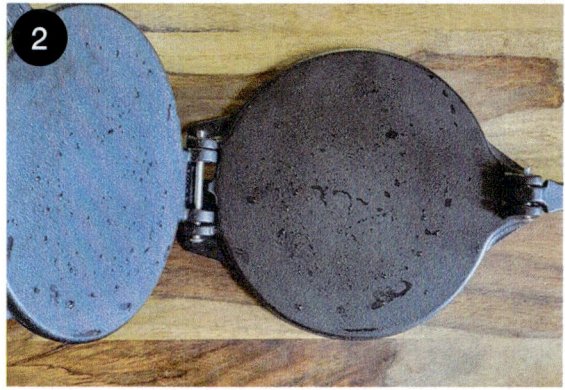

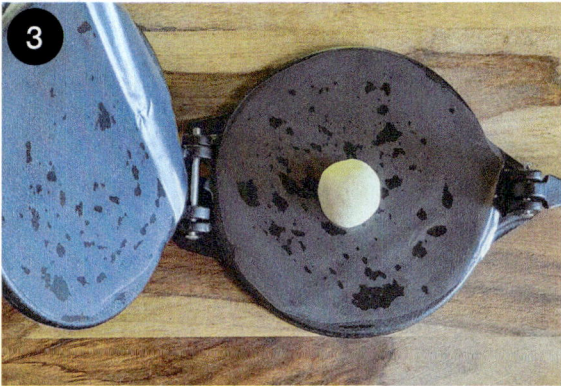

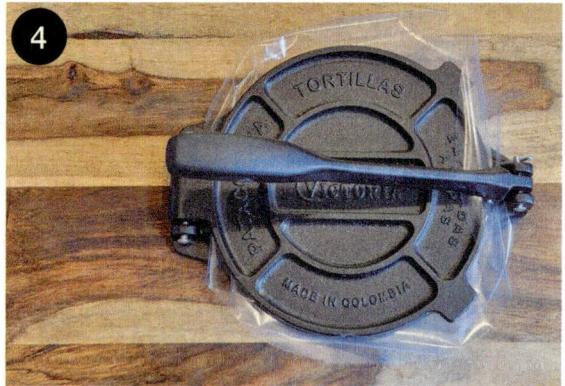

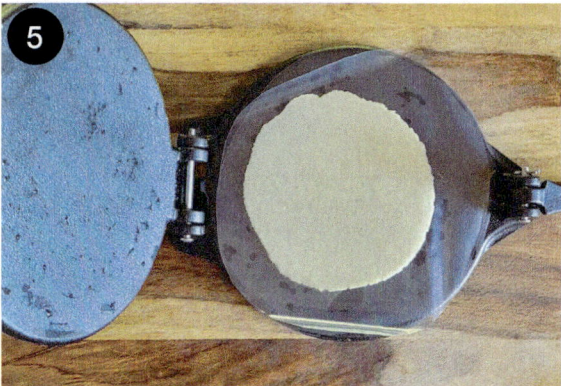

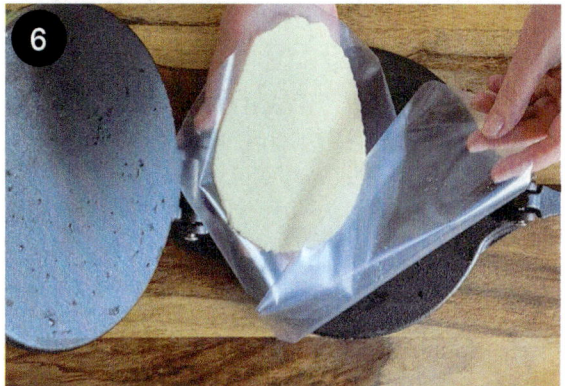

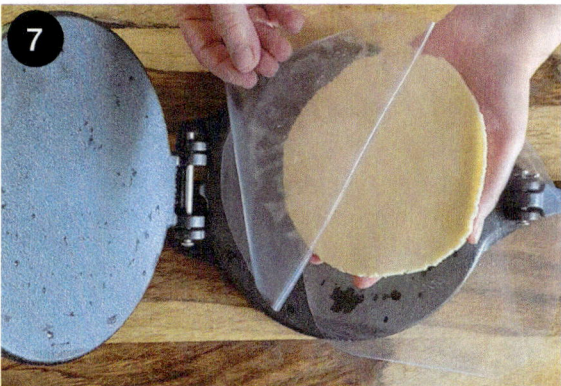

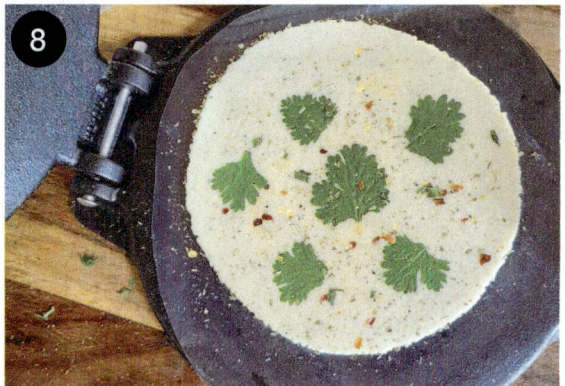

(continued from previous page)

Center the ball on the bottom press surface and close the handle down semi-firmly into a 4-inch (10 cm) round. Open the press and spin the tortilla around 180 degrees. Close the handle and press gently into a 4 1/2-inch (11.25 cm) round that is 1/8-inch (.3 cm) thick. After a few tries you will begin to instinctively feel the right amount of pressure to use.

Peel the top piece of plastic off and lift the tortilla with the bottom plastic stuck to it. Place it dough side down in your hand and peel the plastic away from the dough.

Reduce heat to medium and gently place the tortilla in the pan. Let cook for 1 minute. Flip it with a spatula and cook for 1 minute 30 seconds. Use a paper towel to gently press the tortilla surface down a bit (it may be too hot for fingers) then flip again. Cook for 1 minute and watch for it to poof up and become slightly pillow-y on top. This is how you know you've made a good dough. You may need to flip it a couple more times until it has light brown toasted marks. Place it in a tortilla warmer, wrap with foil, or a clean heavy kitchen towel to keep warm. Cooking times will vary according to your burner and pan.

If the edges are dry and a bit crumbly it means the dough is too dry. If this is the case, add 2 teaspoons of warm water to the dough and knead again to mix. If the dough is too wet it will not peel off of the plastic, in which case add 2 teaspoons of masa and knead into the dough. Do another test or two until you have the right consistency.

Repeat for the remaining tortillas, stacking and covering them as you go.

If you do not have a tortilla press, place a piece of plastic on a work surface and center the dough ball. Cover the top with plastic and press down with a heavy skillet or cutting board. Turn the tortilla 180 degrees and press again for an even thickness. It may not create a perfectly even thickness but you will still have a delicious homemade tortilla!

Now that you have your stack of warm tortillas you can assemble your tacos, huevos rancheros, or any dish requiring a fresh tortilla. They are best eaten as freshly as possible, so plan accordingly.

FOR DECORATIVE CILANTRO & SPICE TORTILLAS

For special occasions, holidays, brunches, or a fancy dinner party, cilantro leaves pressed into the tortillas add a thoughtful touch. Creating scenes and patterns with spices are also fun additions. Edible flowers are an elegant detail, though they have not yet been tested by Monash so best keep a lookout on their app for newly tested foods.

Prepare the dough as usual. Press it to a 4-inch (10 cm) round. Turn it 180 degrees. Peel off the top plastic and place your desired herbs and spices onto the tortilla surface. Return the top plastic into position and close the handle down for the second 4 1/2-inch (11.25 cm) round press.

Peel the plastic from the dough as usual and begin to cook decorative side down, flipping and timing as instructed.

When you plate, place the decorative tortillas to the side of the dish, not covered with sauce or toppings.

Tips: Cilantro leaves of different sizes make an interesting pattern, or one single leaf in the center is a lovely minimalist look.

Other ingredients to craft your designs: minced chives, tiny shavings or cuts of green scallion stalks, pinches of dried oregano, thyme, sage, turmeric, cumin, 5-7 red pepper flakes, pinch of pure mild red chile powder (containing no onion or garlic, the ingredients should list only: red chile. On the Monash App this is called Chilli (chili) red, powdered).

When using turmeric and red chile powder, a little goes a long way so pinch and use sparingly.

When pressing the spices, particularly the turmeric, red chile powder or paprika, you will need to wipe the plastic with a damp paper towel to clean it, or use a new plastic circle before continuing to the next decorative tortilla.

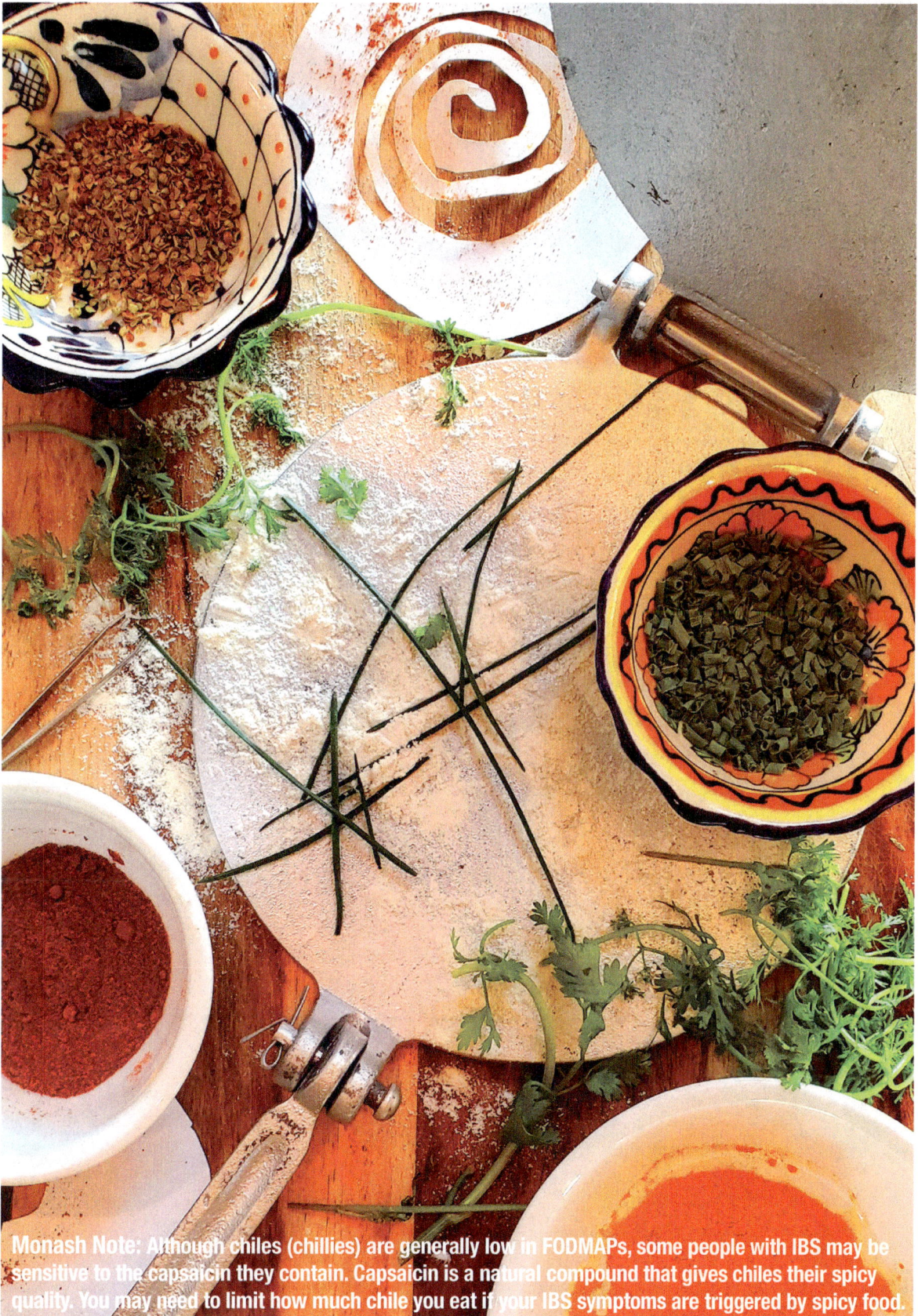

Monash Note: Although chiles (chillies) are generally low in FODMAPs, some people with IBS may be sensitive to the capsaicin they contain. Capsaicin is a natural compound that gives chiles their spicy quality. You may need to limit how much chile you eat if your IBS symptoms are triggered by spicy food.

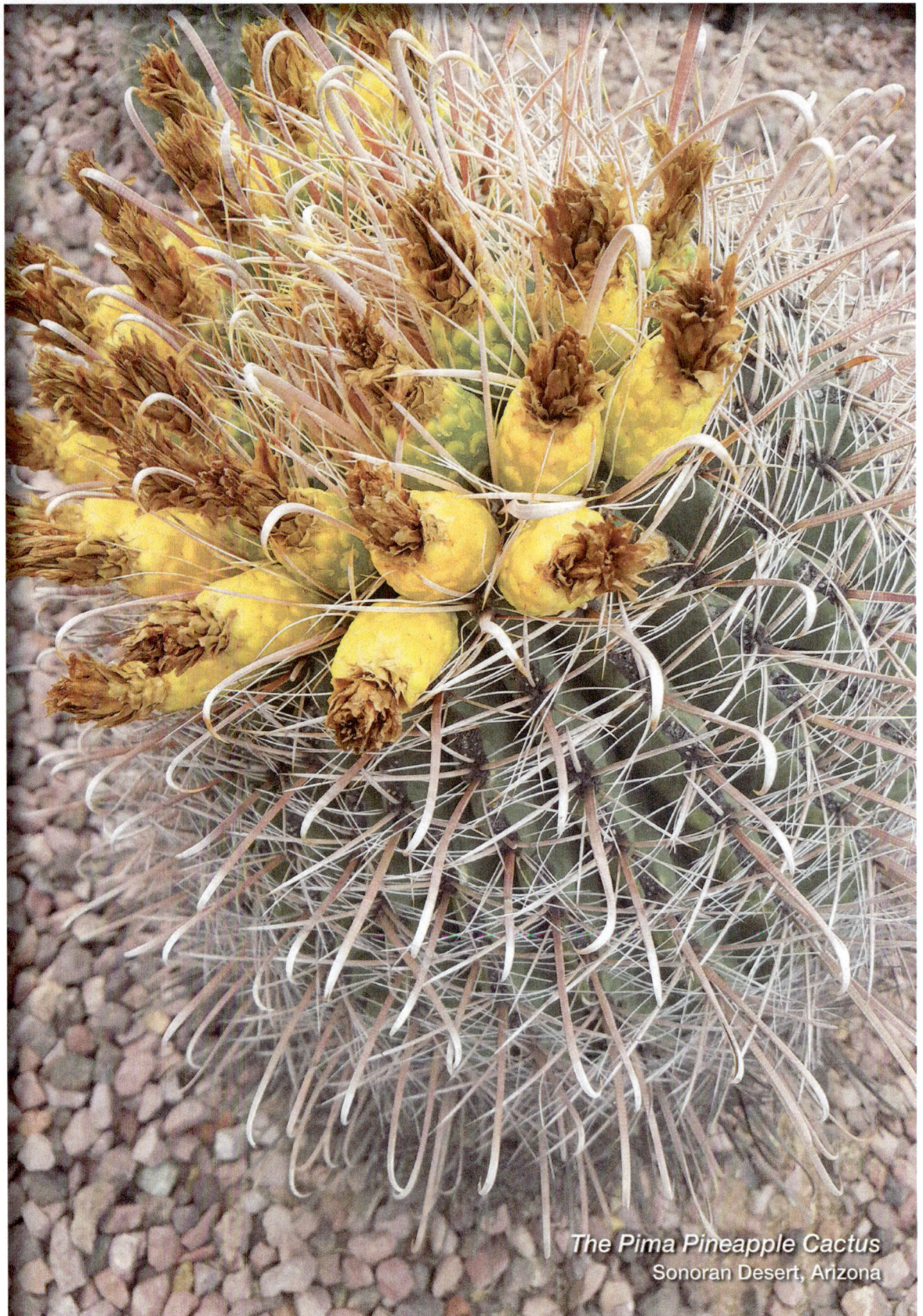

The Pima Pineapple Cactus
Sonoran Desert, Arizona

Lemony Bok Choy

LOW FODMAP ❤ IBS FRIENDLY ❤ GLUTEN-FREE ❤ DAIRY-FREE

Not only is bok choy the perfect swap for HiFO celery, it's also a healthy side dish providing fiber, Vitamins C and K, and other health-promoting nutrients. When available, I buy the more tender baby bok choy and am sure to chop and wash them thoroughly as they typically contain a bit of grit.

MAKES 6 SERVINGS
INGREDIENTS

5 baby (425 g total) bok choy, or one large (425 g)

2 tablespoons (30 ml) Low FODMAP Garlic-Infused Oil (page 50), made with extra virgin olive oil, or plain olive oil is also fine

1/2 scant teaspoon (2 g) fine sea salt

1/4 teaspoon fresh ground black pepper

1/2 cup (120 ml) water

Juice of 1/2 lemon, and the zest if desired

Method: Cut off the leaves and chop them into 1-inch (2.5 cm) pieces. Cut the root ends off and discard. Slice the stems to 1/2-inch (1.25 cm) lengthwise stalks, then cut into 1/2-inch (1.25 cm) pieces. Place the leaves and pieces into a bowl of cool water and swish around with a slotted spoon to wash. The bok choy will float to the top and any grit will sink to the bottom. Use the slotted spoon to move them to a plate.

Pour the oil into a large nonstick skillet over medium high heat until it shimmers. Add the bok choy. Evenly sprinkle with salt and pepper over all.

Add the water and lemon juice. Cook for 6 to 8 minutes, stirring occasionally. This will result in just-tender bok choy that still has some crunch to it. Some people with IBS find that cooking it to very tender is easier to digest, in which case stir for 5 minutes more or until the liquids have evaporated. If they begin to char while cooking, reduce the heat to medium and add a bit more water.

Taste for lemon. If you'd like more zip, sprinkle each serving with a little lemon zest for flavor and garnish. Serve immediately.

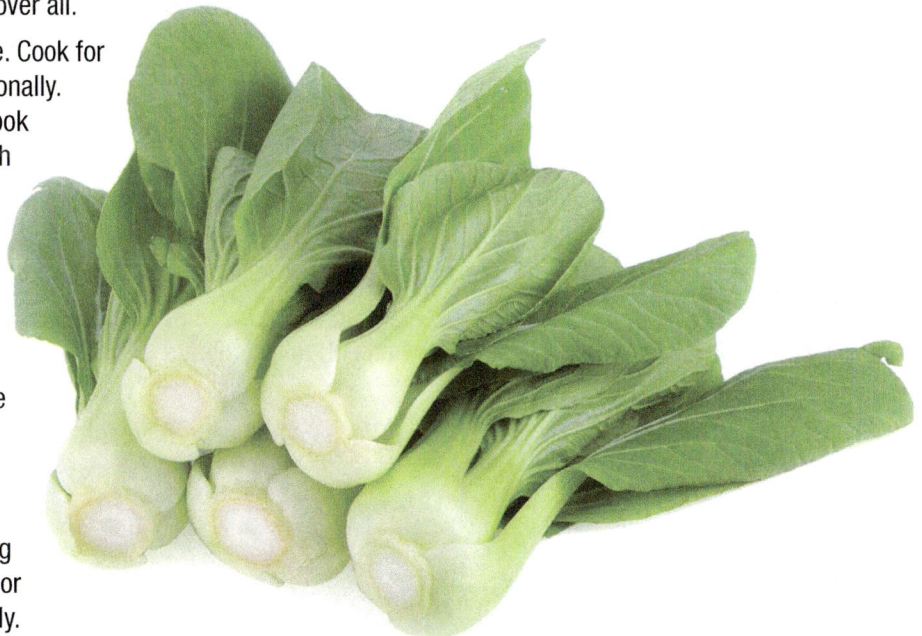

Cilantro Green Rice with Spinach & Lime

LOW FODMAP ❤ IBS FRIENDLY ❤ GLUTEN-FREE ❤ DAIRY-FREE

Variations of green rice are aplenty. Some favorites are purées of tomatillo or green chile salsas blended with rice and herbs. This version features fluffy rice coated with a warm blend of sautéed spinach, scallion greens, cilantro and lime juice. Simple, fresh and pairs well with many main courses.

MAKES 6 SERVINGS
INGREDIENTS

2 3/4 cups (655 ml) Low FODMAP Chicken Stock (page 135), or water

1/2 teaspoon (2.5 g) fine sea salt

1 1/2 cups (285 g) white rice; I use basmati because it's fluffy

2 tablespoons (30 ml) Low FODMAP Garlic-Infused Oil (page 50), made with extra virgin olive oil

1 cup (50 g) fresh baby spinach

1/4 cup (13 g) thin sliced scallions, green parts only

1 cup (16 g) fresh medium packed cilantro, mostly leaves, chopped fine

Juice of 1 lime, plus more to your taste

Method: Bring the stock or water with salt to a boil in a medium saucepan over high heat. Add the rice and boil for 2 minutes. Reduce to simmer and cover with a lid. Simmer for 15 minutes or until the rice is tender and fluffs nicely with a fork. Remove from heat and keep covered.

Pour the oil into a small sauté pan or nonstick skillet over medium high heat until it shimmers. Add the spinach and scallion greens. Stir with a spatula until the spinach is tender. This will take 2 to 3 minutes and the spinach will reduce considerably.

Spoon the spinach and scallions with pan liquid into a blender along with the cilantro and lime juice. Give it a few pulses and scrape down with a spatula. Continue to pulse until everything begins to combine and you have a coarse pesto consistency. If you have a stubborn mixture, add 1 tablespoon (15 ml) of water to get things moving.

Spoon the mixture into the rice. Gently stir and fluff to incorporate. Taste and adjust for salt and lime. Serve immediately.

Stored in an airtight container, green rice will keep up to 3 days in the refrigerator.

Mexican Restaurant Style Rice

LOW FODMAP ❤ IBS FRIENDLY ❤ GLUTEN-FREE ❤ DAIRY-FREE

My favorite step for this recipe is toasting the rice in oil before adding the liquids. It has the most satisfying nutty aroma. The tiny cubed carrots add a little veg and a nice warm color to the rice.

LoFO swaps are simply green parts of scallions in place of white onion, and LoFO garlic-infused oil for the minced garlic cloves.

MAKES 4 SERVINGS
INGREDIENTS

2 tablespoons (30 ml) Low FODMAP Garlic-Infused Oil (page 50), made with canola oil

1 cup (185 g) basmati rice, rinsed and drained well; basmati produces a light fluffy texture, but a short grain white rice is also fine

2 medium (150 g total) carrots, peeled and cut into 1/4-inch (.63 cm) cubes

1/8 cup (7 g) thin sliced scallions, green parts only

3/4 teaspoon (3.75 g) fine sea salt

1/2 teaspoon (1 g) ground cumin

1/2 teaspoon (1 g) pure mild red chile powder (containing no onion or garlic, the ingredients should list only: red chile. On the Monash App this is called Chilli (chili) red, powdered)

1/2 teaspoon dried oregano

1 3/4 cups (414 ml) Low FODMAP Chicken Stock (page 135)

1/4 cup (59 ml) canned plain tomato purée, containing no onion, garlic or other high FODMAPs

Juice of 1/2 lime

1/4 cup (4 g) fresh medium packed cilantro, mostly leaves, finely chopped for garnish

Method: Pour the oil into a heavy-bottom nonstick skillet (that has a lid) over medium heat until it shimmers. Add the rice and carrots. Continually stir with a wooden spoon until the rice begins to smell nutty and turns a light golden color, about 5 to 6 minutes.

Add the scallion greens and spices. Cook and stir 1 minute. Add the stock and tomato purée. Bring to a boil for 4 minutes stirring often.

Reduce the heat to low, cover with lid and simmer for 10 to 15 minutes or until the rice is tender. Drizzle the lime juice evenly over the rice and fluff with a fork. Top with cilantro. Serve immediately.

The rice will keep in the refrigerator for up to 3 days when stored in an airtight container.

Monash Note: Although chiles (chillies) are generally low in FODMAPs, some people with IBS may be sensitive to the capsaicin they contain. Capsaicin is a natural compound that gives chiles their spicy quality. You may need to limit how much chile you eat if your IBS symptoms are triggered by spicy food.

Green Chile Thanksgiving Dressing
(or any day dressing)

LOW FODMAP ❤ IBS FRIENDLY ❤ GLUTEN-FREE ❤ DAIRY-FREE

Easy swaps for dressing are: low FODMAP gluten-free bread in place of high FODMAP bread, making your own garlic oil (page 50), using the green parts of scallions instead of white or yellow onions, bok choy in place of celery, and oyster mushrooms instead of button. Some of Schar brand gluten-free breads have been Monash certified and you can check the Monash App for different types offered. Schar gluten-free baguette is certified low FODMAP. Leaving the bread out overnight to become stale helps create a better texture in the end.

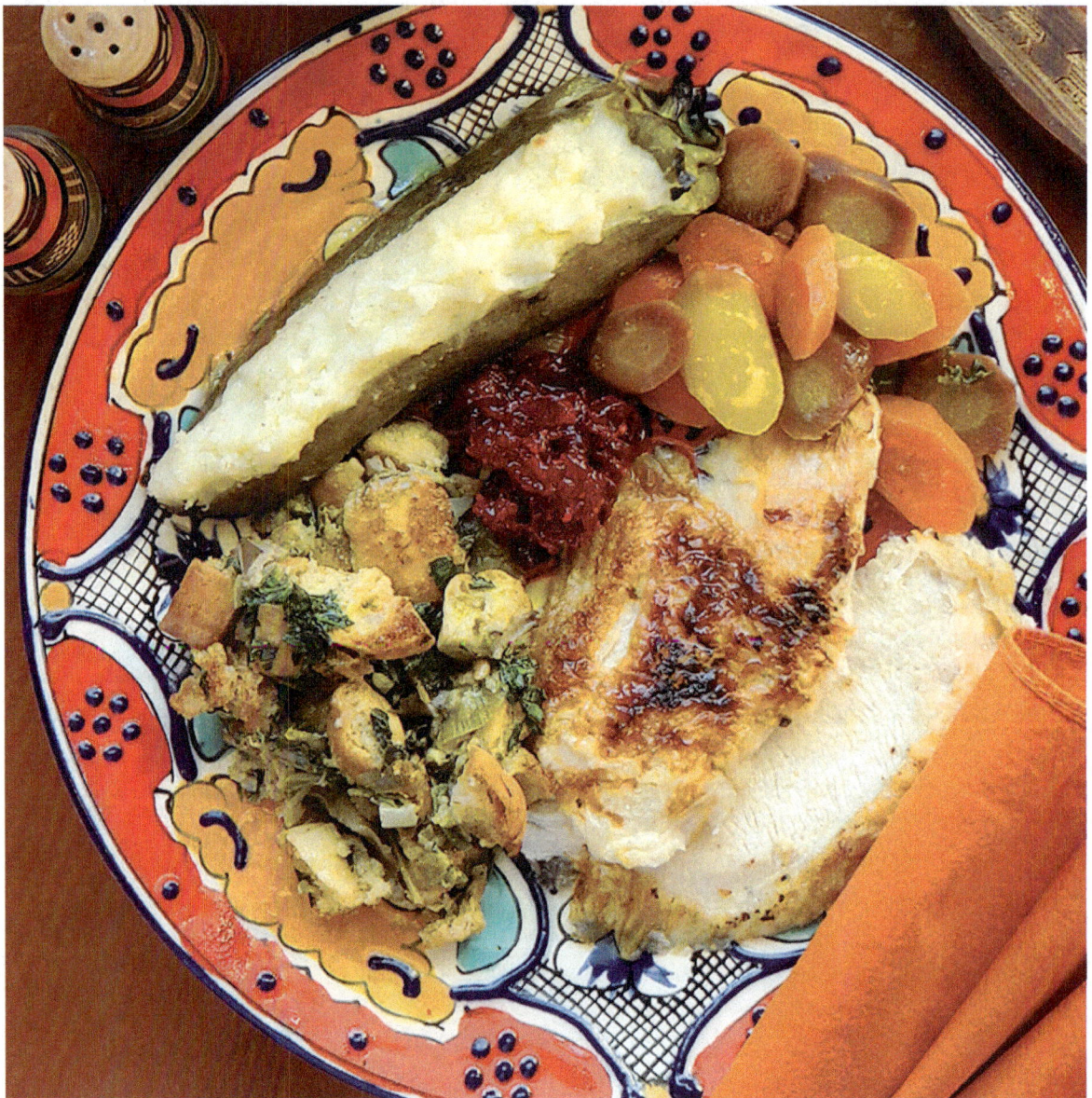

MAKES 4-6 SERVINGS
INGREDIENTS

8 slices (approx. 240 g total) low FODMAP gluten-free white sandwich bread with crusts, 1/2-inch (1.25 cm) cubed, or 240 g low FODMAP baguette, cubed

2 tablespoons (30 ml) Low FODMAP Garlic-Infused Oil (page 50), made with extra virgin olive oil

1/2 cup (25 g) thin sliced scallions, green parts only

1 1/2 cups (115 g) fine chopped bok choy

1 cup (75 g) rough chopped oyster mushrooms; you will need to buy 2 cups (150 g) of mushrooms because the heavy stems are cut from the caps and discarded

1/2 cup (120 ml) Low FODMAP Chicken Stock (page 135)

1, 4-ounce (113 g) can plain chopped mild green chiles (containing no onion, garlic or other high FODMAP ingredients. On the Monash App they are noted as Chilli (chili) green, mild, chopped, canned)
-OR-
5 medium (61 g each) mild fresh green chiles, roasted and prepped (page 46) will yield approx. 5/8 cup (115 g) diced chile meat (on the Monash App they are noted as: Chile, green, peeled, deseeded)

1 large egg

1/4 cup (4 g) fresh fine chopped parsley, mostly leaves as the stems can be bitter

1 teaspoon (2 g) dried sage

1 teaspoon (2 g) dried thyme

1/2 teaspoon (2.5 g) fine sea salt

1/2 teaspoon fresh ground black pepper

Method: Preheat oven to 375 F / 190 C

Coat an 8-inch (20 cm) square or round baking pan with cooking spray oil and evenly distribute the cubed bread.

Pour the oil in a medium nonstick skillet over medium high heat. Add the scallion greens, bok choy and mushrooms. Sauté until the bok choy is just tender. Add to the bread, sprinkling it evenly over the top.

Whisk together the remaining ingredients and pour over the bread. Press everything down with a spatula to remove any air bubbles.

Bake for 25 to 35 minutes or until the center is cooked through but not dry. Remove from the oven and cover with foil to keep warm until ready to serve.

Stored in an airtight container, dressing will keep in the fridge for up to 3 days.

Tip: A Thanksgiving kitchen is always a flurry of activity, with many dishes to prepare and details to remember. If you happen to forget to leave the bread out overnight, dry it out by cutting it into cubes, placing on a baking sheet to bake at 375 F / 190 C for 15 minutes until slightly brown around the edges.

Monash Note: Although chiles (chillies) are generally low in FODMAPs, some people with IBS may be sensitive to the capsaicin they contain. Capsaicin is a natural compound that gives chiles their spicy quality. You may need to limit how much chile you eat if your IBS symptoms are triggered by spicy food.

No Beans Refried "Beans"

LOW FODMAP ❤ IBS FRIENDLY ❤ GLUTEN-FREE ❤ DAIRY-FREE

Beans are high in FODMAPs and their LoFO portion amounts are not enough required for a side dish. By combining root vegetables, canned lentils and spices including pure red chile powder, the texture and color are spot-on. This faux recipe has all of the flavor of refried beans without the beans!

MAKES 6 SERVINGS – 1/4 CUP (APPROX. 60 G) EACH, DEPENDING HOW MUCH THE BEANS ARE REDUCED
INGREDIENTS

3/4 cup (113 g) small diced, peeled sweet potato

1 1/4 cups (213 g) large diced, peeled russet potato

2 3/4 cups (650 ml) Low FODMAP Chicken Stock (page 135) containing no garlic, onion or other high FODMAP ingredients

1 teaspoon (2 g) minced fresh epazote, optional

1 teaspoon (2 g) pure, mild red chile powder (containing no onion or garlic, the ingredients should list only: red chile. On the Monash App this is called Chilli (chili) red, powdered)

3/4 teaspoon (3.75 g) fine sea salt

1/2 teaspoon (1 g) ground cumin

1/2 teaspoon dried oregano

1/4 teaspoon fresh ground black pepper

3 slices bacon

1/2 cup (92 g) canned, rinsed and drained brown lentils

2 tablespoons (7 g) thin sliced scallions, green parts only, plus more for garnish

Juice of 1/2 lime

Method: Place the sweet and russet potatoes in a medium saucepan. Cover with 1-inch (2.5 cm) of water to completely submerge. Bring to a boil for 15 to 20 minutes until very tender. By cutting the more dense sweet potato smaller they will cook to tender in time with the russet. Drain the potatoes and spoon into a blender. Add the stock, epazote, red chile powder, salt, cumin, oregano and pepper. Blend into a smooth purée, about 1 minute. Set aside.

In a large nonstick skillet, cook the bacon to crisp. Reserve 2 tablespoons (30 ml) of the bacon drippings in the pan. (The bacon pieces are a snack for the cook!). Pour in the lentils and cook for 2 to 3 minutes over medium heat. Mash with a wooden spoon or spatula as they cook, but not too much as you want good texture for the "beans."

Pour the blended purée into the skillet of lentils, add the scallion greens and lime juice. Cook over medium heat for 3 to 4 minutes, stirring as it bubbles and reduces to the desired consistency of not too soupy or too thick.

Taste and adjust for salt and lime. Garnish with sliced scallion greens.

Refried "beans" will keep up to 3 days in the refrigerator when stored in an airtight container.

Tip: Microwave the lime for 10 seconds before squeezing to release more juices.

Vegetarian Option: Replace the bacon drippings with Low FODMAP Garlic-Infused Oil (page 50), made with canola oil. And swap in water for the chicken stock.

Monash Note: Although chiles (chillies) are generally low in FODMAPs, some people with IBS may be sensitive to the capsaicin they contain. Capsaicin is a natural compound that gives chiles their spicy quality. You may need to limit how much chile you eat if your IBS symptoms are triggered by spicy food.

Garlic Olive Oil & Chive Mashed Potatoes

LOW FODMAP ❤ IBS FRIENDLY ❤ GLUTEN-FREE ❤ DAIRY-FREE

For many years, I whipped together a lavish blend of potatoes with heavy cream, sour cream or cream cheese, mashed garlic, and a variety of grated cheeses. While LoFO is not a dairy-free diet, I still have issues with lactose and all those garlic cloves. That's why I adore this recipe with aromatic LoFO garlic-infused oil, a mixture of coconut and plain almond milk, and pop of fresh chives. This is calm tummy home-sweet-home in a bowl!

MAKES 4 SERVINGS
INGREDIENTS

2 large russet potatoes (745 g total), peeled and cut into 1-inch (2.5 cm) cubes

1 teaspoon (5 g) fine sea salt, plus 1/2 teaspoon (2.5 g) more for seasoning

2 tablespoons (30 ml) Low FODMAP Garlic-Infused Oil (page 50), made with extra virgin olive oil

1/3 cup (80 ml) canned full-fat coconut milk for cooking, containing no inulin, well-stirred

2 tablespoons (30 ml) plain, unsweetened almond milk, plus 1/8 to 1/4 cup (30-60 ml) more if needed for a smooth creamy consistency

2 teaspoons (2 g) fresh minced chives

1/4 teaspoon fresh ground black pepper

Method: Bring 6 cups (1.4 L) water to a rolling boil in a large pot. Add the potatoes and 1 teaspoon salt. Reduce to medium heat and boil for 20 minutes or until very tender. Drain, then spoon into a mixing bowl.

Add the garlic oil, milks, chives, 1/2 teaspoon salt and 1/4 teaspoon pepper. Use a hand or immersion blender and whip until smooth. Taste and adjust for salt and pepper. Serve immediately.

Stored in an airtight container, mashed potatoes will keep in the fridge for up to 3 days.

Tip: If you are able to tolerate, blend 2 tablespoons (28 g) butter in with the final ingredients for a silky finish.

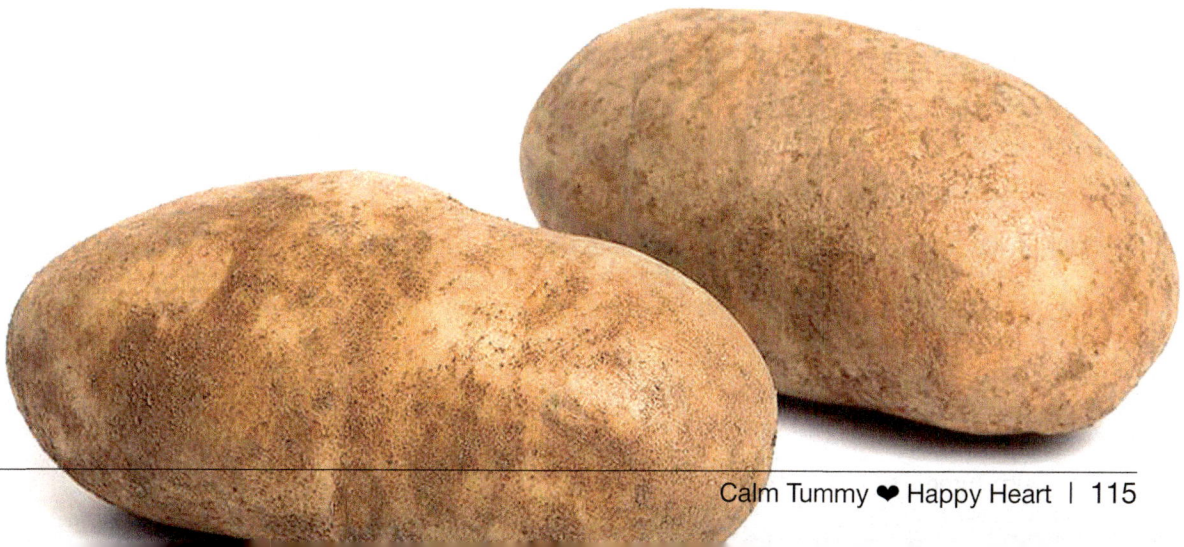

Fiesta Slaw

LOW FODMAP ❤ IBS FRIENDLY ❤ GLUTEN-FREE ❤ DAIRY-FREE

This bright multi-color slaw brings the party to the table! The flavors blend for a surefire crowd pleaser that's even better the next day after the ingredients have infused and chilled in the fridge.

MAKES 6-8 SERVINGS
SLAW INGREDIENTS

2 large (200 g total) carrots, peeled

1 large (164 g) fresh red bell pepper, stemmed, seeds and ribs removed

3 1/2-ounces (100 g) red cabbage

5.3-ounces (150 g) jicama, peeled

1/2 cup (8 g) fresh medium packed cilantro, mostly leaves, rough chopped

3/4 cup (38 g) thin sliced scallions, green parts only

DRESSING INGREDIENTS

1/4 cup (56 g) mayonnaise, containing no onion or garlic

1/4 cup (60 ml) red wine vinegar

2 teaspoons (10 ml) maple syrup

3/4 teaspoon (4 g) fine sea salt

Juice of 1 lime

2 tablespoons (30 ml) Low FODMAP Garlic-Infused Oil (page 50), made with canola oil, cooled

Method

Slaw: Cut the carrots, red bells, cabbage, and jicama into slices that will fit into a food processor feed tube. Fit the processor with the shredding blade. Shred them and place in a medium mixing bowl. Add the chopped cilantro and scallion greens. Stir to combine.

Dressing: Whisk the ingredients and pour over the shred. Stir and toss well to coat. Taste and adjust for salt or additional vinegar.

Stored in an airtight container, slaw will keep in the fridge overnight.

Tips: Place the lime in the microwave on high for 10 seconds to release more juices before squeezing. If you happen to get a dry lime and have a lemon on hand, it will do just fine.

If you don't have a food processor, a box grater also works well.

Monash Note: Although chiles (chillies) are generally low in FODMAPs, some people with IBS may be sensitive to the capsaicin they contain. Capsaicin is a natural compound that gives chiles their spicy quality. You may need to limit how much chile you eat if your IBS symptoms are triggered by spicy food.

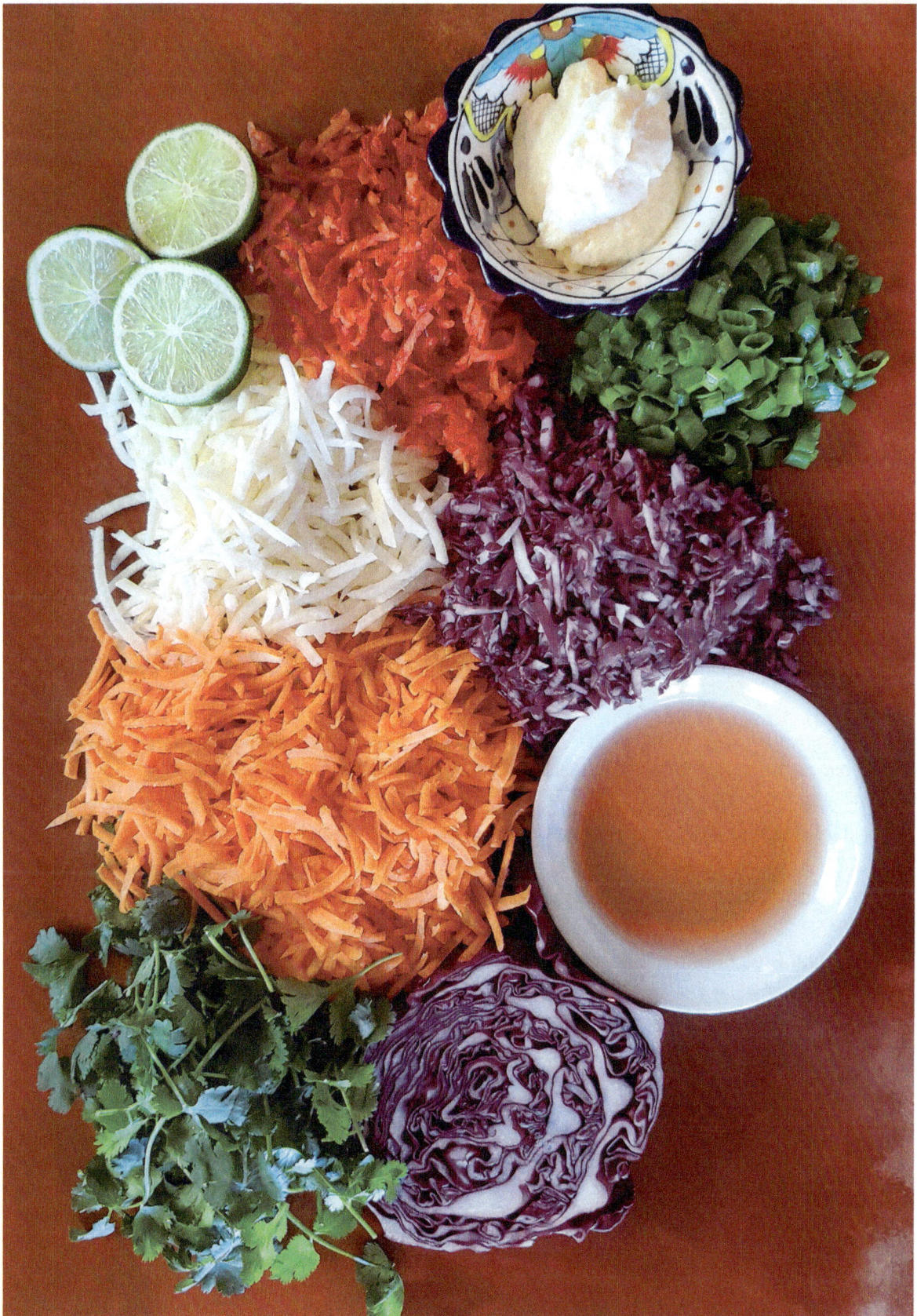

Fresh Green Chiles Rellenos with Mashed Potatoes

LOW FODMAP ❤ IBS FRIENDLY ❤ GLUTEN-FREE ❤ DAIRY-FREE

One of my most craveable side dishes is a fresh roasted green chile filled with mashed potatoes. It pairs with steak, roasted chicken, pork tenderloin, ribs, meatloaf, and as a holiday side dish. One green chile has as much vitamin C as 5 oranges, and the creamy mashed potatoes infuse with the charred chile flavor very nicely.

If you are not familiar with banana-shaped green chiles, see page 44 for identifying different chile shapes and sizes. Green Chiles are known by names such as: Hatch, Anaheim, Colorado Green, New Mexican, and Chiles Verde Del Norte.

MAKES 6 SERVINGS
CHILES INGREDIENTS
6 medium sized 5.5-inch (14 cm) (61 g) each fresh mild green chiles, roasted and prepped (page 46) leaving the stems intact and cutting a pocket per instructions for rellenos (on the Monash App they are noted as: Chile, green, peeled, deseeded)

POTATO FILLING INGREDIENTS
Follow the recipe for Garlic Olive Oil and Chive Mashed Potatoes on page 115, warm and ready to use. They are divine!

Method: Using a small spoon, fill the prepped chiles with mashed potatoes. Serve immediately, or place them on a serving platter and cover with foil to keep warm until ready to serve.

The mashed potatoes can be made a day in advance and re-heated for serving, however, I find that the chiles taste and hold together better when prepared the same day.

Tip: If you are able to tolerate dairy, place the rellenos in a heatproof baking pan. Top each with 1 tablespoon (7 g) shredded cheddar, queso fresco or Manchego cheese. Place under the broiler for 1 to 2 minutes to melt the cheese.

For Breakfast Green Chiles Rellenos: Fill each chile with plain scrambled eggs, 2 pieces crisp crumbled bacon, and 2 tablespoons Pico de Gallo (page 64). If tolerated, use the cheeses listed above and broil.

Monash Note: Although chiles (chillies) are generally low in FODMAPs, some people with IBS may be sensitive to the capsaicin they contain. Capsaicin is a natural compound that gives chiles their spicy quality. You may need to limit how much chile you eat if your IBS symptoms are triggered by spicy food.

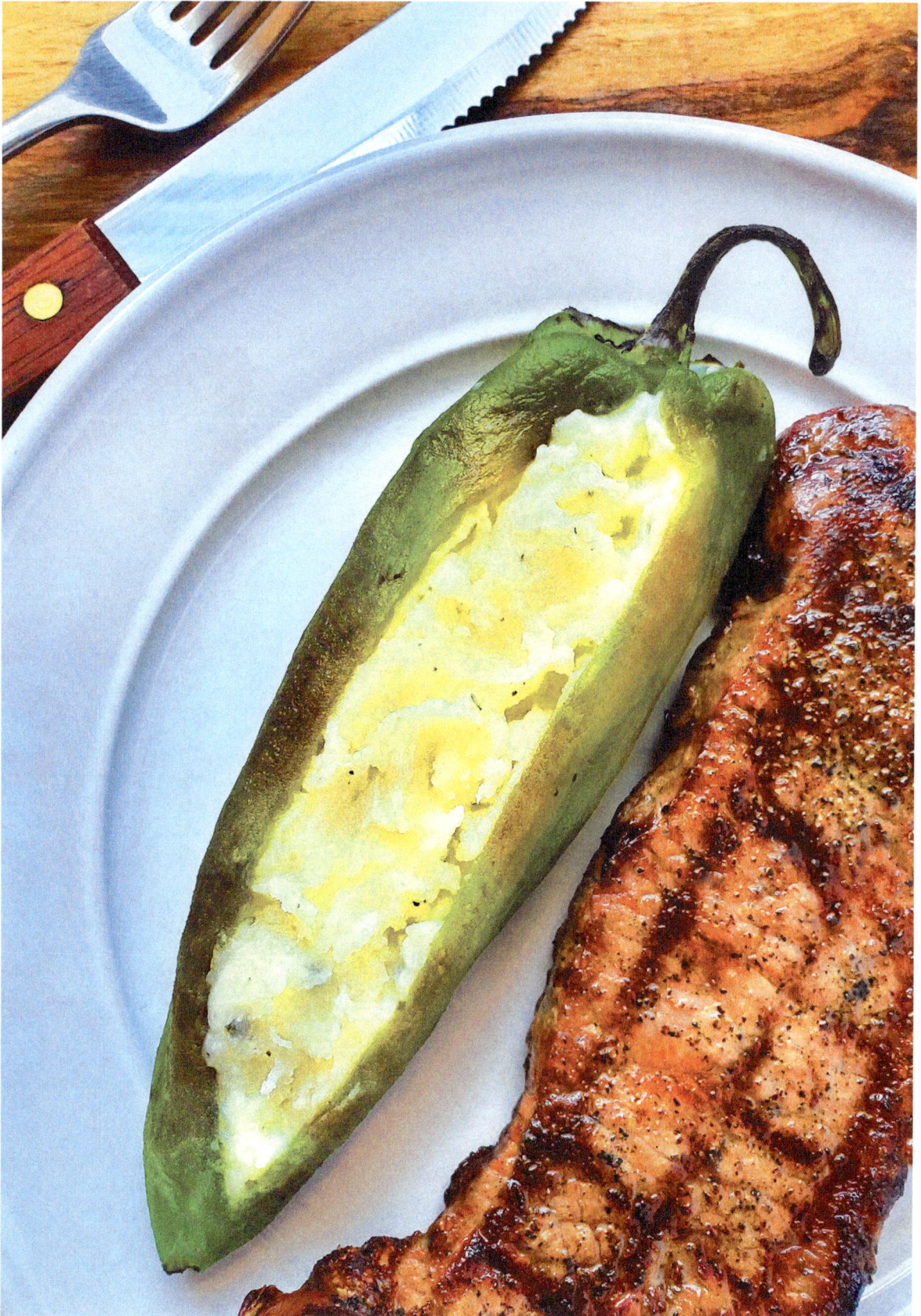

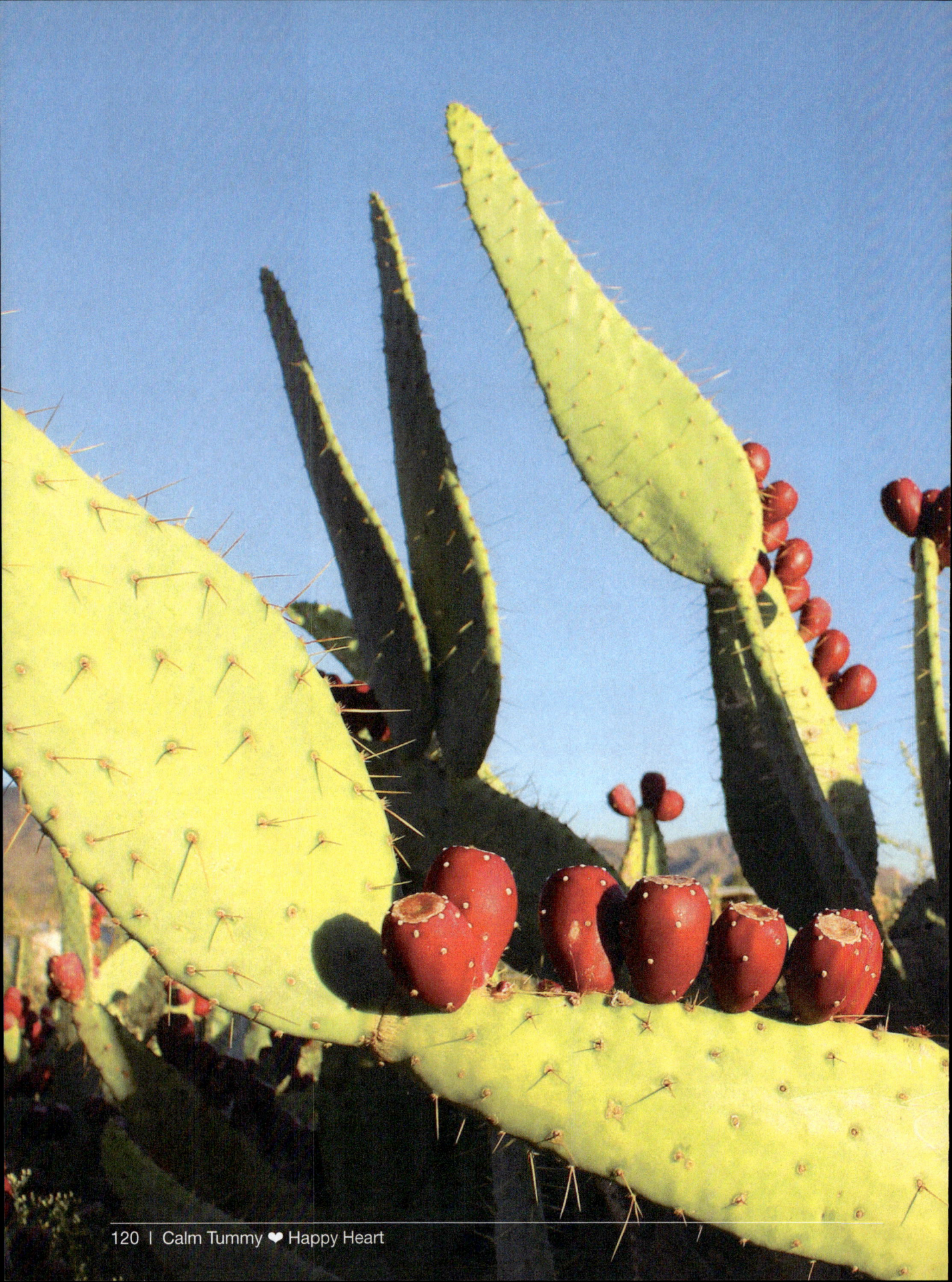

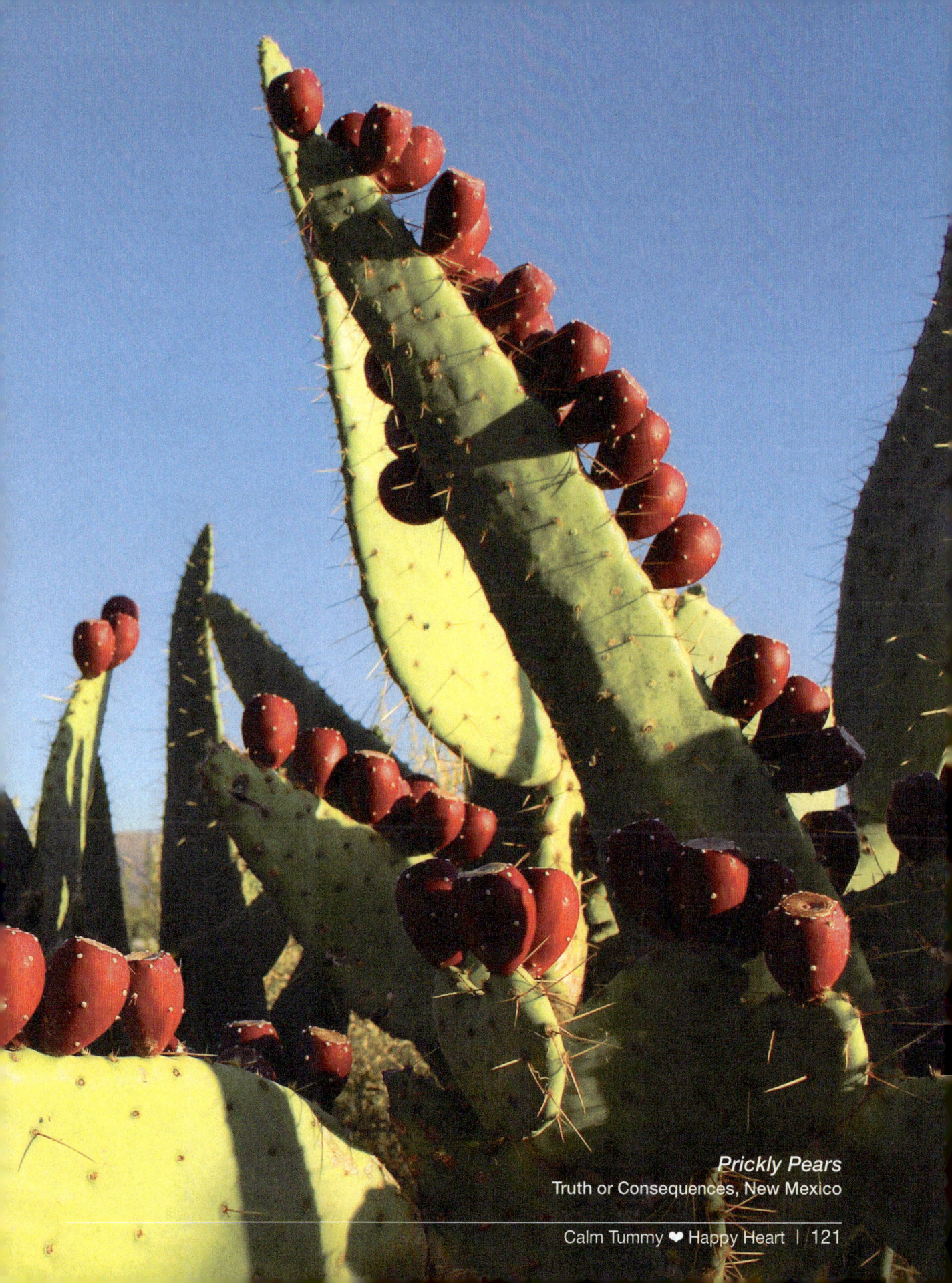

Prickly Pears
Truth or Consequences, New Mexico

Salads, Chilis & Soups

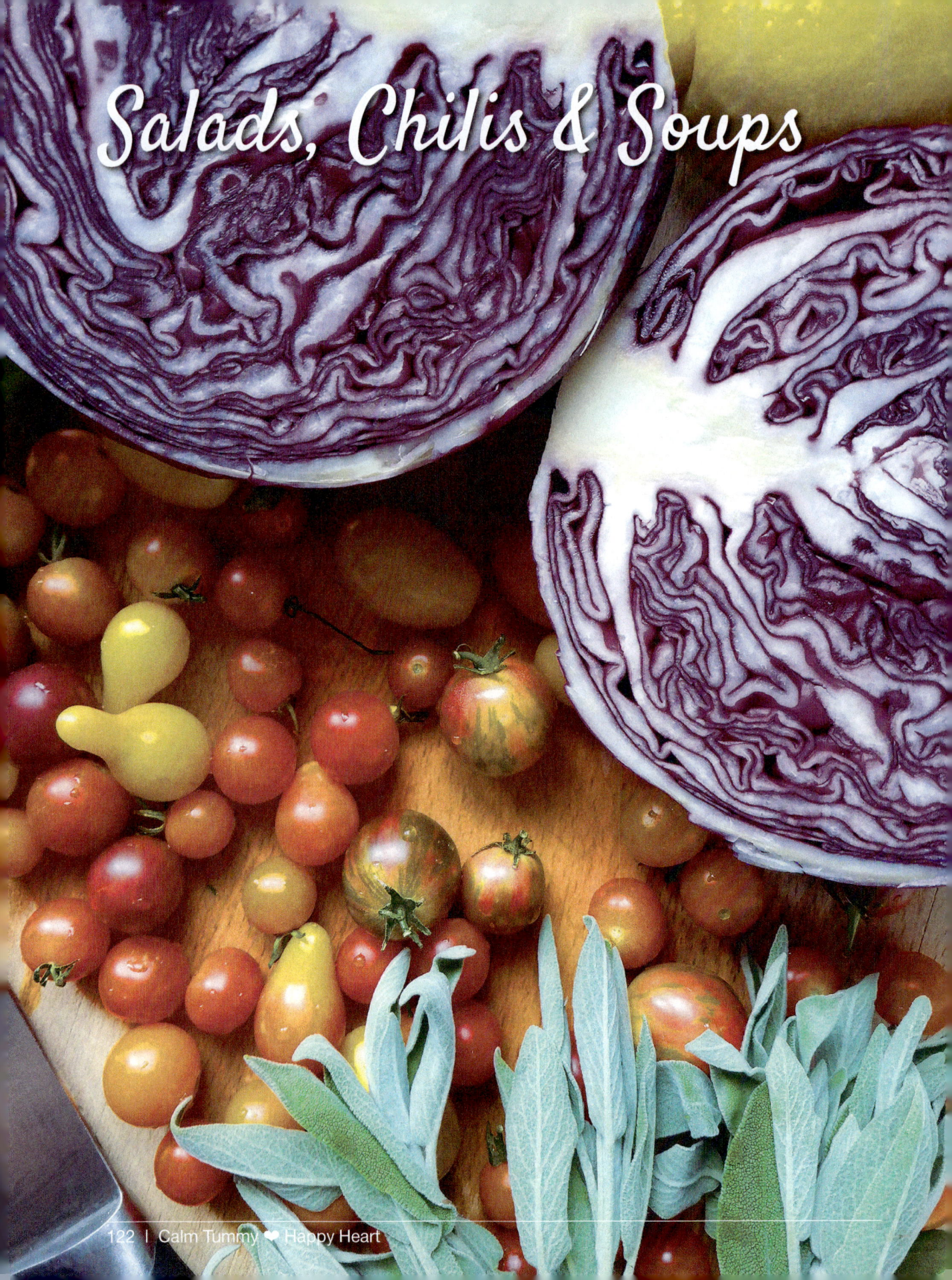

- ❤ **Calm Tummy Happy Heart Salad**

- ❤ **Pulled Pork Caesar Salad
  with Lemon Vinaigrette & Red Chile Croutons**

- ❤ **Grilled Romaine Taco Salad**

- ❤ **Grilled Chicken Chile Macaroni Salad**

- ❤ **Low FODMAP Chicken Stock**

- ❤ **Mesa Verde Masa Beef Chili**

- ❤ **Green Chile Pork Pozole (Stew)**

- ❤ **Chicken Tortilla Soup**

- ❤ **Ma's Gazpacho**

- ❤ **All Seasons Carrot Soup with Jalapeño Essence**

Food brand names are sometimes listed within a recipe, and this means they are Monash Certified. For more brand options we use and love, please visit **Fodifylt.com**

Monash Note: Although chiles (chillies) are generally low in FODMAPs, some people with IBS may be sensitive to the capsaicin they contain. Capsaicin is a natural compound that gives chiles their spicy quality. You may need to limit how much chile you eat if your IBS symptoms are triggered by spicy food.

Calm Tummy Happy Heart Salad

LOW FODMAP ❤ IBS FRIENDLY ❤ GLUTEN-FREE ❤ DAIRY-FREE

In the "My Story" chapter I share about a point in my life when I gave up searching for answers about my symptoms. Even though I was exhausted and the expenses for testing and treatments had piled up, it was a huge mistake to discontinue my search to be properly diagnosed with a proven treatment plan. During this time I would make big salads at the beginning of each week so I didn't have to think about food every day. For someone with ironclad digestion, the ingredients I used would have been perfectly fine to eat and go about their day. For me it was a mine field of trigger foods like: black and pinto beans, cauliflower, wheat pasta,

asparagus, red onions, loads of sweet corn, peas, garlic croutons, button mushrooms, all drizzled with garlic-based dressing, and oftentimes wrapped in a flour tortilla. My symptoms had never been worse.

This dish, the Calm Tummy Happy Heart Salad, is one of the first recipes I converted into low FODMAP and this is why I chose to name my cookbook after it. A hearty, filling salad with garden fresh flavors, salmon, and creamy citrus red chile dressing, this is a complete meal with several protein suggestions in the Tips section. Here's to a calm tummy and happy heart!

MAKES 1 SALAD
SALMON INGREDIENTS

1, 3 - 4 ounce (84 - 112 g) wild caught salmon fillet

1/4 teaspoon (.5 g) ground cumin

1/4 scant teaspoon (1 g) fine sea salt

1/8 teaspoon fresh ground black pepper

1 1/2 tablespoons (45 ml) Low FODMAP Garlic-Infused Oil (page 50), made with extra virgin olive oil

DRESSING INGREDIENTS

2 teaspoons (10 ml) fresh squeezed orange juice

2 teaspoons (9 g) mayonnaise, containing no onion or garlic

1 teaspoon (5 ml) red wine vinegar

1/4 teaspoon (1.25 g) plain, prepared yellow mustard, containing no onion or garlic

1/4 teaspoon (.5 g) pure mild red chile powder (containing no onion or garlic, the ingredients should list only: red chile. On the Monash App this is called Chilli (chili) red, powdered.

1/8 teaspoon maple syrup

2 fresh chive threads, minced

Pinch of fine sea salt

SALAD INGREDIENTS

3/4 cup (56 g) thinly sliced crisp Romaine lettuce

1/4 cup (39 g) cooked quinoa

1/8 cup (19 g) peeled, 1/2-inch (1.25 cm) cubed yam; steamed, boiled, or pan cooked in a bit of extra virgin olive oil

4 canned, pitted and sliced ripe black olives

1/4 small (20 g) fresh Roma tomato, small diced

2 (20 – 30 g total) red radishes, sliced thin

1 scallion, green part only, sliced thin

2 teaspoons (6 g) piñon nuts, lightly pan toasted

Microgreens for garnish

Method

Salmon: Dust the salmon with cumin, salt and black pepper. Pour the oil into a medium nonstick skillet over medium high heat. Cook the salmon for 4 minutes, flip and cook 4 to 5 minutes longer or to desired doneness. Drain on a paper towel and flake into chunks with a fork.

Dressing: Whisk the dressing ingredients in a small bowl until creamy and fully blended.

Assembly: Choose your favorite salad bowl and arrange the salmon and salad ingredients as you like. Drizzle with dressing. Top with the toasted piñons and microgreens. Serve immediately.

Tips: Other protein options: plain shredded or grilled sliced chicken, pulled pork, cod, halibut, or flank steak, all prepared as the salmon in this recipe with no onion, garlic or other high FODMAP ingredients. When preparing flank steak, be sure to slice it very thin against the grain for a tender bite.

This is a great salad for topping baked potatoes or a low FODMAP gluten-free pizza or flatbread.

At the writing of this cookbook, microgreens had not yet been tested for FODMAPs. You may find that they are not a trigger food for you. Meanwhile let's keep an eye on Monash postings for newly tested foods.

Monash Note: Although chiles (chillies) are generally low in FODMAPs, some people with IBS may be sensitive to the capsaicin they contain. Capsaicin is a natural compound that gives chiles their spicy quality. You may need to limit how much chile you eat if your IBS symptoms are triggered by spicy food.

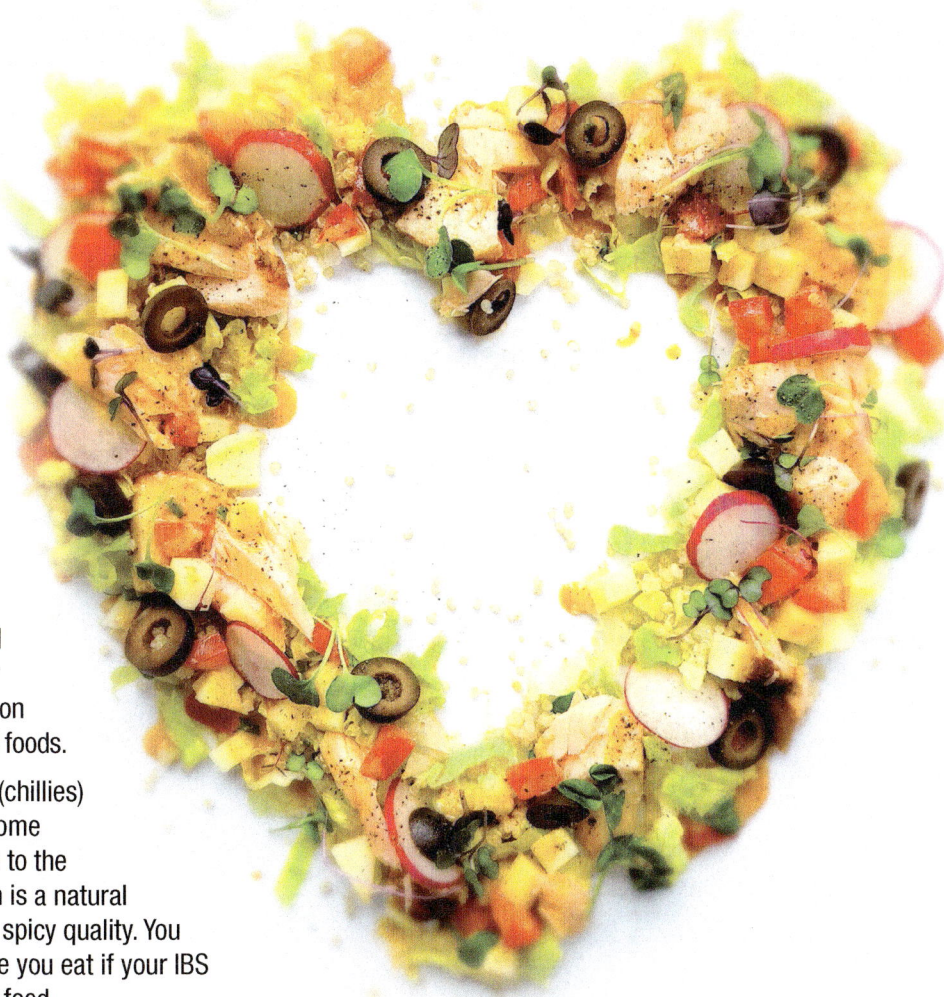

Pulled Pork Caesar Salad with Lemon Vinaigrette & Red Chile Croutons

LOW FODMAP ❤ IBS FRIENDLY ❤ GLUTEN-FREE ❤ DAIRY-FREE

Caesar Salad is a favorite restaurant go-to because it's easy to swap out the high FODMAPs. Preparing it at home is even better because you make it just like you like it.

This version has the crisp Romaine you'd expect, and is topped with slow-roasted pulled pork, diced tomato, LoFO gluten-free crunchy red chile croutons, and a bright lemon, olive oil, Dijon dressing. Slow Oven-Roasted Pulled Pork (page 80) requires 8+ hours of slow roasting. If you're short on time and your local bbq joint prepares their pork with only salt and pepper, with no onion, garlic, bbq sauce or other HiFO ingredients, pick up a to-go order of 6-ounces (170 g) and you're good to go.

MAKES 2 SALADS
CROUTON INGREDIENTS

2 slices low FODMAP gluten-free white bread, or 1 Schar brand gluten-free ciabatta roll (Monash certified)

2 teaspoons (10 ml) extra virgin olive oil

1/2 teaspoon (1 g) (plus another 1/2 teaspoon to your taste) pure mild red chile powder (containing no onion or garlic, the ingredients should list only: red chile. On the Monash App this is called Chilli (chili) red, powdered)

1/8 teaspoon fine sea salt, plus a pinch more if you like

1/8 teaspoon fresh ground black pepper

DRESSING INGREDIENTS

2 teaspoons (10 ml) fresh lemon juice (microwave for 10 seconds before squeezing to yield more juice)

2 teaspoons (10 ml) extra virgin olive oil

1/2 teaspoon (3 g) prepared Dijon mustard, containing no onion or garlic

1/2 teaspoon Worcestershire sauce

1/4 teaspoon fine sea salt

1/4 teaspoon fresh ground black pepper

PORK AND TOPPINGS INGREDIENTS

6-ounces (170 g) Slow Oven-Roasted Pulled Pork (page 80)

2 teaspoons (10 ml) extra virgin olive oil

1 whole head (200 g) Romaine lettuce, washed, cored and finely chopped, patted dry with a paper towel

1/2 (100 g) common tomato, diced

Method: Preheat the oven to 375 F / 190 C

(continued on next page)

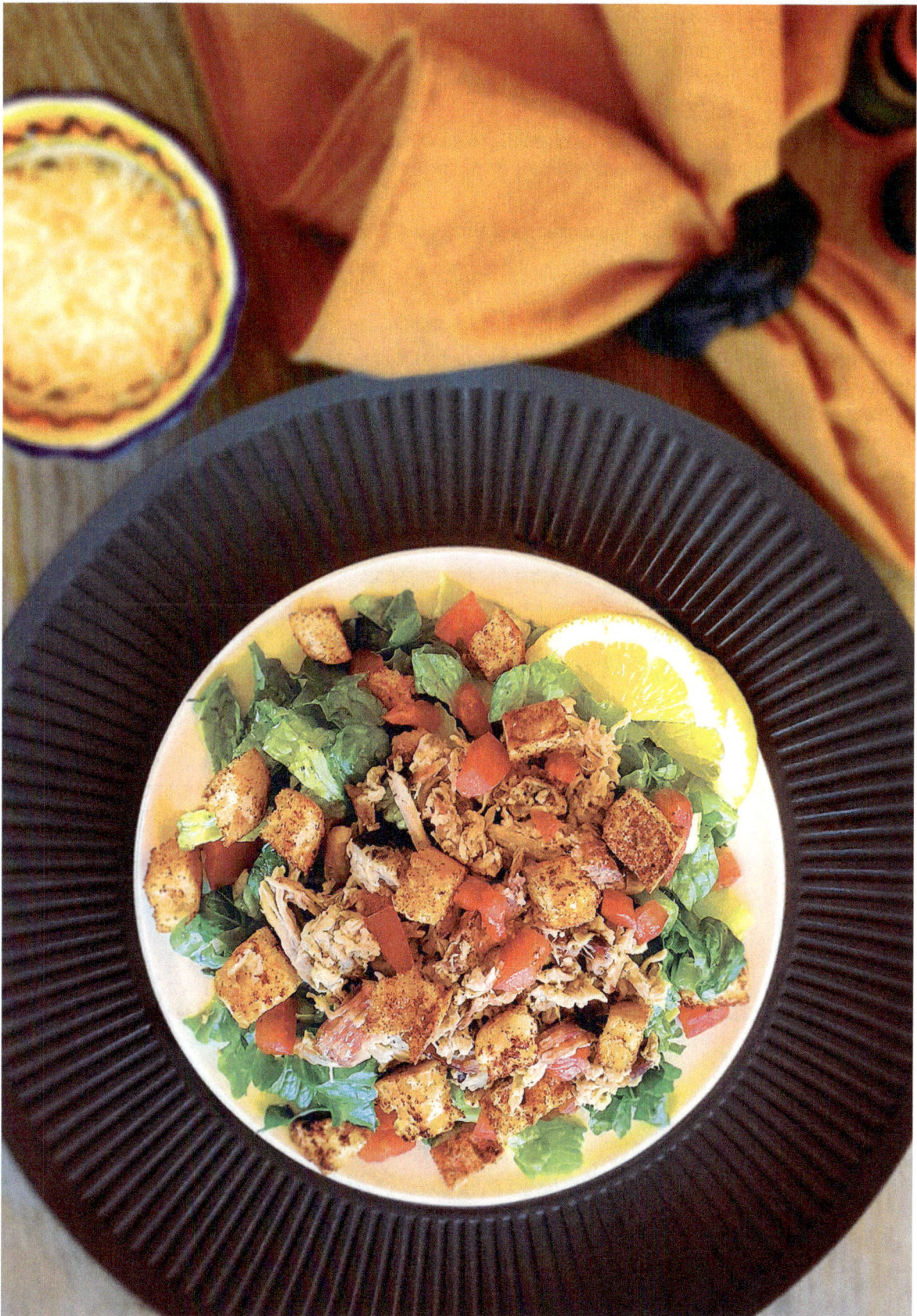

(continued from previous page)

Croutons: Lightly coat a rimmed baking sheet with cooking spray oil. Cut the bread into 1/2-inch (1.26 cm) pieces and spread them out on the pan. Drizzle with 2 teaspoons (10 ml) oil. Use your hands to toss and coat them. Sprinkle with chile powder, salt and pepper. Again, use your hands to thoroughly coat.

Bake for 5 minutes. Pull out of the oven and use a spatula to roll and flip them around the pan. Bake 3 to 5 minutes more until crunchy. Ovens differ, so keep an eye on them as they will burn quickly. Slide them onto paper towels and set aside to cool.

Dressing: Place all of the dressing ingredients in a small bowl. Whisk vigorously and set aside.

Pork: If you are re-heating the pulled pork, pour 2 teaspoons (10 ml) extra virgin olive oil in a small nonstick skillet over medium high heat. Stir a bit until the meat is fully warmed. Oftentimes I like to form the meat into loose patties and get a really good sear on them for a crispy bite.

Toppings & Assembly: Use your hands or two spoons to mix and coat the chopped lettuce with the dressing in a mixing bowl. Fill two salad bowls or plates with the lettuce, top with the warm pork, add the croutons and tomato.

Two lemon slices are a nice garnish, and have a pepper mill on hand to add a few turns of fresh ground black pepper if desired. Serve immediately.

Tips: If you are able to tolerate, divide 4 teaspoons (10 g) shredded or fine grated parmesan or Manchego cheese to top the salads.

Grilled chicken breasts and pan seared salmon with salt, pepper and a spritz of lemon also pair very well with this salad.

When cooking with red chile powder it is always a good idea to read the label for any onion, garlic or HiFO ingredients. See page 48 for more information about chile with an 'e' vs. chili with an 'i.'

When taking the time to slow roast a pork shoulder (also called Boston Butt), I like to shred it and then freeze in 4 to 6-ounce portions in heavy, tightly sealed freezer baggies. It will keep frozen up to 4 to 5 months.

Monash Note: Although chiles (chillies) are generally low in FODMAPs, some people with IBS may be sensitive to the capsaicin they contain. Capsaicin is a natural compound that gives chiles their spicy quality. You may need to limit how much chile you eat if your IBS symptoms are triggered by spicy food.

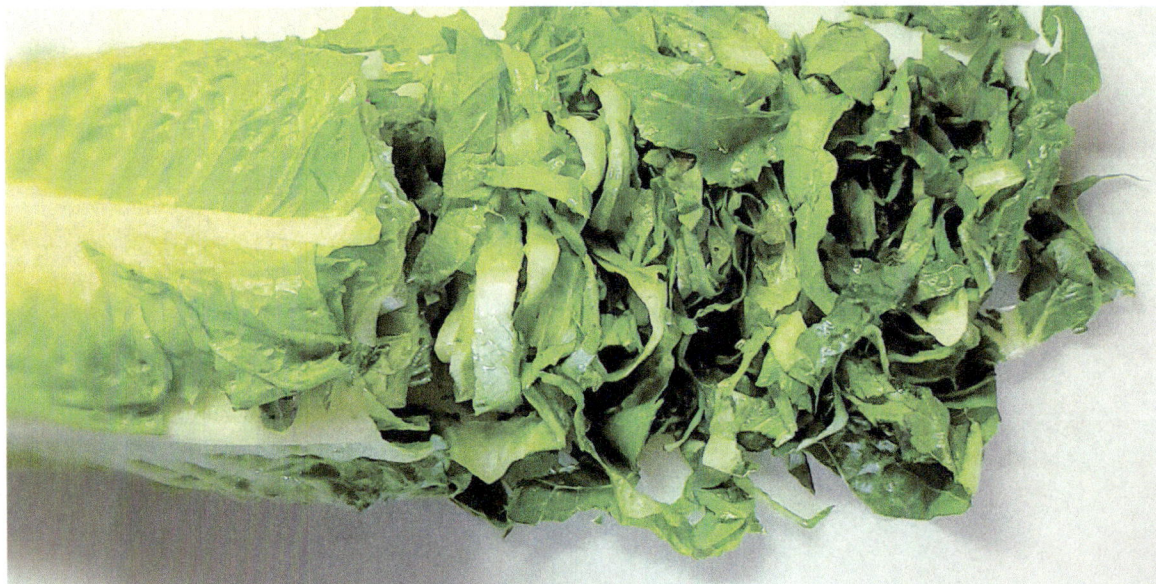

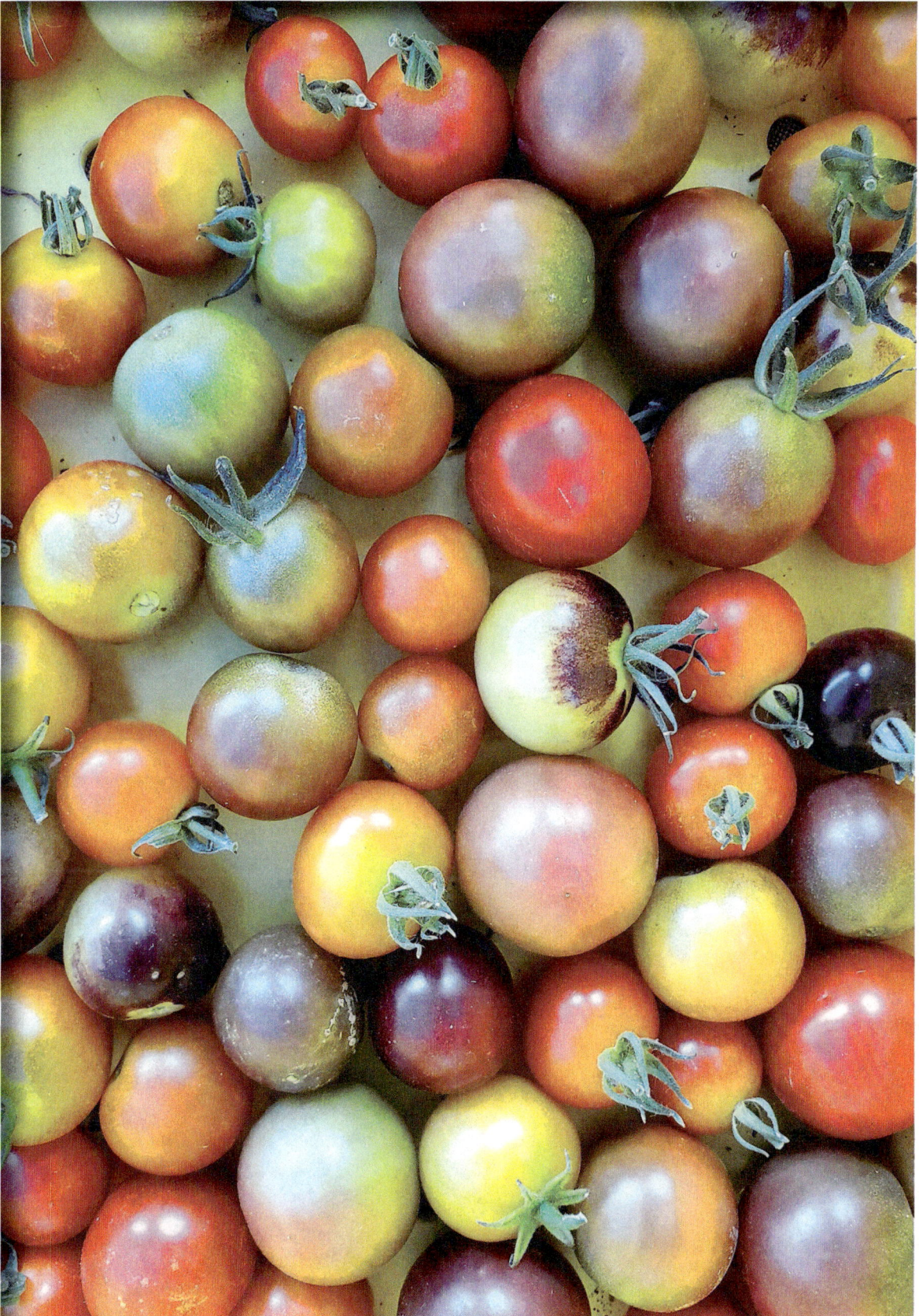

Grilled Romaine Taco Salad

LOW FODMAP ❤ IBS FRIENDLY ❤ GLUTEN-FREE ❤ DAIRY-FREE

There are many versions of Taco Salad. I grew up with the large, deep fried flour tortilla bowls with lots of ground beef, diced onions, refried beans, sour cream, garlic-based taco sauce and assorted toppings. This grilled version has all of the taco flavors, minus the fried bowl, for a zesty robust lunch or dinner complete meal salad.

MAKES 2 SALADS

TACO SEASONING MIX INGREDIENTS

1/2 teaspoon (1 g) ground cumin

1/2 teaspoon (1 g) pure mild red chile powder (containing no onion or garlic, the ingredients should list only: red chile. On the Monash App this is called Chilli (chili) red, powdered)

1/2 teaspoon (1 g) smoked paprika

1/2 teaspoon dried oregano

1/2 teaspoon (2.5 g) fine sea salt

1/4 teaspoon fresh ground black pepper

DRESSING INGREDIENTS

Juice of 1/2 lime

1 tablespoon (18 g) plain, dairy-free, unsweetened coconut yogurt

1 teaspoon (5 g) mayonnaise, containing no onion, garlic or other high FODMAPs

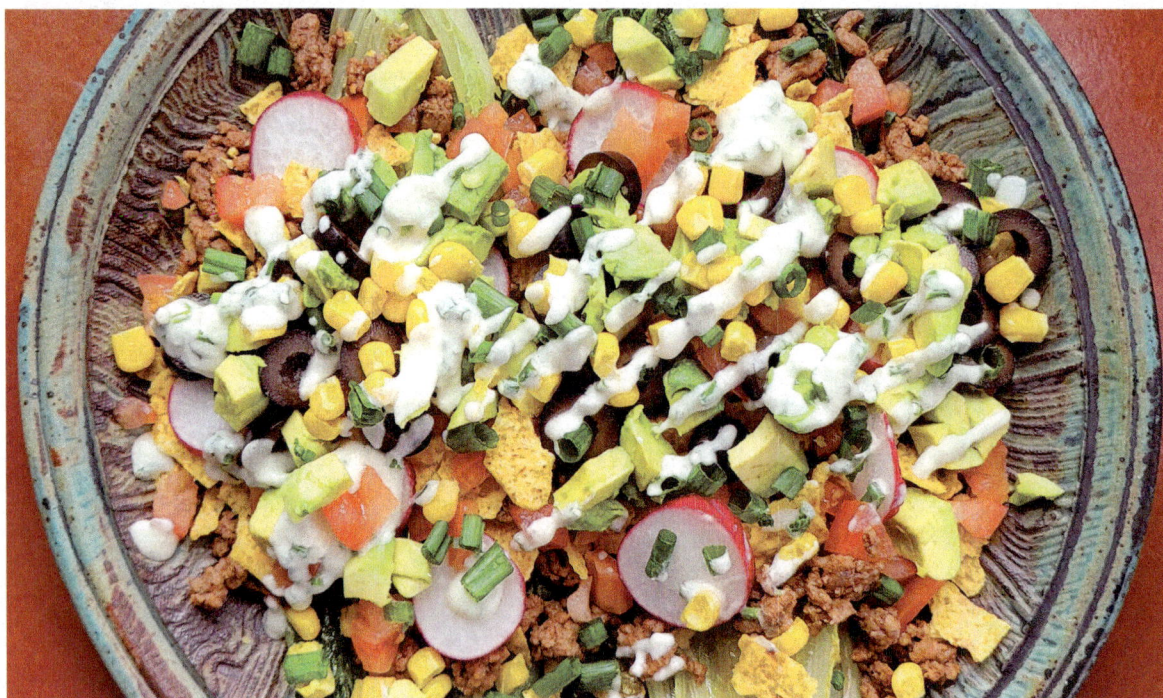

1 teaspoon (5 ml) extra virgin olive oil

1 teaspoon (1 g) minced chives

SALAD INGREDIENTS

1/2-pound (227 g) ground beef, 80/20, grass fed if available

1 teaspoon (2 g) masa harina

2 tablespoons (30 ml) water

1 small head of Romaine lettuce, (150 g total) sliced in half lengthwise, washed and patted dry with a clean kitchen towel

2 tablespoons (19 g) canned corn kernels, drained

1 small (50 g) fresh Roma tomato, diced or sliced

Approx. 10 gluten-free corn tortilla chips (30 g), crushed

2 large (40 g total) red radishes, sliced thin

8 canned, pitted ripe black olives, halved

1.76 ounces (50 g) avocado, cut into small chunky pieces

4 scallions, green parts only, sliced thin

Cooking spray oil, salt and pepper

Method

Taco Seasoning: Whisk the mix ingredients in a small bowl. Set aside.

Dressing: Whisk the dressing ingredients in a small bowl. Set aside.

Salad: Place the ground beef in a medium nonstick skillet over medium high heat. Cook until the meat is browned, stirring often with a wooden spoon, breaking up the meat into small pieces as you cook. Drain and return to the skillet.

Add the seasoning mix, masa harina and water. Over medium heat, stir for 2 to 3 minutes. Taste and adjust for salt. Set aside, covered to keep warm.

Heat your bbq grill or stovetop grill pan to medium high.

Lightly coat the Romaine with cooking spray oil. Sprinkle with a light dusting of salt and pepper. Place the Romaine cut side down on the grill grates.

Let the lettuce grill until slightly charred, only on the cut side. This takes about 8 to 10 minutes.

Assembly: Place the Romaine on two plates or one platter to share. Top with the taco beef, tomato, crushed chips, radishes, black olives, avocado, dressing, scallion greens and corn. Serve immediately.

Tips: If you are able to tolerate, add a dollop of conventional or lactose-free sour cream, or plain dairy-free, unsweetened coconut yogurt on top, and 1 tablespoon fresh grated cheddar cheese per salad.

For a veggie version, swap the beef with plain firm tofu (not silken) 2/3 cup (170 g) cubed per serving, pan seared in extra virgin olive oil to crisp, then coated with the taco seasoning.

Monash Note: Although chiles (chillies) are generally low in FODMAPs, some people with IBS may be sensitive to the capsaicin they contain. Capsaicin is a natural compound that gives chiles their spicy quality. You may need to limit how much chile you eat if your IBS symptoms are triggered by spicy food.

Grilled Chicken Chile Macaroni Salad

LOW FODMAP ❤ IBS FRIENDLY ❤ GLUTEN-FREE ❤ DAIRY-FREE

This simple mac salad is in my fridge all summer long and definitely on the menu for picnics by the pond. The smoky grilled chicken, buttery chiles and lemon juice with zest will have you and yours loving every bite of this delightful, fresh flavor combo!

Plan to have the macaroni cooked and ready. The chiles and chicken are grilled together, and then the chiles need prepping as instructed on page 46, as their skins are inedible. Fresh poblanos or green chiles are the way to go here. If you are not familiar with chile varieties, see page 45 for descriptions. Also, I generally don't use canned chiles for this dish as many brands tend to be salty. That, with the zesty lemon tartness, would very likely pucker your picnickers' palates.

SERVES 4
CHICKEN & CHILE INGREDIENTS

Canola oil to grease the grill grates

1 pound (16-ounces / 454 g) boneless, skinless chicken breasts (generally 2 - 3 breasts)

2 tablespoons (30 ml) extra virgin olive oil

1/2 teaspoon (2.5 g) fine sea salt

1/2 teaspoon (1 g) fresh ground black pepper

4 medium (97 g each) fresh poblano peppers, roasted and prepped as instructed on page 46, will yield 1 cup (180 g) chile meat, diced
-OR-
8 medium (61 g each) mild fresh green chiles, roasted and prepped as instructed on page 46, will yield 1 cup (180 g) diced chile meat (on the Monash App they are noted as: Chile, green, peeled, deseeded)

DRESSING INGREDIENTS

1/2 cup (115 g) mayonnaise containing no onion or garlic

Zest and juice of 1 lemon (organic if available)

1/4 teaspoon pure mild red chile powder (containing no onion or garlic, the ingredients should list only: red chile. On the Monash App this is called Chilli (chili) red, powdered)

1/4 teaspoon ground cumin

1/4 teaspoon fresh ground black pepper

SALAD INGREDIENTS

4 cups (580 g) cooked gluten-free elbow macaroni, cooked according to package directions for al dente, drained

(continued on next page)

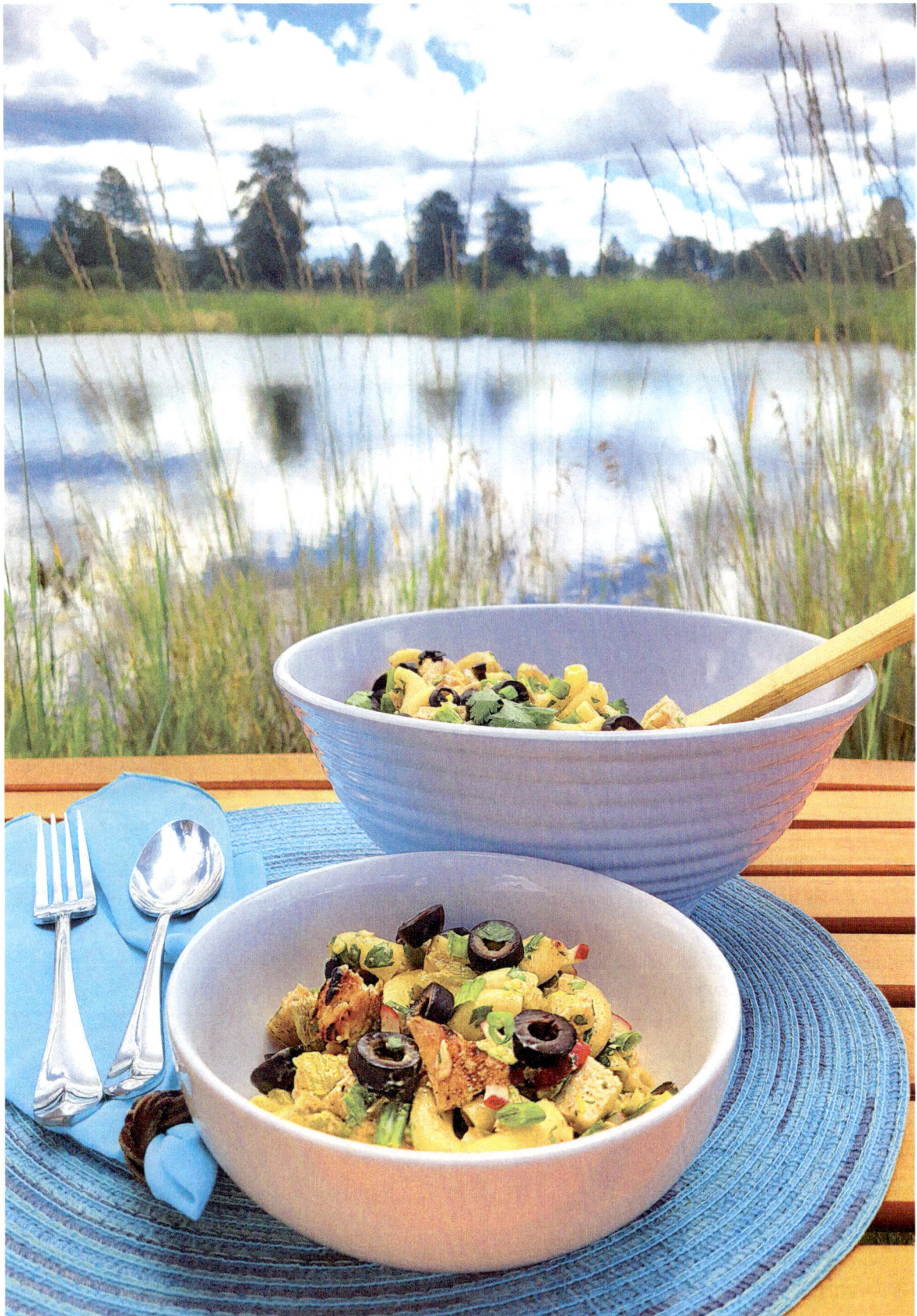

(continued from previous page)

1 cup (16 g) fresh medium packed cilantro, mostly leaves, finely chopped, plus more cilantro leaves for garnish

3/4 cup (38 g) thin sliced scallions, green parts only, plus more for garnish

6 (60 g total) red radishes, matchstick cut

1/2 cup (60 g) canned, pitted ripe black olives, sliced

Method

Chicken: Bring the grill to medium high heat. Using metal tongs and a paper towel doused with a bit of canola oil, grease the grates.

Butterfly cut the chicken by placing your hand flat on top of one breast and cut into the side lengthwise to divide in half, stopping at 1-inch (2.5 cm) before slicing all the way through. Open the fillet flat and it will be heart-shaped. Repeat for the second breast. Cut away any fatty pieces. Make sure your knife is nice and sharp, otherwise the meat will shred as you slice into it. Coat the fillets evenly with the olive oil and dust with salt and pepper on both sides.

Place the chicken and chiles on the grill.

Grill the chicken for 4 minutes and flip with tongs. Grill 4 to 5 minutes longer or until cooked through and showing no pink in the centers. Place on a cutting board and dice

Chiles: While the chicken grills, turn to rotate the chiles with metal tongs to blister and char on all sides. Refer to page 46 for instructions on prepping the chiles after grilling/roasting. When you have the beautiful green chile fillets, cut them into a large dice.

Dressing: Whisk the dressing ingredients together until creamy and smooth.

Assembly: Place the macaroni, chicken, chiles, cilantro, scallion greens and radishes in a large mixing bowl. Spoon and gently stir in the dressing to combine. Scoop the salad into a large serving dish. Garnish the top with fresh cilantro leaves, scallion greens and the sliced black olives. Chill covered in the fridge until ready to serve.

Tips: Microwave the lemon for 10 seconds to release more juices. Zest the lemon first, then squeeze.

Stored in a tightly sealed container, the salad will keep for 3 days in the fridge.

You'll never be a-loney when you make this macaroni! (so, sooo sorry, I could not resist :-)

Monash Note: Although chiles (chillies) are generally low in FODMAPs, some people with IBS may be sensitive to the capsaicin they contain. Capsaicin is a natural compound that gives chiles their spicy quality. You may need to limit how much chile you eat if your IBS symptoms are triggered by spicy food.

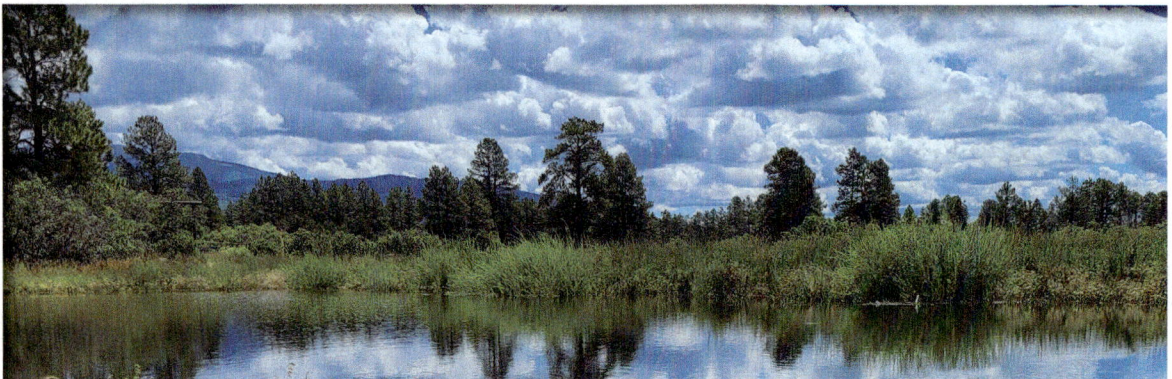

Low Fodmap Chicken Stock

LOW FODMAP ❤ IBS FRIENDLY ❤ GLUTEN-FREE ❤ DAIRY-FREE

Some stock recipes call for simmering the chicken uncovered for 2 or more hours, but I find that the stock evaporates and I'm adding more and more water to the pot every 30 minutes or so. This method – covering the pot with a lid and simmering for 3 hours – always results in a rich, golden stock. Just be sure to check it now and again, as you may need to add a little water, but it will not require a significant amount.

MAKES 8 CUPS (2 L)
INGREDIENTS

4-pounds (1.8 kg) chicken wings

4 quarts (16 cups) (3.8 L) water

6 scallions, green parts only, rough chopped

1 carrot (75 g) peeled and cut into 1-inch (2.5 cm) pieces

2 tablespoons (2 g) fresh parsley leaves, without stems as they can be bitter

1 teaspoon whole black peppercorns

Method: Bring the chicken and water to a rolling boil in a large stockpot. Boil for 10 minutes. Use a slotted spoon to skim off any foam from the surface. Reduce to a simmer and cook for 2 hours, covered with a lid. Check every 30 minutes and add hot water if the stock has reduced a bit.

Add the remaining ingredients and simmer for 1 hour, again checking for added water. Pour the stock through a fine mesh metal strainer into a large bowl and discard the solids. Skim off any foam or fat from the surface.

Let cool completely, about 30 minutes. Refrigerate or freeze immediately. Stock will last in the refrigerator for up to 2 days and can be frozen in airtight freezer containers for 2 to 3 months.

Tip: The cooked carrots are a nice snack for the chef!

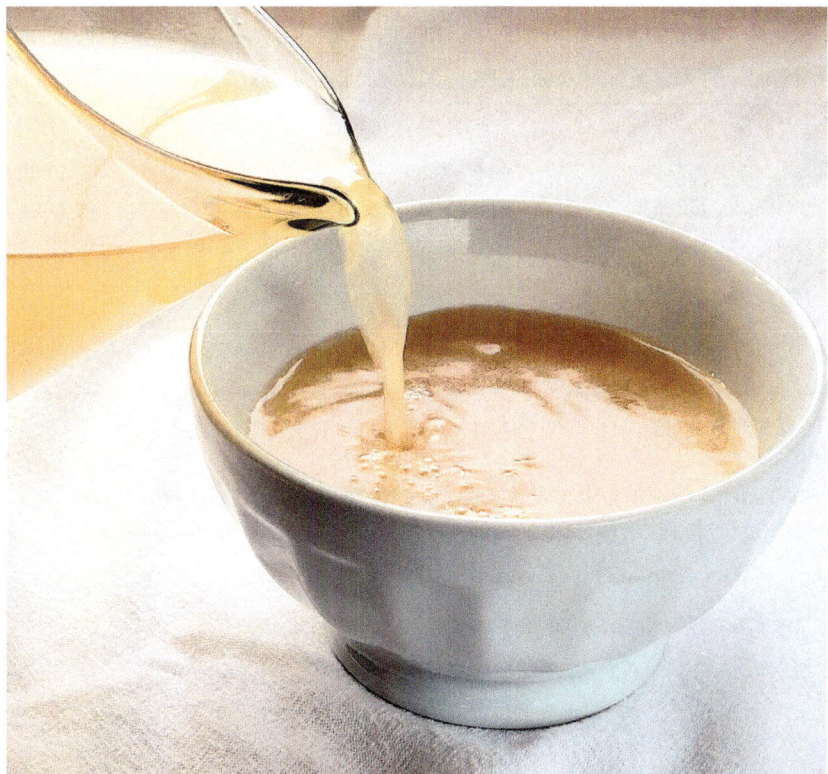

Mesa Verde Masa Beef Chile

LOW FODMAP ❤ IBS FRIENDLY ❤ GLUTEN-FREE ❤ DAIRY-FREE

Southwesterners take their chili very seriously. The stories you've heard about chili contest judges who receive sirens-a-blazin' police escorts to make it in time for a competition is a real thing. Sometimes the judges are pulled over for speeding. They explain to the officer that they're running late, dozens of chili cook-off contestants have had no sleep for 48 hours preparing secret family heirloom recipes that are kept under lock and key, pots are simmering as they speak, and judging is minutes away. The officer — a die-hard chili lover who proudly wears an "Everybody Digs My Chili" t-shirt underneath his uniform — recognizes the gravity of the situation and commands "follow me!" The judge reaches the venue on time and the officer is asked to sit in as an honorary taste tester. Awards and prizes are handed out. Moments like these can make even the most cantankerous cowboy shed a tear.

I've made this LoFO masa harina thickened beef chili for years and no one, not even a chili judge or two, has guessed that it's low FODMAP. It's not difficult at all. The trick is to use the green parts of scallions instead of white onion, LoFO garlic-infused extra virgin olive oil instead of chopped garlic cloves, leave out the beans, and thicken it with masa harina.

This is blue ribbon worthy.

MAKES 4 SERVINGS
INGREDIENTS

2 tablespoons (30 ml) Low FODMAP Garlic-Infused Oil (page 50), made with extra virgin olive oil

1 1/2-pounds (680 g) ground beef 80/20, grass fed if available

1/2 cup (25 g) thin sliced scallions, green parts only

2 teaspoons (4 g) pure mild red chile powder (containing no onion or garlic, the ingredients should list only: red chile. On the Monash App this is called Chilli (chili) red, powdered)

1 teaspoons (2 g) ground cumin

2 teaspoons (7 g) medium packed light brown sugar

1, 15-ounce (425 g) can plain, peeled Roma tomatoes, with juices

1, 4-ounce (113 g) can plain mild chopped green chiles (containing no onion, garlic or other high FODMAP ingredients. On the Monash App they are noted as Chilli (chili) green, mild, chopped, canned)
-OR-
5 medium (61 g each) mild fresh green chiles, roasted and prepped (page 46) will yield approx. 5/8 cup (115 g) diced chile meat (On the Monash App they are noted as: Chile (chili), green, peeled, deseeded)

2 cups (475 ml) Low FODMAP Chicken Stock (page 135) or water, plus extra if needed

3 tablespoons (17 g) masa harina, plus more depending on how thick you like your chili

2 teaspoons (10 ml) red wine vinegar, plus 1 more teaspoon per your taste

(continued on next page)

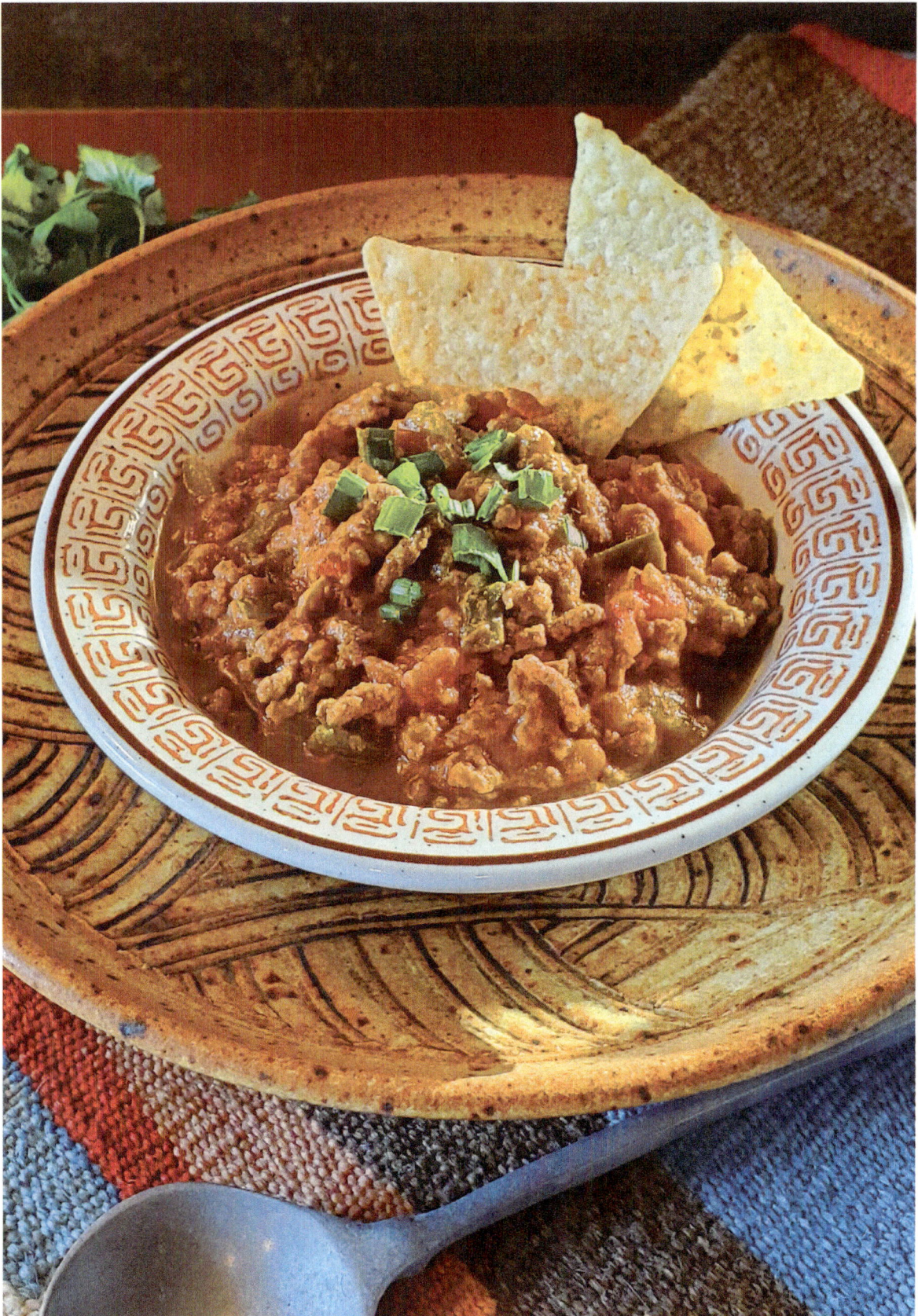

(continued from previous page)

1 teaspoon (10 g) plain, prepared yellow mustard, containing no onion or garlic

1 teaspoon (5 g) fine sea salt

1/2 teaspoon (1 g) fresh ground black pepper

1/4 or 1/2 teaspoon cayenne powder, optional

GARNISHES

Green parts of scallions, sliced thin

Cilantro leaves

3 crushed gluten-free corn tortilla chips per bowl

Method: Pour the garlic infused oil into a large soup pot over medium high heat. Add the beef and stir to brown. A wooden spatula works well to crush-crumble the meat as it cooks. Add the scallion greens, red chile powder, cumin and brown sugar. Stir for 2 minutes.

Add the tomatoes, chopped green chiles, stock, masa harina, vinegar and remaining chili ingredients. Use the spatula to crush and break up the tomatoes into small pieces. Give the chili a good stir. Allow to bubble for 5 minutes. Reduce heat to simmer uncovered for 15 minutes or reduced to desired thickness. Stir often.

If the chili is too chunky to your liking, use a hand-held immersion blender for desired smoothness. Or, ladle half of the chili into a blender. Place the lid and cover with a heavy, clean kitchen towel to avoid splatters. Blend for 30 seconds and pour back into the chili pot. Stir to combine.

Garnish with desired toppings. Serve immediately.

Tips: If you are able to tolerate, top each bowl with 1 tablespoon conventional or lactose-free sour cream, or plain, dairy-free unsweetened coconut yogurt, and/ or 1 tablespoon (7 g) each shredded cheddar cheese.

A simple salad of arugula or Romaine lettuce with sliced radish and common cucumber, sliced green parts of scallions, and red wine vinegar with olive oil is a fresh side to pair with this dish.

Monash Note: Although chiles (chillies) are generally low in FODMAPs, some people with IBS may be sensitive to the capsaicin they contain. Capsaicin is a natural compound that gives chiles their spicy quality. You may need to limit how much chile you eat if your IBS symptoms are triggered by spicy food.

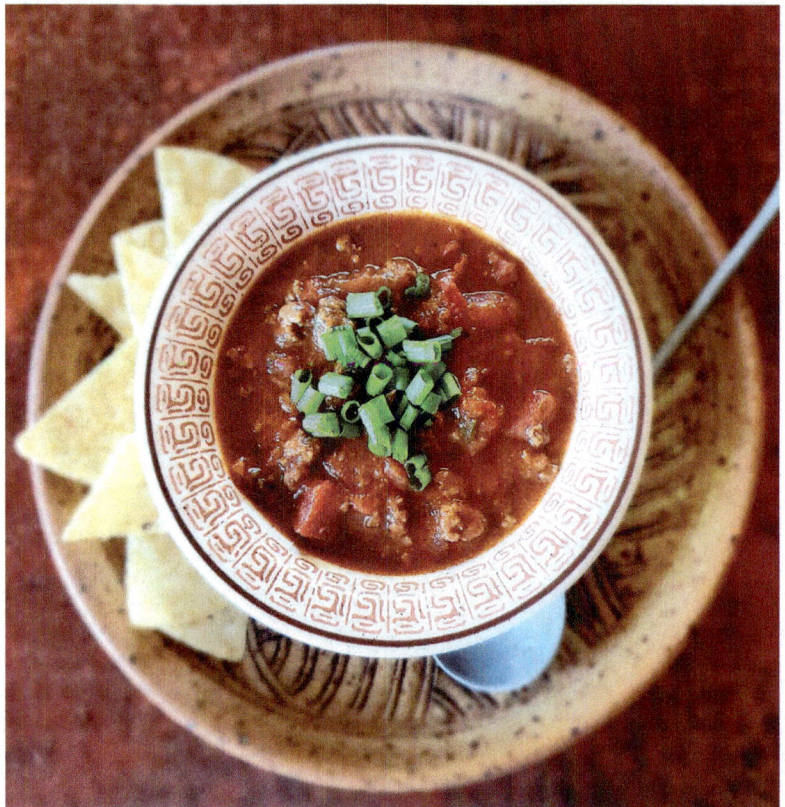

Green Chile Pork Pozole (Stew)

LOW FODMAP ❤ IBS FRIENDLY ❤ GLUTEN-FREE ❤ DAIRY-FREE

It is a rare day when Jim passes on the opportunity to order this traditional Mexican pork, pozole and chile stew, particularly the peppery-buttery green chile version. This is why I've spent many moons in the kitchen testing swaps and ingredient amounts to replicate the tender pork with just the right amounts of seasoning and bits of creamy pozole (hominy). I make this all year long, even in the hot Southwest summer months. It's that good!

MAKES 8 SERVINGS
INGREDIENTS

2-pounds (907 g) boneless pork loin, or boneless thick cut pork chops, cut into 1-inch (2.5 cm) cubes

1 teaspoon (5 g) fine sea salt, plus extra as needed

2 teaspoons (4 g) freshly ground black pepper, divided, plus extra

3 tablespoons (45 ml) Low FODMAP Garlic-Infused Oil (page 50), made with extra virgin olive oil, divided

1 large (380 g) russet potato, peeled and cut into 1/4-inch (.63 cm) cubes

3 medium zucchinis (500 g total) trimmed, sliced into 1/2–inch (1.25 cm) circles and quartered

1/2 cup (25 g) thin sliced scallions, green parts only

7 cups (1.7 L) Low FODMAP Chicken Stock (page 135)

2 cups (330 g) canned plain pozole (hominy), drained

3, 4-ounce cans (340 g total) plain mild chopped green chiles (containing no onion, garlic or other high FODMAP ingredients. On the Monash App they are noted as Chilli (chili) green, mild, chopped, canned)

1 teaspoon (2 g) pure mild red chile powder (containing no onion or garlic, the ingredients should list only: red chile. On the Monash App this is called Chilli ((chili) red, powdered)

1/2 teaspoon (1 g) pure chipotle powder containing no onion, garlic or other high FODMAP ingredients

1 teaspoon (2 g) ground cumin

1 teaspoon dried oregano

2 tablespoons (15 g) cornstarch

2 tablespoons (30 ml) cold water

Juice of 1/2 lime

TOPPINGS

24 (72 g) gluten-free store-bought corn tortilla chips, crushed

8 scallions, green part only, sliced thin

8 lime wedges

Method: Spread the cubed pork out on your cutting board and evenly dust with 1 teaspoon salt and 1 teaspoon pepper.

Pour 2 tablespoons oil in a large heavy-bottom soup pot over medium high heat. Brown the pork on all sides, but do not completely cook the meat as it will finish in the simmering process. Transfer to a plate. (continued on next page)

(continued from previous page)

To the same pot, add 1 tablespoon oil and set the heat to medium. Add the potato and zucchini. Sauté for 4 minutes or until the potatoes are just becoming tender. Add 1/2 cup (120 ml) chicken stock and cook 4 more minutes, stirring often.

Add the scallion greens, remaining stock, pozole, green chile, red chile powder, pure chipotle powder, cumin, oregano, and 1 teaspoon black pepper. Spoon the browned pork back into the pot and bring to a low boil for 5 minutes. Reduce to simmer for 20 minutes, covered.

Make a slurry by stirring cornstarch and cold water together in a small bowl. Drizzle into the pot and stir gently for 3 to 4 minutes or until the stew is slightly thickened.

Add the lime juice, stir well and taste; adjust salt and pepper as desired.

Ladle into soup bowls. Garnish with desired toppings.

This stew will keep up to 3 days when stored in an airtight container in the refrigerator.

Tips: If tolerated, top each bowl with 1 tablespoon (7 g) grated cheddar cheese. Also per your tolerance, top each serving with 1 tablespoon (15 g) conventional or lactose-free sour cream.

Canned green chiles are oftentimes heavily salted, so best to taste before adding more salt.

Monash Note: Although chiles (chillies) are generally low in FODMAPs, some people with IBS may be sensitive to the capsaicin they contain. Capsaicin is a natural compound that gives chiles their spicy quality. You may need to limit how much chile you eat if your IBS symptoms are triggered by spicy food.

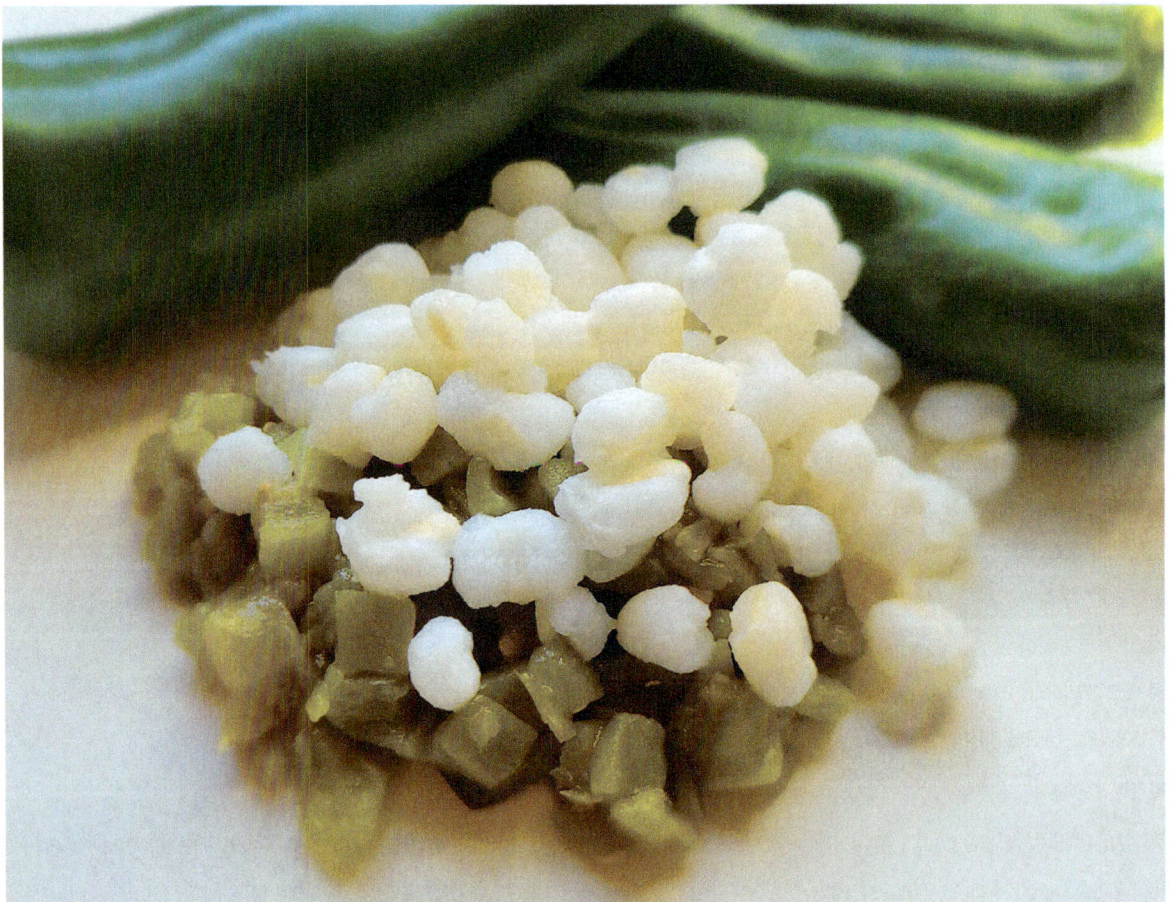

Chicken Tortilla Soup

LOW FODMAP ❤ IBS FRIENDLY ❤ GLUTEN-FREE ❤ DAIRY-FREE

Chicken Tortilla Soup is the remedy for any ailment or life's uncertainty. Feeling sniffles of a cold coming on? Chicken Tortilla Soup. One of those days when you feel like a walking blooper reel? Chicken Tortilla Soup. Someone erroneously broke your heart? Chicken Tortilla Soup, and a love milagro (charm) in your pocket to find new romance.

This low FODMAP version offers all of the flavor and warmth to provide these comforts. And as far as uncertainties go, one thing I know for sure is that a finish of lime and lemon juice add an enchanting sparkle to this bowl of savory magic.

Please review the Poached Chicken Breasts recipe (pg 83) calling for a few ingredients that infuse into the pot liquor and chicken as it poaches. Also, you will need 3 tablespoons of Low FODMAP Garlic Infused Oil (page 50) for your sauté.

MAKES 6 SERVINGS: 10 CUPS (2.4 L) – APPROX. 1 3/4 CUPS (414 ML) PER SERVING

INGREDIENTS

2 pounds (907 g total) skinless boneless chicken breasts, trimmed of fat

3 tablespoons (45 ml) Low FODMAP Garlic-Infused Oil (page 50), made with olive or canola oil in a large nonstick skillet, ready to use

4 medium (300 g total) carrots, peeled and sliced thin on the diagonal

1 cup (75 g) fine chopped bok choy with leaves, washed to remove any grit

1/2 cup (25 g) thin sliced scallions, green parts only, plus more for garnish

2 medium (62 g total) fresh jalapeños, stems, seeds and ribs removed, minced

2 teaspoons (4 g) pure mild red chile powder (containing no onion or garlic, the ingredients should list only: red chile. On the Monash App this is called Chilli (chili) red, powdered)

2 teaspoons dried oregano

1 teaspoon (2 g) ground cumin

1/2 teaspoon (2.5 g) fine sea salt, plus 1/2 teaspoon more if needed

1/2 teaspoon (1 g) smoked paprika

1/2 teaspoon (1 g) fresh ground black pepper

7-ounces (200 g) canned, plain whole peeled Roma tomatoes, drained and rough chopped

Juice of 1 lime

Juice of 1/2 lemon

24 corn tortilla chips, store-bought, 4 per serving

(continued on next page)

(continued from previous page)

GARNISHES

Fresh cilantro leaves

Lime wedges

6-ounces (180 g) avocado, sliced or cubed

Method: Poach the chicken breasts as instructed on page 83 in a large soup pot. Pour the broth through a fine mesh metal strainer into a large bowl. Remove and discard the poaching peppercorns, scallion greens and parsley. The carrot pieces are a snack for the cook! Let the chicken rest on a cutting board.

The poaching recipe calls for 8 cups (2 L) of water. After poaching you will have approx. 6 1/2 cups (1.5 L) of pot liquor (broth) for your soup. Using a measuring cup, make a note of how many cups you have as you pour it back into the soup pot. Add water to yield 8 cups (2 L).

When the chicken is cool enough to handle, shred it with your hands. Set aside.

Heat the garlic oil in a nonstick skillet over medium high heat. Add the carrots, bok choy, scallion greens and jalapenos. Sauté for 6 minutes, adding a splash of water if the sauté becomes too dry. Add the red chile powder, oregano, cumin, salt, paprika and pepper. Stir for 1 minute. Spoon the sauté into the pot of stock. Bring to a boil, then reduce heat to low. Cover and simmer for 10 minutes. Add the tomatoes and shredded chicken. Cover and simmer for 10 more minutes. Finish by stirring in the lime and lemon juices. Taste and adjust for salt.

Assembly: Ladle into 6 bowls. Top with 4 crushed tortilla chips each, sliced scallion greens, fresh cilantro leaves, lime wedges and 1-ounce (30 g) avocado per bowl. Serve immediately.

Monash Note: Although chiles (chillies) are generally low in FODMAPs, some people with IBS may be sensitive to the capsaicin they contain. Capsaicin is a natural compound that gives chiles their spicy quality. You may need to limit how much chile you eat if your IBS symptoms are triggered by spicy food.

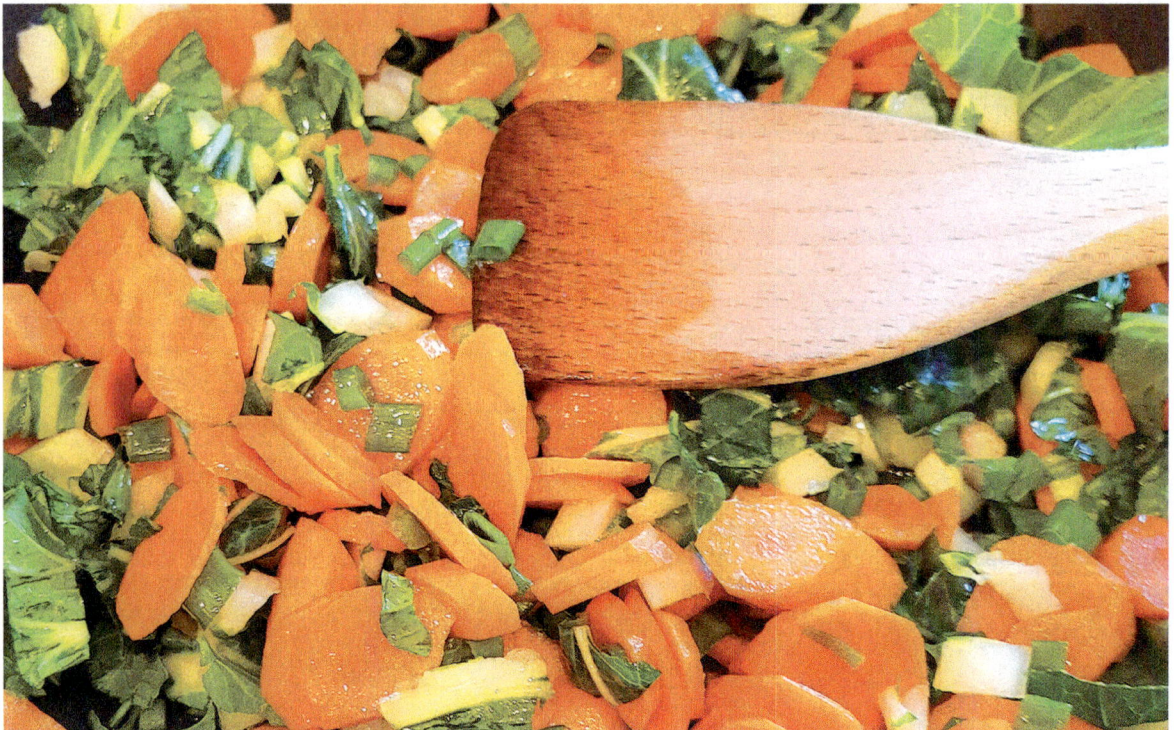

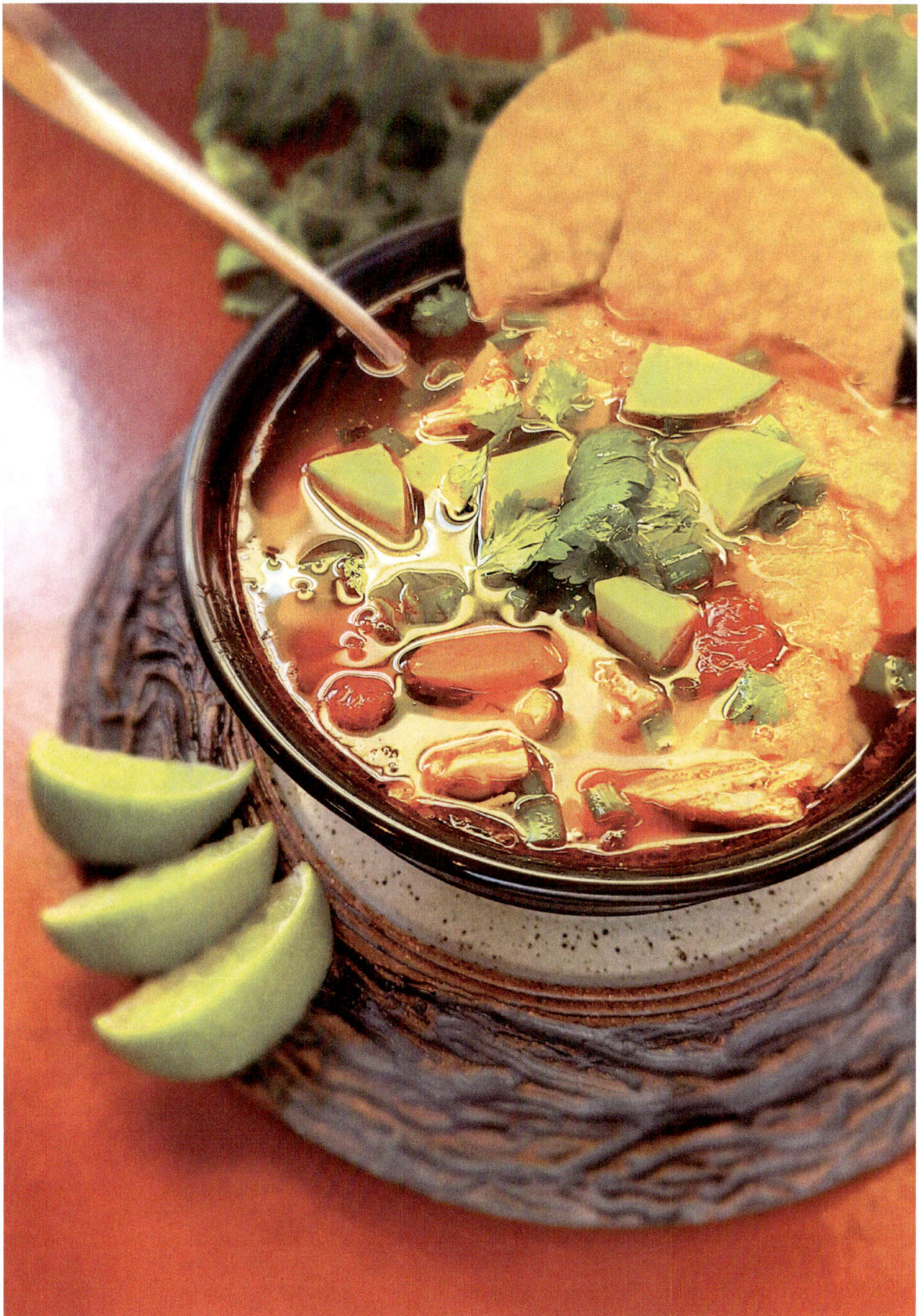

Ma's Gazpacho

LOW FODMAP ❤ IBS FRIENDLY ❤ GLUTEN-FREE ❤ DAIRY-FREE

This is an adapted recipe given to me by my Ma. I have wonderful memories of her making cold "salsa soup" on hot summer days. For special occasions, she would serve it topped with grilled shrimp or crab. This green gazpacho with green chiles, cucumbers and cilantro is puréed with scallion green parts and tangy ingredients for that lovely gazpacho zing! And you won't need to be precise with your knife cuts, as it all goes into the blender.

This recipe requires at least 6 hours to infuse in the refrigerator; the flavors will improve immensely. Plan for making the LoFO Garlic Infused oil (page 50) and prepping the green chiles, as their skins are inedible (page 46).

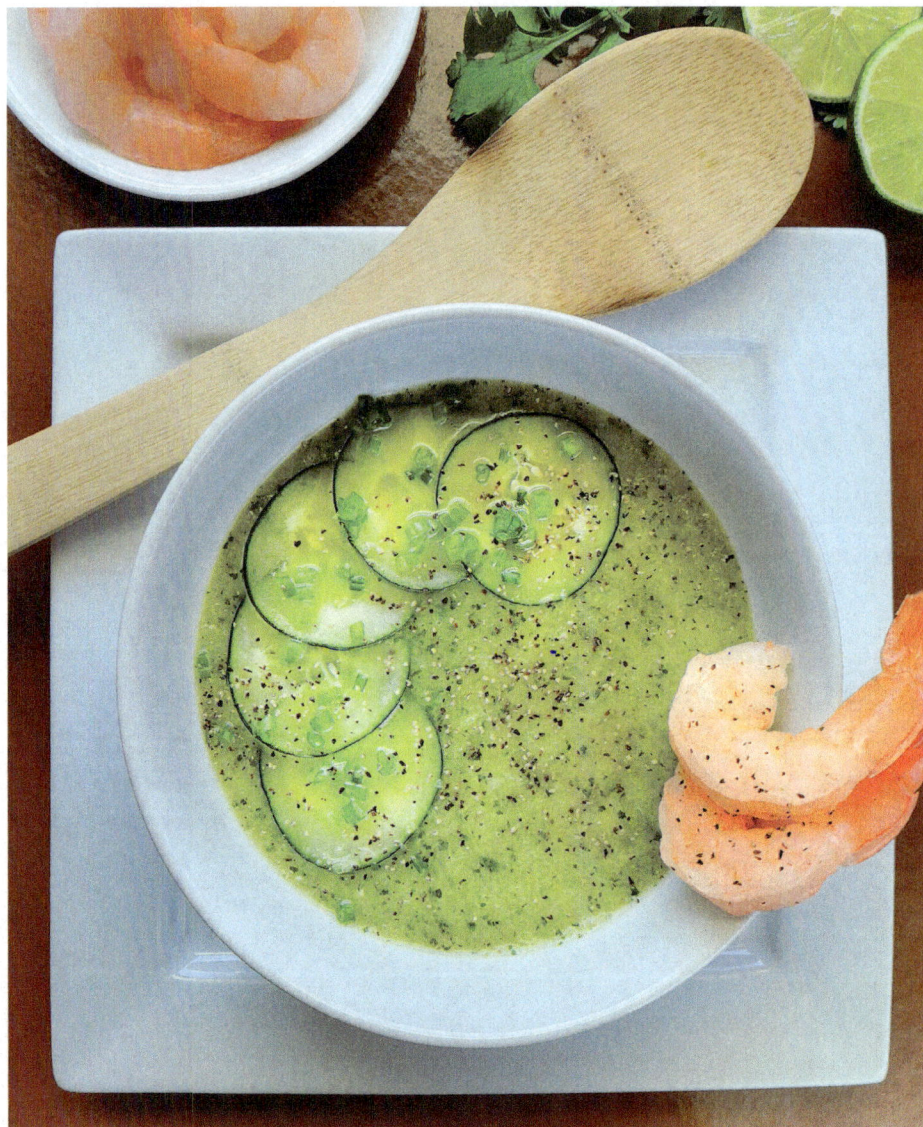

MAKES 6 SERVINGS – 5 CUPS (1.183 L) TOTAL
INGREDIENTS

3 medium (6.5-ounces / 183 g total) mild, fresh green chiles, roasted and prepped as shown on page 46, will yield 3/8 cup (69 g) chile meat (on the Monash App they are noted as: Chile, green, peeled, deseeded)

1/4 cup (59 ml) Low FODMAP Garlic-Infused Oil (page 50), made with canola oil, cooled and ready to use

3 cups (450 g) peeled, diced common cucumbers, plus more for paper-thin sliced rounds for garnish

2 cups (473 ml) cold water

3/4 cup (12 g) fresh medium packed cilantro, mostly leaves, rough chopped, plus more for garnishes

1/2 cup (25 g) thin sliced scallions, green parts only, plus more for garnish

2 tablespoons (45 ml) apple cider vinegar

Juice of 2 limes

1/2 teaspoon (2.5 g) fine sea salt

1/4 teaspoon ground cumin

1/4 teaspoon fresh ground black pepper

1/8 teaspoon sugar

8-ounces (228 g) plain, dairy-free unsweetened coconut yogurt

Lime wedges for garnish

SUGGESTED PROTEINS FOR TOPPING

2 cups (900 g) cooked crab meat, picked over for shells or cartilage

1-pound (454 g) plain cooked deveined medium shrimp, shelled and tails removed

Method: Use the roasting method on page 46 to remove the skins and prep the green chiles. Cut the chile meat into 1/4-inch (.63 cm) pieces and place in a large bowl.

Add the garlic oil, cucumber, water, cilantro, scallion greens, vinegar, lime juice, salt, cumin, pepper and sugar to the bowl. Give it a good stir to mix, then pour the gazpacho into a blender. Purée for 1 minute. Pour back into the bowl, stir with a spoon and taste to adjust for salt or vinegar. Cover with plastic wrap and place in the refrigerator for at least 6 hours to allow the flavors to meld and improve. Depending on the size of your blender, you may need to purée the soup in batches.

Just before serving, whisk in the yogurt to fully incorporate.

Assembly: Ladle into serving bowls. If desired, top with a mound of crab or 3 to 4 shrimp each. Garnish with cucumber rounds, and sprinkle with cilantro and sliced scallion greens. Place a lime wedge by each bowl. Serve cold.

Gazpacho will keep up to 3 days when stored in an airtight container in the fridge. If the gazpacho contains crab or shrimp, it will also keep up to 3 days when stored and refrigerated properly.

Tip: The dairy-free yogurt I prefer has a creamy coconut-base that gives only the slightest hint of coconut flavor. If you are able to tolerate, use a lactose-free or conventional cow's milk plain yogurt.

Monash Note: Although chiles (chillies) are generally low in FODMAPs, some people with IBS may be sensitive to the capsaicin they contain. Capsaicin is a natural compound that gives chiles their spicy quality. You may need to limit how much chile you eat if your IBS symptoms are triggered by spicy food.

All Seasons Carrot Soup
With Jalapeño Essence

LOW FODMAP ❤ IBS FRIENDLY ❤ GLUTEN-FREE ❤ DAIRY-FREE

Aside from the convenience of making this all year long, hot or chilled, the beauty of this recipe is that the jalapeño cooks and simmers with the soup and is removed just before blending, leaving the most delicate peppery essence. This technique is also used when cooking certain rice dishes by infusing with a whole chile pepper and removing it just before serving.

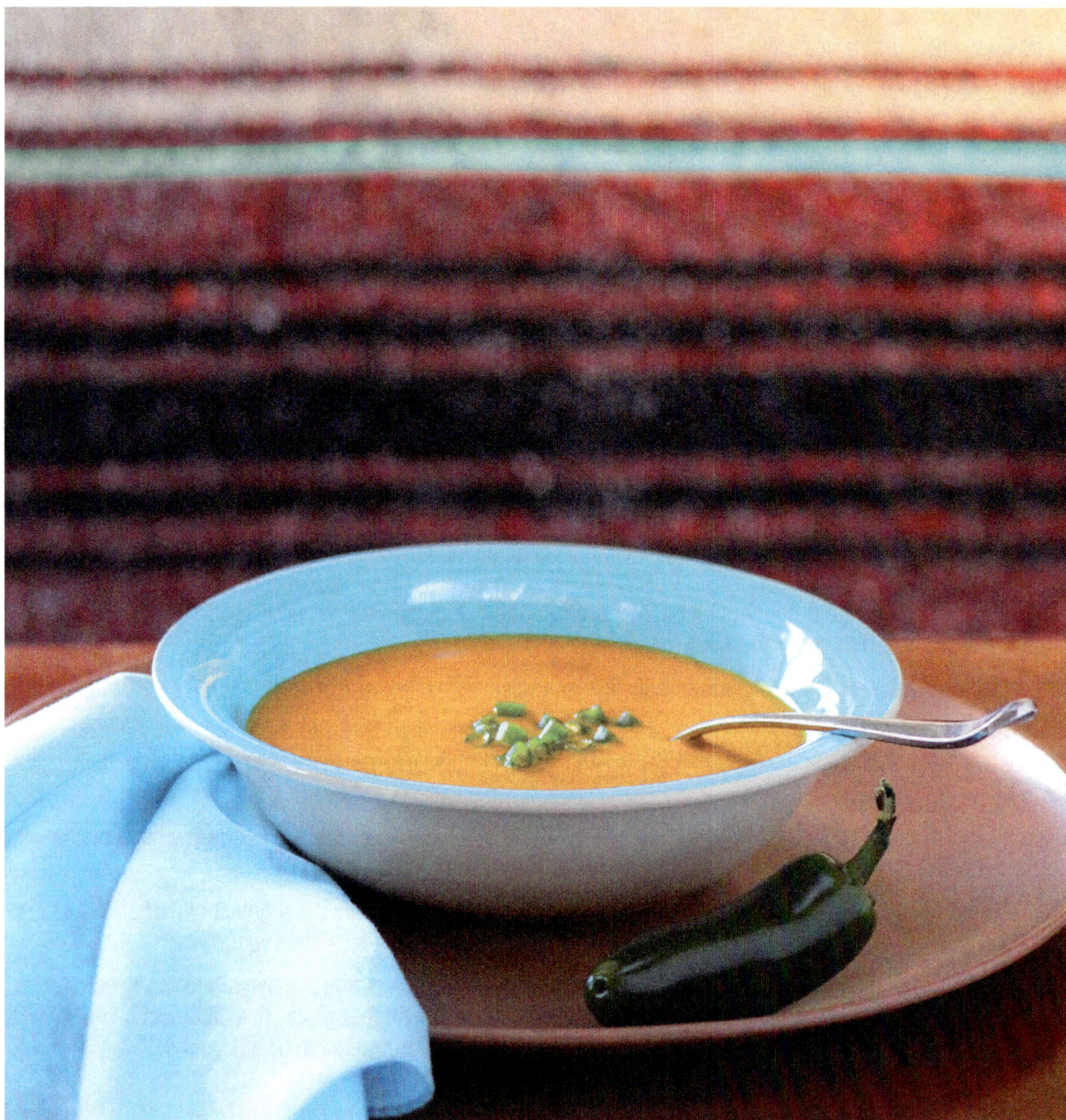

MAKES 4 SERVINGS
INGREDIENTS

2 tablespoon (30 ml) Low FODMAP Garlic-Infused Oil (page 50), made with extra virgin olive oil, divided

1 (41 g) fresh medium jalapeño, cut in half lengthwise, stemmed, seeded, leave membrane intact

2 tablespoons (7 g) thin sliced scallions, green parts only, plus more for garnish

4 1/2 cups (1.07 L) Low FODMAP Chicken Stock (page 135)

1/3 cup (80 ml) canned plain tomato purée

2 tablespoons (30 ml) canned full-fat coconut milk for cooking, containing no inulin, well-stirred

2 teaspoons (60 ml) maple syrup

1 teaspoon (2 g) ground cumin

1/2 teaspoon (2.5 g) fine sea salt

1/4 teaspoon fresh ground black pepper

10 medium (750 g total) carrots, peeled and cut into 1/2-inch (1.25 cm) pieces

Juice of 1/2 lime, or more if desired

Method: Pour 1 tablespoon oil into a large nonstick skillet over medium high heat. Add the jalapeño halves and scallion greens. Stir for 1 minute.

Add the remaining ingredients and bring to a boil for 5 minutes. Stir, cover with a lid and reduce heat to simmer for 20 to 25 minutes. Once the carrots are fork tender, remove the skillet from heat and allow the soup to cool for 5 minutes, uncovered.

Remove the jalapeño. Carefully ladle the soup into a blender. Cover with the lid and a heavy clean kitchen towel to avoid hot splatters. Purée until smooth.

If the soup is too thick add a bit more stock or water and blend. If too thin, place back in the saucepan at medium heat and allow to reduce, stirring often.

Taste to adjust for salt, lime juice or a bit more maple syrup if desired.

Pour the soup into 4 bowls. Top with scallion greens and drizzle each with the remaining garlic oil. Serve immediately.

This soup will keep in the refrigerator up to 3 days when stored in an airtight container.

Tip: For a hot brunch dish, place 1 poached egg in the center and 1 slice crisp crumbled bacon over each.

Monash Note: Although chiles (chillies) are generally low in FODMAPs, some people with IBS may be sensitive to the capsaicin they contain. Capsaicin is a natural compound that gives chiles their spicy quality. You may need to limit how much chile you eat if your IBS symptoms are triggered by spicy food.

A few things to love...

The Grand Canyon and sunset at the South Rim Watchtower

Finding an authentic carniceria with homemade corn tortillas

That first summer day when green chile harvest begins

Listening to Jim play the piano

Saying "hello again beautiful" to the silhouette of Mesa Verde

People who stop to save lost dogs

Red earth and rock art

Santa Fe, New Mexico any time any day

Steam train whistles

The otherworldly beauty of Southern Utah, Moab,
Bisti / De-na-zin Wilderness and Arizona ribboned slot canyons

Big ranches with good-hearted people and lots of dogs

Snowy winters in Taos beside a roaring kiva fireplace

Quiet of the desert where all you hear are the twinkling of stars

The history lessons of driving and walking the Santa Fe Trail

Adobe houses, historic adobe churches, and Earthships

Connecting with people who share their stories

Walking through a green chile or lavender farm

Standing at The Mittens of Monument Valley

Small town art fairs, farmer's markets and street dances

Waking up each morning feeling grateful and knowing
that Jim and the people in my life feel the same

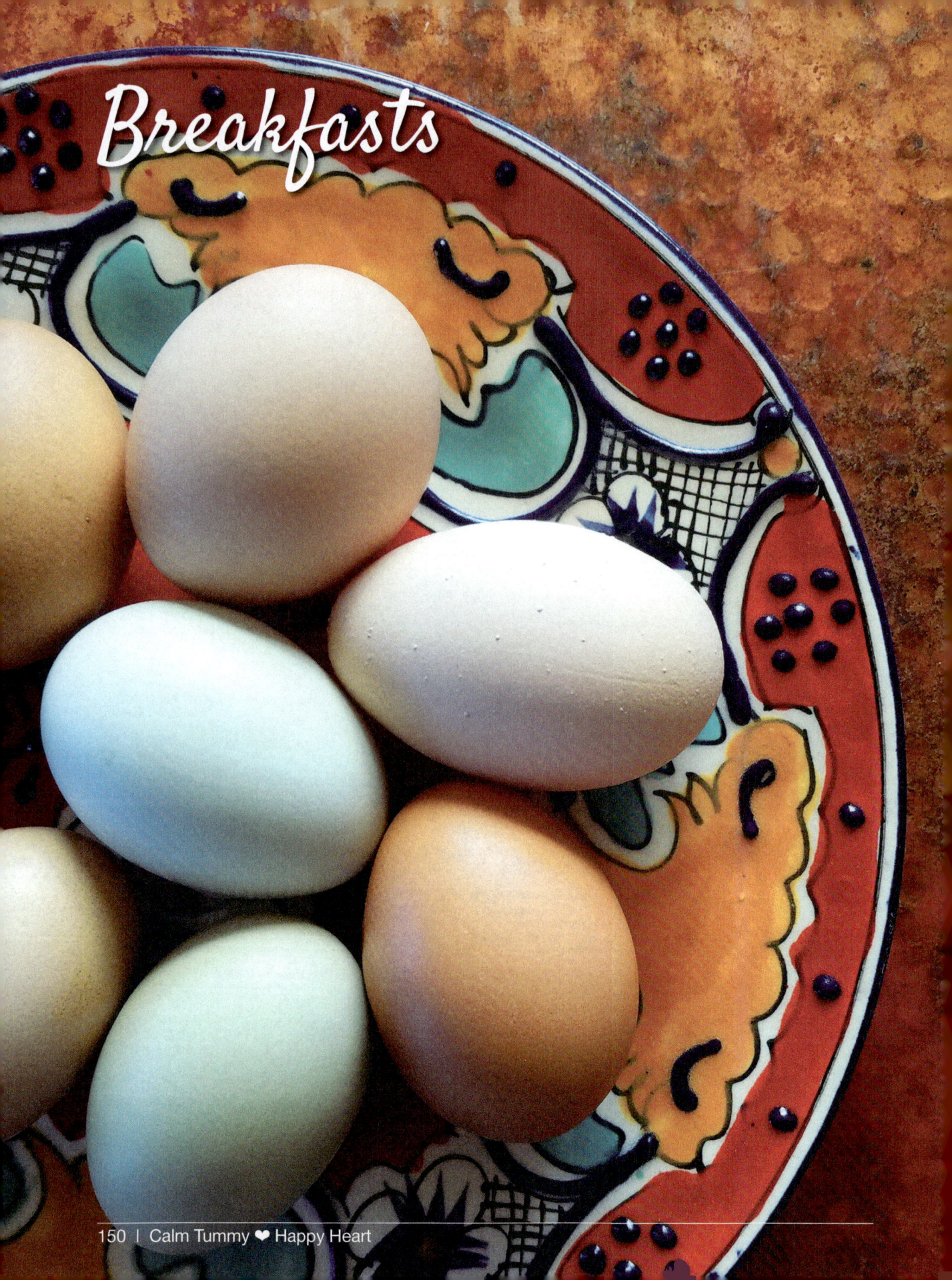

Breakfasts

- **Chilaquiles with Bacon & Fried Eggs**
- **Simple Huevos Rancheros**
- **Green Eggs & Ham Southwest Style**
- **Cornmeal Pancakes with Pulled Pork, Tangy Sauce, & Cinnamon Maple Syrup**
- **Cimarron Steak & Eggs**
- **Eggs From Hell**
- **Chorizo Frittata**

Food brand names are sometimes listed within a recipe, and this means they are Monash Certified. For more brand options we use and love, please visit **FodifyIt.com**

Monash Note: Although chiles (chillies) are generally low in FODMAPs, some people with IBS may be sensitive to the capsaicin they contain. Capsaicin is a natural compound that gives chiles their spicy quality. You may need to limit how much chile you eat if your IBS symptoms are triggered by spicy food.

Chilaquiles With Bacon & Fried Eggs

LOW FODMAP ❤ IBS FRIENDLY ❤ GLUTEN-FREE ❤ DAIRY-FREE

Every cook in the Southwest has their own version of Chilaquiles – corn tortilla chips coated in a warm red spicy sauce with toppings and a fried egg. This dish, with layers of flavor and textures, makes it the perfect breakfast greeting for guests visiting the Southwest for the first time.

The New Mexican dried red chile pods normally used to re-hydrate and blend into the traditional sauce have not yet been tested for FODMAPs, however some dried chiles have been found to contain high FODMAPs and so I suspect that red chile pods may also contain high amounts of fructose. Not to worry! This version with a quick salsa reduced with chicken stock, then mixed into the chips is fresh and delectable. Topped with crisp bacon strips, cilantro, scallion green parts, radishes, avocado, and fried eggs – this is a delicious, memorable platter.

If you have time to make the salsa and LoFO chicken stock (page 135) for the sauce one day in advance it will free your time from chopping and prepping in the morning. However, the cooking and coating of the chips must be done just before serving or they will be too soggy.

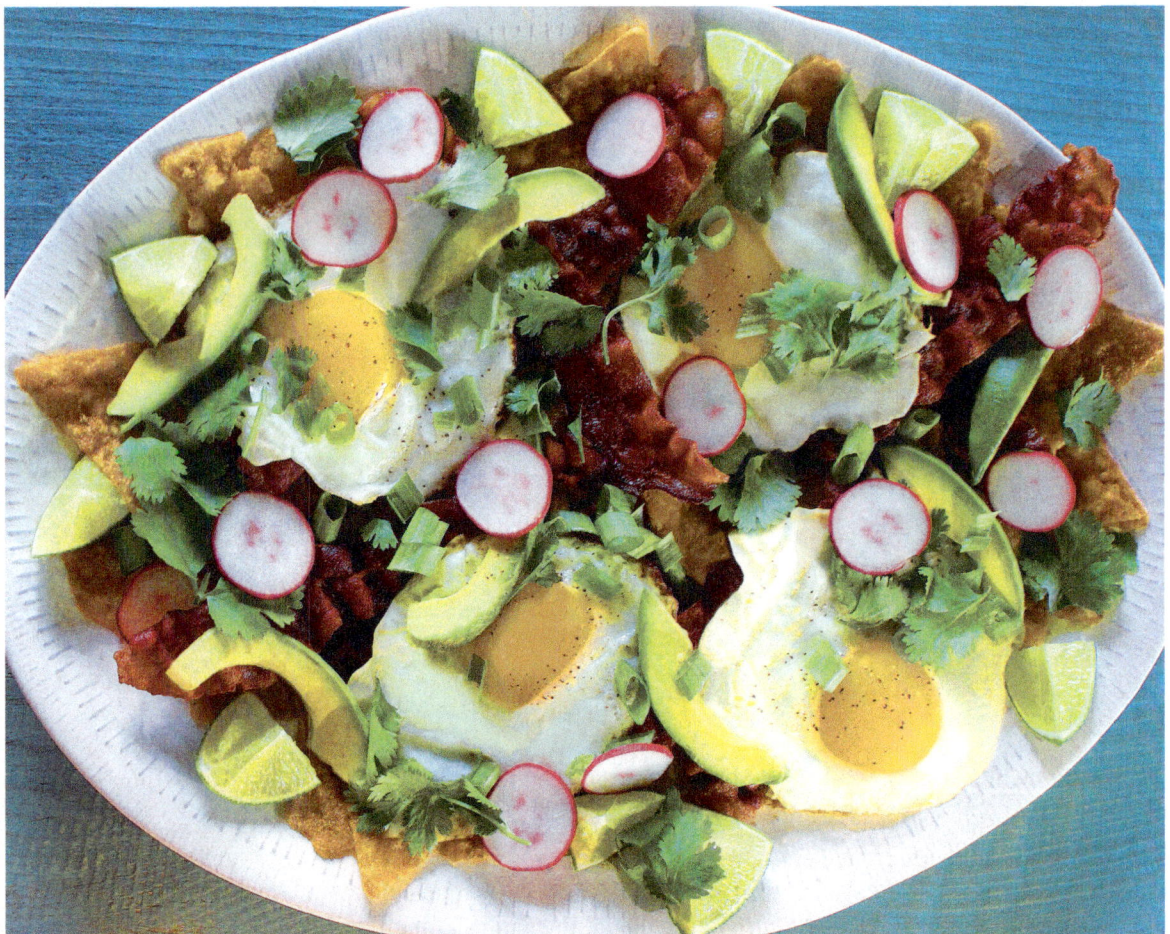

MAKES 4 SERVINGS

SALSA SAUCE INGREDIENTS

10.5-ounces (300 g) plain, canned whole Roma tomatoes, drained and rough chopped

3/4 cup (180 ml) Low FODMAP Chicken Stock (page 135)

1 tablespoon (15 ml) Low FODMAP Garlic-Infused Oil (page 50), made with extra virgin olive oil

2 fresh Serrano chiles (28 g each) stemmed, seeded and rough chopped (or leave the seeds and inner ribs for more heat)

2 tablespoons (2 g) fresh medium packed cilantro, mostly leaves, rough chopped

1/2 teaspoon (1 g) ground cumin

1/2 teaspoon (2.5 g) fine sea salt (if the chips you are using are very salty, add only 1/4 teaspoon or no salt at all)

2 tablespoons (7 g) thin sliced scallions, green parts only

Juice of 1/2 lime

BACON & EGGS INGREDIENTS

12 slices bacon

4 large eggs

CHIPS & TOPPING INGREDIENTS

4 1/4-ounces (120 g) unsalted or low salt store-bought corn tortilla chips

4-ounces (120 g) cubed avocado, divided into 4 portions

1 lime cut into 8 wedges

4 (40 g total) red radishes, thin sliced

1/4 cup (4 g) medium packed cilantro leaves

2 tablespoons (7 g) thin sliced scallions, green parts only

Method

Salsa Sauce: Place the metal blade in a food processor. Add the sauce ingredients. Pulse/blend to a consistency that still has some texture. You want some bits of chile and cilantro to come through rather than a completely smooth sauce. The juice from the tomatoes will make for a soupy consistency that you will reduce.

Pour the sauce into a large nonstick skillet. Bring to a low boil over medium heat. Cook for 5 minutes, stirring occasionally to reduce to the consistency of tomato sauce. If it should reduce to a very thick consistency it won't properly coat the chips, so add more LoFO chicken stock or water to thin it a bit. Set the pan aside, covered to keep the sauce warm.

Bacon: Cook the bacon to crispy in a large nonstick skillet over medium high heat. Turn them once or twice for even cooking. Place on paper towels to drain. Drain the bacon fat reserving 2 tablespoons (30 ml) in the pan to cook your eggs.

Eggs: Heat the pan drippings over medium heat. Break the eggs into the skillet and place a lid or piece of foil over the pan. Check after 3 minutes. Cook to desired doneness with opaque whites. Remove from heat and cover to keep warm.

At this point you will want to call everyone to breakfast, as the assembly and quick delivery to the table is a must. Ring that dinner triangle because chilaquiles wait for no one!

(continued on next page)

(continued from previous page)

Chips & Assembly: If the sauce has cooled to lukewarm, place the pan over medium high heat until the sauce is just bubbly and hot. Add the chips and gently stir and fold with a spatula to coat. Remove from the heat and spoon onto a large serving platter.

Place the bacon strips criss-crossed over the chips. Use a spatula to nestle the eggs between the bacon. Top with the avocado, lime wedges, radishes, and a sprinkling of cilantro and scallion greens.

Serve immediately.

Tips: Suggested Proteins To Add:

Plain Shredded Chicken: See recipe on page 82 for Whole Poached Chicken for Shredding & Stock.

Shrimp: Shelled, deveined, tails removed, lightly sautéed in extra virgin olive oil with a light dusting of salt and fresh ground black pepper

If you are able to tolerate, cheese is traditionally served over chilaquiles: Shredded Monterey Jack: 1 scant 1/2 cup (40 g) per serving. Or feta (similar to Cotija) 3 tablespoons (21 g) per serving. At the writing of this cookbook, Cotija cheese has not yet been tested. You may find that it is not a trigger for you, and be sure to check the Monash App and social media for updates on newly tested foods.

If you prefer, make plain scrambled eggs in place of fried.

Monash Note: Although chiles (chillies) are generally low in FODMAPs, some people with IBS may be sensitive to the capsaicin they contain. Capsaicin is a natural compound that gives chiles their spicy quality. You may need to limit how much chile you eat if your IBS symptoms are triggered by spicy food.

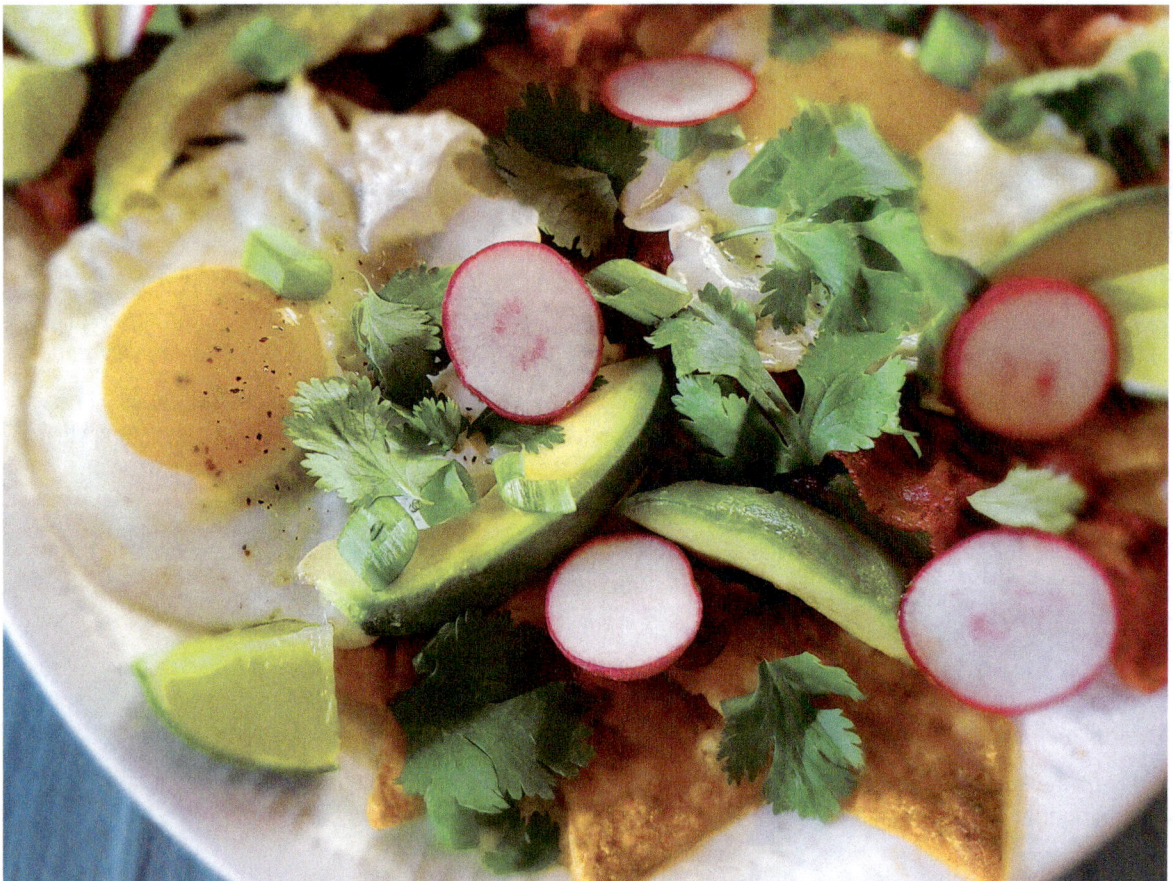

Simple Huevos Rancheros

LOW FODMAP ❤ IBS FRIENDLY ❤ GLUTEN-FREE ❤ DAIRY-FREE

One of those perfect dishes, like a taco plate or green chile burger that delivers just the right combination of ingredients. Warm corn tortillas with eggs, Pico de Gallo, Green Chile Sauce and Refried Beans – I would be stunned to find a SW cafe where it was not offered!

This recipe requires a double batch of Green Chile Sauce (page 60) and 2 servings of No Beans Refried "Beans" (page 114), ready to use.

(continued on next page)

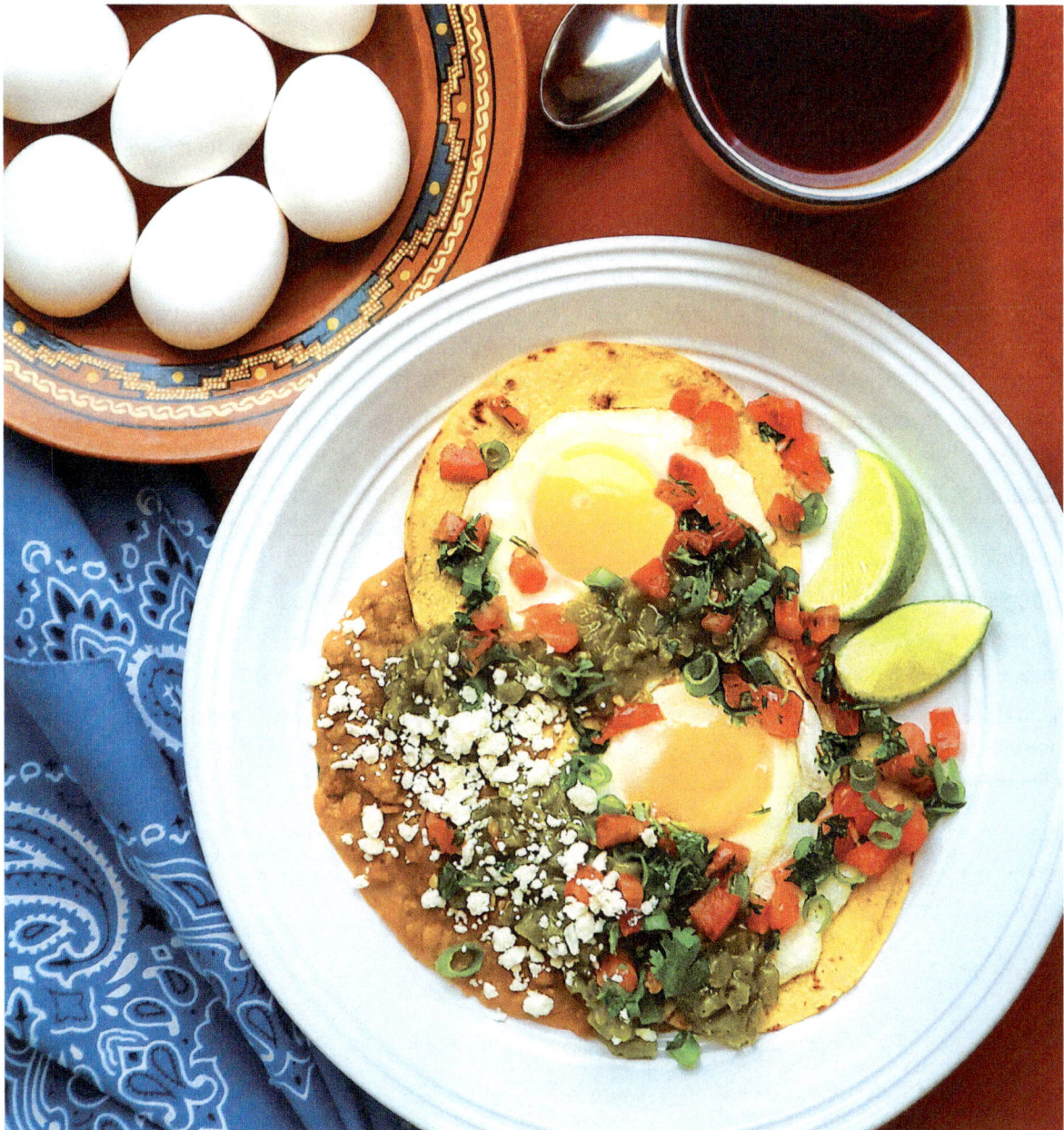

(continued from previous page)

MAKES 2 SERVINGS

PICO DE GALLO INGREDIENTS

1/2 small (60 g) common tomato, cored and diced

4 scallions, green parts only, sliced thin

1/4 cup (4 g) fresh medium packed cilantro, mostly leaves, rough chopped, plus a few whole leaves for garnish

Juice of 1/4 - 1/2 lime, per your tangy preference

TORTILLAS & EGGS INGREDIENTS

4, 6-inch (15 cm) low FODMAP gluten-free yellow corn tortillas, or 4 homemade tortillas (page 104)

4 large eggs

1 tablespoon (15 ml) canola oil

1 double batch Green Chile sauce (page 60), warm

2 servings No Beans Refried "Beans" (page 114), warm (extra "beans" may be used for tomorrow's taco platter or for dipping with tortilla chips)

Method

Pico de Gallo: Stir the ingredients in a small bowl and chill in the refrigerator.

Tortillas: Lightly coat a large nonstick skillet with spray cooking oil over medium high heat. Place the tortillas in the pan and warm them for 30 seconds to 1 minute. Flip and warm the other side 30 seconds until just toasted. Wrap them in a heavy clean kitchen towel, foil, or stack in a tortilla warmer.

Eggs: Add 1 tablespoon (15 ml) oil to the skillet over medium heat. Add the 4 eggs and cook sunny side up to your liking. I oftentimes cover the pan with a lid or sheet of foil so they cook evenly and quicker.

Assembly: Place 2 tortillas per plate. Top with 2 eggs each. Spoon on the Green Chile Sauce, then the Pico de Gallo. Spoon No Beans Refried "Beans" to the side of the tortillas. Garnish with cilantro leaves and lime wedges if desired. Serve immediately.

Tips: Homemade tortillas will take a bit longer to pan toast, but are definitely worth it.

If you are able to tolerate, top the "beans" with 2 teaspoons crumbled feta or queso fresco per serving. Cotija cheese has not yet been tested by Monash so let's keep a lookout for new testing results.

Monash Note: Although chiles (chillies) are generally low in FODMAPs, some people with IBS may be sensitive to the capsaicin they contain. Capsaicin is a natural compound that gives chiles their spicy quality. You may need to limit how much chile you eat if your IBS symptoms are triggered by spicy food.

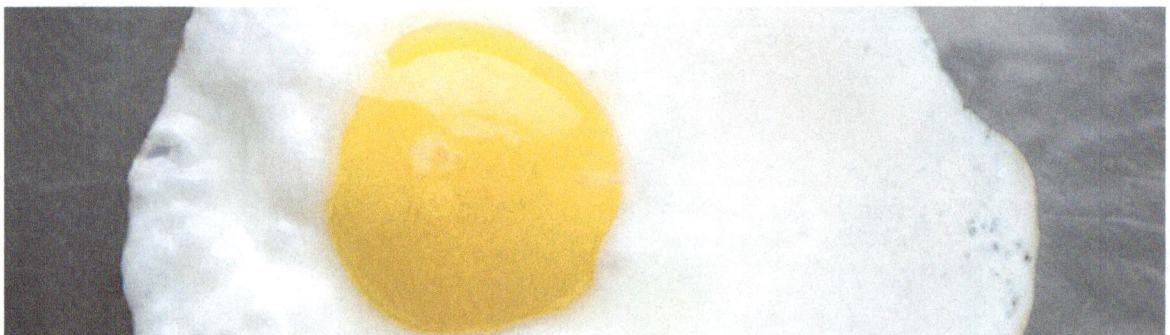

Green Eggs & Ham Southwest Style

LOW FODMAP ❤ IBS FRIENDLY ❤ GLUTEN-FREE ❤ DAIRY-FREE

A Southwest twist on the classic children's story dish, this luscious version starts with a creamy low FODMAP Hollandaise Sauce, with fresh spinach and sides to enhance the green. Think of it as an Eggs Benedict sandwich.

This recipe requires Green Chile Hollandaise Sauce (page 68). No changes or additions required, but you will need to keep it warm and ready to use, so plan accordingly.

MAKES 4 SERVINGS
INGREDIENTS

2 teaspoons (10 ml) extra virgin olive oil

4, 1/4-inch (.63 cm) thick slices low FODMAP baked ham, containing no honey, garlic, onion or other high FODMAP ingredients

1/2 cup (25 g) fresh baby spinach

2 low FODMAP gluten-free sandwich rolls; Schar gluten-free ciabatta rolls (50 g each) are Monash certified

2 teaspoons (10 ml) white or cider vinegar

4 large eggs

4 slices (60 g total) common tomato, cut crosswise into 1/4-inch (.63 cm) thick circles

GARNISHES

Green Chile Hollandaise Sauce, warm

4 leafy sprigs fresh cilantro

2 scallions, green parts only, sliced thin

4 slices (approx.150 g total) peeled kiwi

4 small bunches green grapes (3 grapes per bunch)

Method: Pour the oil into a medium nonstick skillet over medium high heat. Sear the ham on both sides and let drain on paper towels. Place the spinach leaves in the hot pan and let wilt for 1 minute. Drain on paper towels with the ham.

Cut the rolls in half and toast until just golden browned and crisp. Place them open-faced on two plates.

Coat the bottom of the skillet with cooking spray oil. Bring 2 inches (5 cm) water to a low boil. Add 2 teaspoons (10 ml) vinegar. Crack the eggs into the water. Reduce heat to low and let poach for 3 to 5 minutes, or until the whites are completely opaque and yolks are done to your liking. Leave them in the water, off heat.

Assembly: Place the tomato slices on the open-faced buns followed by the ham and spinach. Use a slotted spoon to carefully lift the eggs, one at a time, out of the water. Rest them for 15 seconds on a paper towel to absorb excess water, then place over the ham. Spoon on the Green Chile Hollandaise. Garnish the tops with cilantro and scallion greens. Place sides of kiwi and green grapes next to the buns. Serve immediately with forks and sharp steak knives.

Monash Note: Although chiles (chillies) are generally low in FODMAPs, some people with IBS may be sensitive to the capsaicin they contain. Capsaicin is a natural compound that gives chiles their spicy quality. You may need to limit how much chile you eat if your IBS symptoms are triggered by spicy food.

Cornmeal Pancakes with Pulled Pork, Tangy Sauce & Cinnamon Maple Syrup

LOW FODMAP ❤ IBS FRIENDLY ❤ GLUTEN-FREE ❤ DAIRY-FREE

Fluffy pancakes with sweet cinnamon syrup, strawberries – and a tangy sauce? Yep, and it's delicious! It has a fabulous sweet and savory flavor, and the juicy pulled pork sends it right over the top.

Please note that this recipe calls for Slow Oven-Roasted Pulled Pork (page 80) that requires 8+ hours to slow cook, so be sure to plan accordingly.

MAKES 4 SERVINGS – 2 PANCAKES EACH
PANCAKE INGREDIENTS

3/4 cup (180 ml) plain, unsweetened almond milk, plus extra as needed

1/3 cup (80 ml) canned full-fat coconut milk for cooking, containing no inulin, well-stirred

1 large egg

1/2 teaspoon (.25 cm) vanilla extract (essence)

2/3 cup (140 g) low FODMAP medium grind whole grain yellow cornmeal

1/3 cup (46 g) low FODMAP gluten-free all-purpose baking flour, containing xanthan gum (page 55)

2 teaspoons (8 g) sugar

1/2 teaspoon (2 g) baking powder; use gluten-free if following a gluten-free diet

1/4 teaspoon (1 g) baking soda

1/4 teaspoon (1.25 g) fine sea salt

2 teaspoons (10 ml) canola oil for greasing the pan, more if needed

TANGY SAUCE & PORK INGREDIENTS

1/4 cup (60 ml) low FODMAP prepared ketchup, containing no onion, garlic or other high FODMAP ingredients, see page 71 for homemade tomato ketchup

1/4 cup (60 ml) pan drippings from the Pulled Pork, or water

3 tablespoons (45 ml) apple cider vinegar

2 teaspoons (7 g) medium packed light brown sugar

1 teaspoon (5 g) plain, prepared yellow mustard, containing no onion or garlic

1 teaspoon (5 ml) Worcestershire sauce

1 teaspoon (2 g) pure chipotle powder

12-ounces (340 g) Slow Oven-Roasted Pulled Pork (page 80), ready to use and hot

(continued on next page)

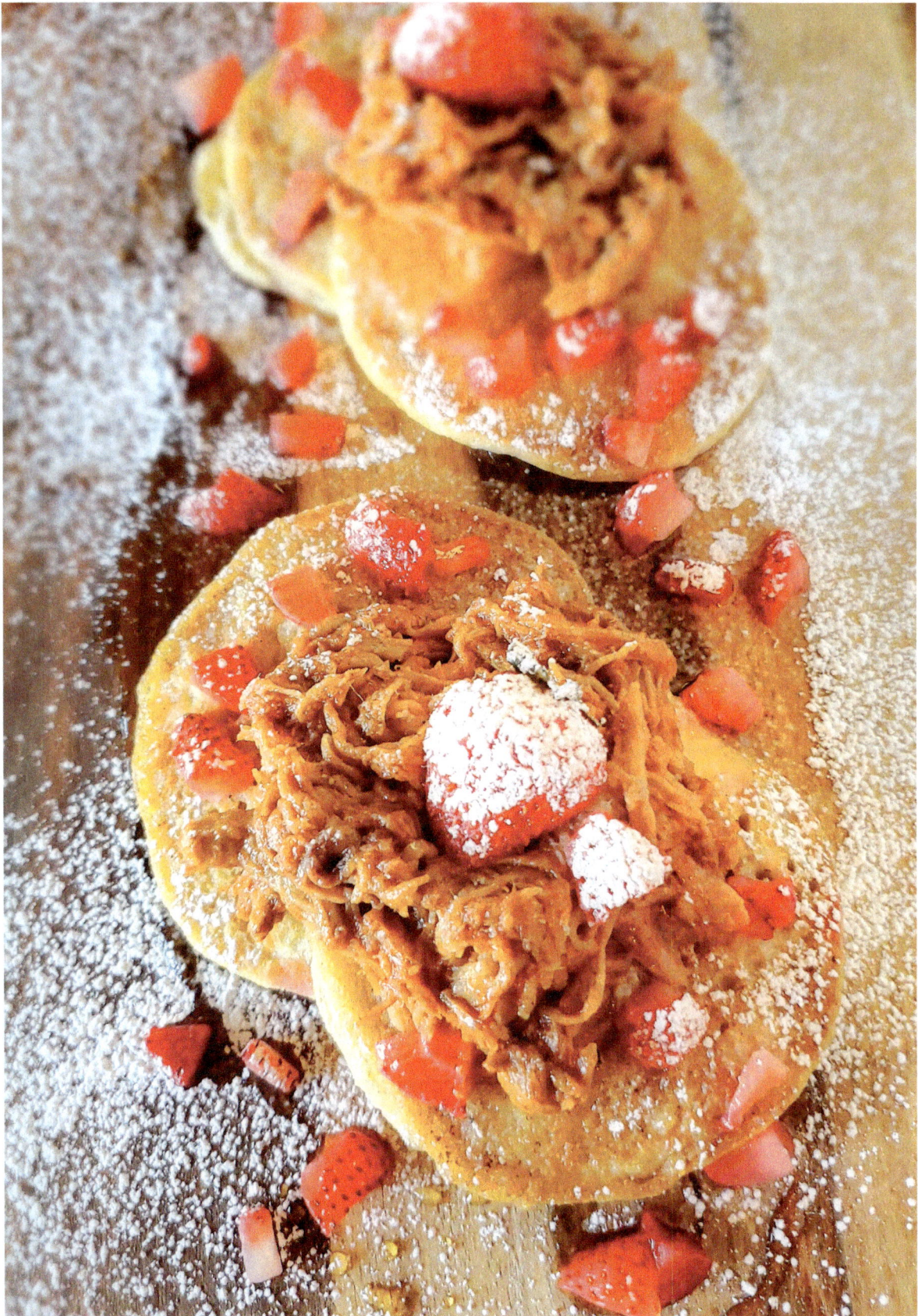

(continued from previous page)

CINNAMON SYRUP & TOPPING INGREDIENTS

Scant 1/2 cup (120 ml) maple syrup

1/2 teaspoon (2 g) ground cinnamon

8 (105 g) fresh ripe strawberries, hulled and sliced or large diced

3 teaspoons (7 g) confectioners' sugar (sieved for dusting as the final touch)

Method

Pancakes: Whisk together the 3/4 cup (180 ml) plain unsweetened almond milk, coconut milk, egg and vanilla in a small mixing bowl.

In a separate medium bowl, whisk together the cornmeal, flour, sugar, baking powder, baking soda and salt. Add the milk mixture and whisk to combine. It's okay if there are a few small lumps of cornmeal. Cover the bowl with a clean kitchen towel and let rest for 20 minutes.

Check the batter consistency. It will be slightly thicker than a regular pancake batter, but not so thick as to not be able to scoop with a measuring cup and pour into the pan. If too thick, add 1 tablespoon (15 ml) more almond milk at a time until scoop-able and shapeable.

Use a paper towel to evenly coat a large nonstick skillet surface with 1 teaspoon oil (5 ml) over medium low heat. Using a 1/4 measuring cup (60 ml), scoop 3 pancakes into the pan and use a spatula to gather the edges and shape them into 4-inch (10 cm) cakes.

Let them cook without disturbing until the edges begin to set and the surface of the pancakes begin to bubble, about 2 minutes. Using a spatula, lift up an edge of one cake and see if it holds well to flip. Flip the 3 cakes and cook 2 minutes more or until golden brown on the undersides. Move to a plate and cover with foil, or keep in a tortilla warmer. Repeat for the remaining pancakes.

Tangy Sauce: Mix the sauce ingredients in a medium saucepan. Bring to a low boil and add the pulled pork. Stir gently to coat and heat the pork. Turn off the heat, cover with a lid and set aside.

Syrup: Mix the maple syrup and cinnamon in a small saucepan over medium heat, stirring until the cinnamon melts into the syrup, about 2 minutes. Turn off the heat and allow to cool so it will thicken a bit, about 4 minutes. As it cools, this is a good time to slice or chop the strawberries.

Assembly: Place two pancakes on each plate. Spoon on the pulled pork. Drizzle with syrup, top with strawberries and use a fine mesh metal strainer to dust with confectioners' sugar. Serve immediately.

Tip: When roasting pulled pork, I buy a large 8 to 10-pound (3.6 kg – 4.5 kg) pork shoulder (Boston Butt) to roast and pull. Any leftovers are portioned in airtight containers or freezer baggies to thaw later as needed. Pulled pork will keep up to 3 days in the fridge and will last 2 to 3 months in the freezer.

Monash note: Although chiles (chillies) are generally low in FODMAPs, some people with IBS may be sensitive to the capsaicin they contain. Capsaicin is a natural compound that gives chiles their spicy quality. You may need to limit how much chile you eat if your IBS symptoms are triggered by spicy food.

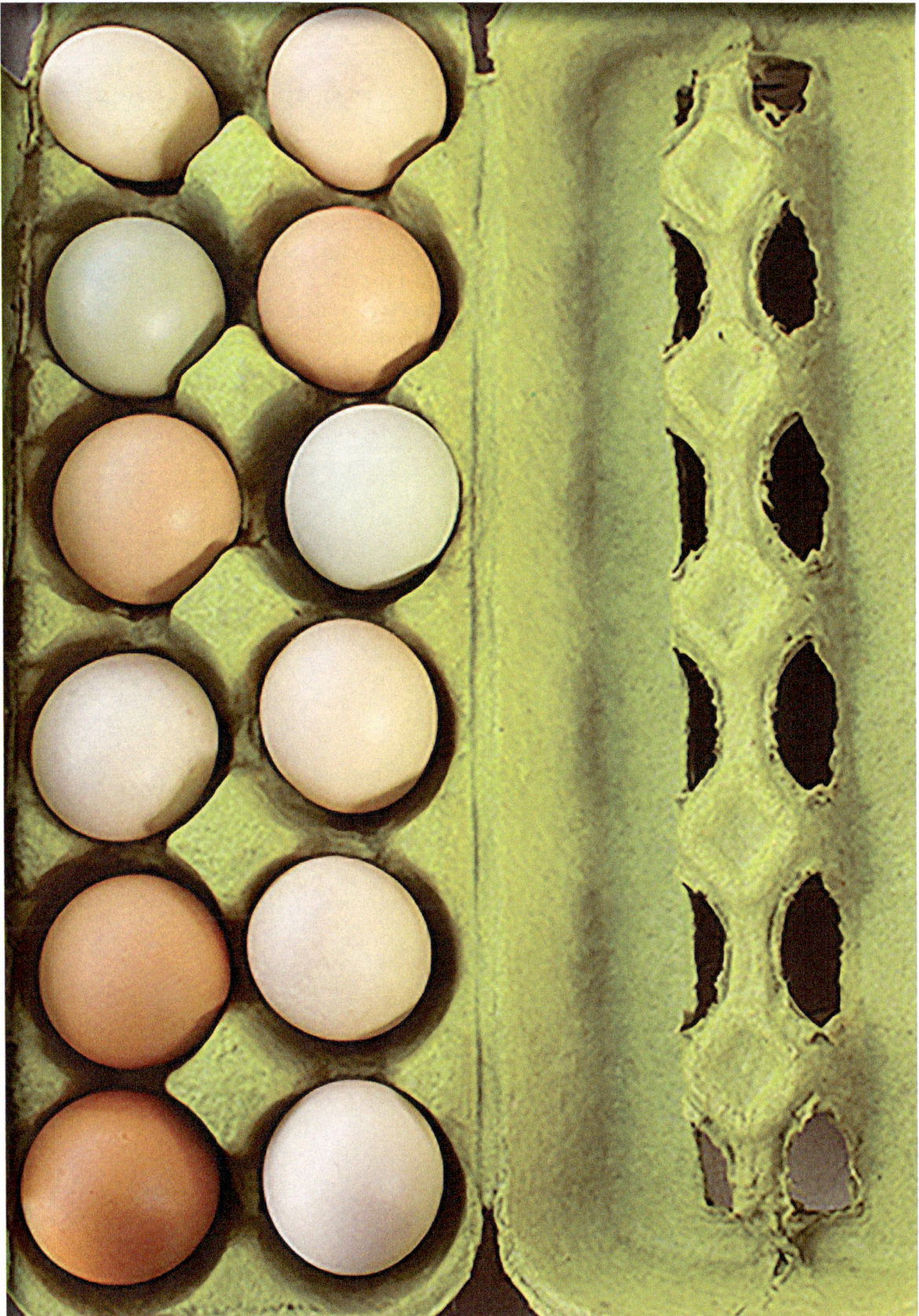

Cimarron Steak & Eggs

LOW FODMAP ❤ IBS FRIENDLY ❤ GLUTEN-FREE ❤ DAIRY-FREE

Steak and Eggs for breakfast is a campfire favorite that is also easy to prepare in your kitchen. A flank steak coated in seasoning rub, grilled or pan cooked is full of flavor, and when thin-sliced against the grain becomes very tender. This recipe also works well with 4 petit filet mignon or 4 small ribeyes (4 to 6-ounces/114 - 170 g) each.

Onion powder has been swapped out and replaced with minced chives, and LoFO Garlic Infused Oil subs for garlic cloves. Pure red chile powder and cumin add earthy warmth, and the campfire wraps it all in smoky goodness.

Please note, the steak requires a 30 minute dry rub infusion.

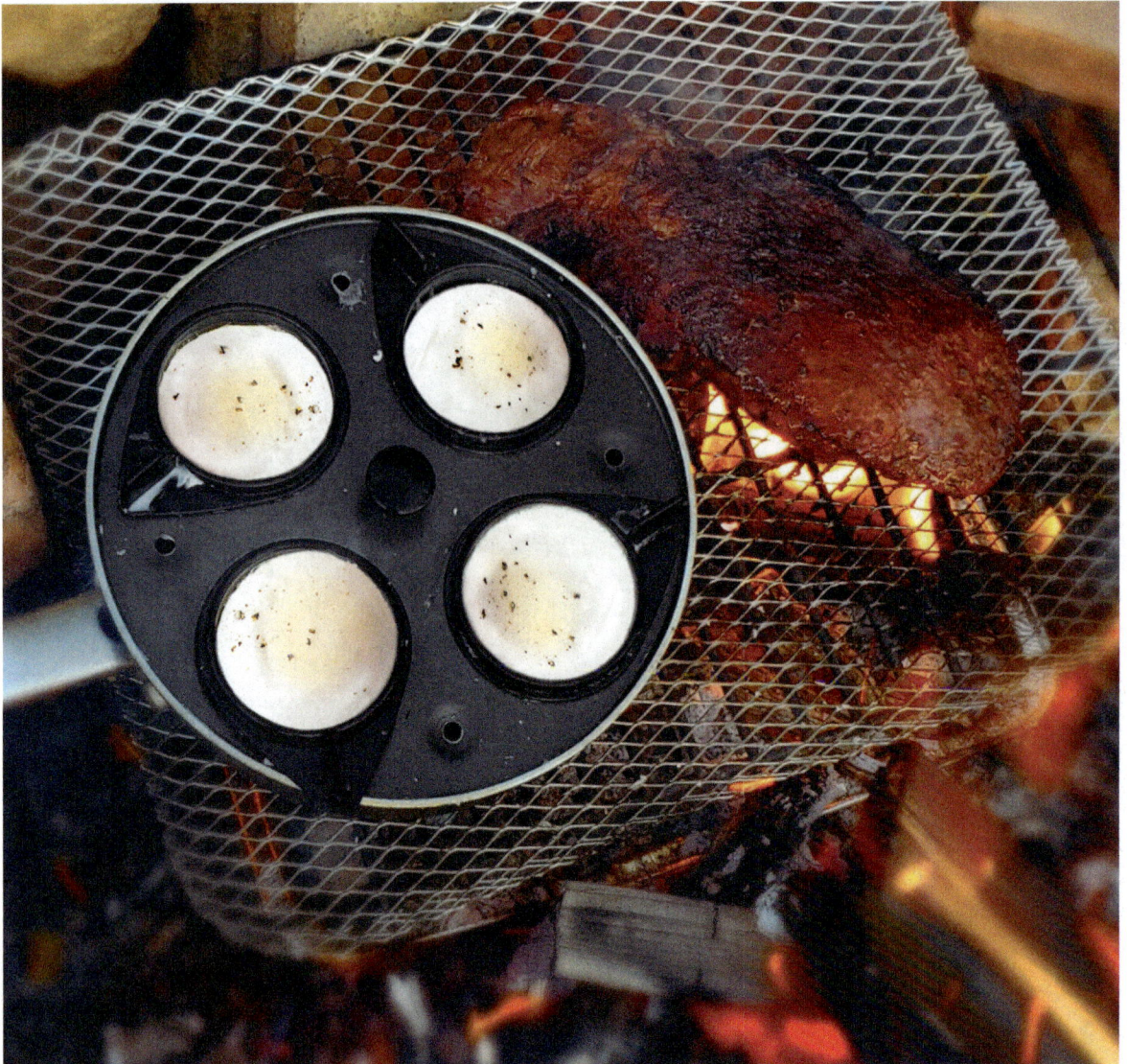

MAKES 4 SERVINGS
DRY RUB INGREDIENTS

2 teaspoons (4 g) pure mild red chile powder (containing no onion or garlic, the ingredients should list only: red chile. On the Monash App this is called Chilli (chili) red, powdered). Use smoked paprika if pure red chile powder is not available.

1 teaspoon (2 g) ground cumin

2 teaspoons (2 g) minced chives

1 teaspoon (5 g) fine sea salt

1/2 teaspoon fresh ground black pepper

STEAK & EGGS INGREDIENTS

1-pound (454 g) flank steak

3 tablespoons (45 ml) Low FODMAP Garlic-Infused Oil (page 50), made with extra virgin olive oil, cooled before coating the steak

8 large eggs (poached, sunny side up or scrambled, your preference)

Method

Rub: Whisk the dry rub ingredients in a small bowl.

Steak: Place the flank steak in a large plastic baggie or shallow baking dish. Use your hands to coat with oil on both sides. Sprinkle the seasoning rub all over and massage gently into the meat. Seal the baggie or plastic wrap the dish and infuse for 30 minutes.

Bring your bbq grill, stovetop grill or lightly oiled skillet to medium high heat. Sear the steak for 1 minute, flip and sear the other side for 1 minute. Reduce heat to medium. If cooking over a campfire, move the steak off direct heat / flames. Cook for 4 minutes, flip and cook 4 more minutes. Use a meat thermometer to check for desired doneness. Transfer to a plate, tent with foil and let rest for 10 minutes or until your eggs are ready.

Eggs: Cook the eggs to your liking and plate them. (I use a 4-cup egg poacher pan with lid, filled with water just below the bottom of the egg cups).

Slice the steak against the grain into thin 1/4-inch (.63 cm) strips. Plate with the eggs and serve immediately.

Tip: For a fresh touch, spoon one serving of Pico de Gallo (page 64) over the sliced steak.

Monash Note: Although chiles (chillies) are generally low in FODMAPs, some people with IBS may be sensitive to the capsaicin they contain. Capsaicin is a natural compound that gives chiles their spicy quality. You may need to limit how much chile you eat if your IBS symptoms are triggered by spicy food.

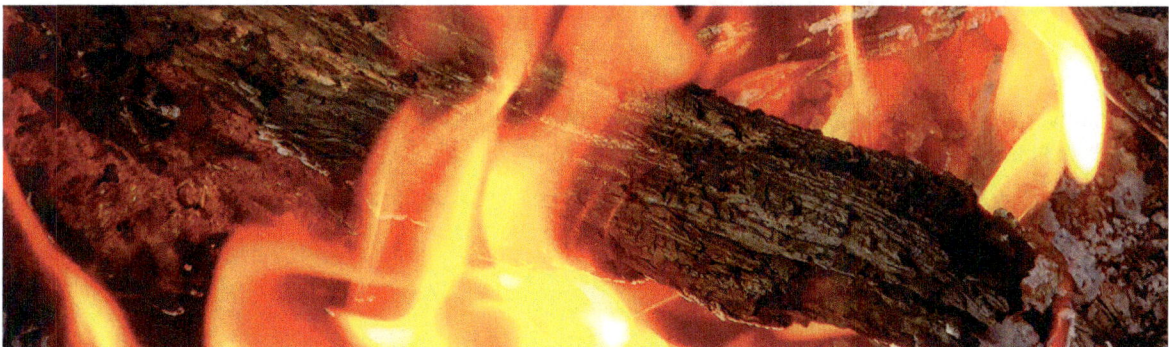

Eggs From Hell

LOW FODMAP ❤ IBS FRIENDLY ❤ GLUTEN-FREE ❤ DAIRY-FREE

This is a simple recipe, not at all hellish to prepare. The name comes from the Serrano and cayenne heat that is oh so sinfully warming on a chilly morning.

MAKES 2 SERVINGS

INGREDIENTS

1 tablespoon (15 ml) Low FODMAP Garlic-Infused Oil (page 50), made with extra virgin olive or canola oil

4 scallions, green parts only, sliced thin

1 Serrano chile pepper (28 g), stem removed, fine diced (plus another half (14 g) Serrano depending on your heat preference)

5.3-ounces (150 g) plain, canned peeled Roma tomatoes, drained and chopped into small pieces

1 tablespoon (15 g) tomato paste, containing no high fructose corn syrup or other high FODMAP ingredients

2 teaspoons (10 ml) red wine vinegar

1 teaspoon (2 g) smoked paprika

1/4 teaspoon (.5 g) cayenne, or 1/2 – 1 teaspoon (1 - 2 g) to really kick things up!

1/2 cup (90 g) cooked brown rice, white or basmati rice

1/2 cup (120 ml) Low FODMAP Chicken Stock (page 135)

Pinch of fine sea salt, to your taste

4 large eggs

1/2 lime cut into 4 wedges

2 tablespoons (2 g) fresh medium packed cilantro, mostly leaves, rough chopped

Method: Pour the oil into a small nonstick skillet over medium high heat. Add the scallion greens and Serrano. Sauté 2 to 3 minutes. Add the tomatoes, tomato paste, vinegar, smoked paprika, cayenne, rice and stock. Gently stir to incorporate and cook for 4 minutes or until bubbly and hot. Use a spoon to scoop a small bit from the pan, let it cool and taste to adjust for additional cayenne and salt.

Allow to bubble and cook, stirring often until just thick enough to make your egg wells. This should take about 3 minutes, depending on how juicy the tomatoes are.

Use a spoon to create 4 evenly spaced wells in the spicy mixture. Crack an egg into each well. Cover the pan with a lid and reduce heat to simmer. Cook for 5 minutes undisturbed. Check that the whites are cooked to fully opaque, and the yolks are as you like them. If not quite done, cover with the lid and check them every 45 seconds until they're just right.

Assembly: Scoop into 2 bowls. Garnish with 2 lime wedges each and sprinkle the tops with cilantro. Or, share the pan. Serve with LoFO gluten-free toast if desired.

Tips: The amount of cayenne you add will depend on how hot your Serrano is. Be sure to taste as you add cayenne, 1 pinch at a time.

If tolerated, top with 1 tablespoon (7 g) each of crumbled feta cheese. Cotija cheese goes well with this dish, though at this time it has not yet been tested for FODMAPs. You may find that it is not a trigger for you.

If your small skillet does not come with a lid, cover the pan with a piece of foil.

Monash Note: Although chiles (chillies) are generally low in FODMAPs, some people with IBS may be sensitive to the capsaicin they contain. Capsaicin is a natural compound that gives chiles their spicy quality. You may need to limit how much chile you eat if your IBS symptoms are triggered by spicy food.

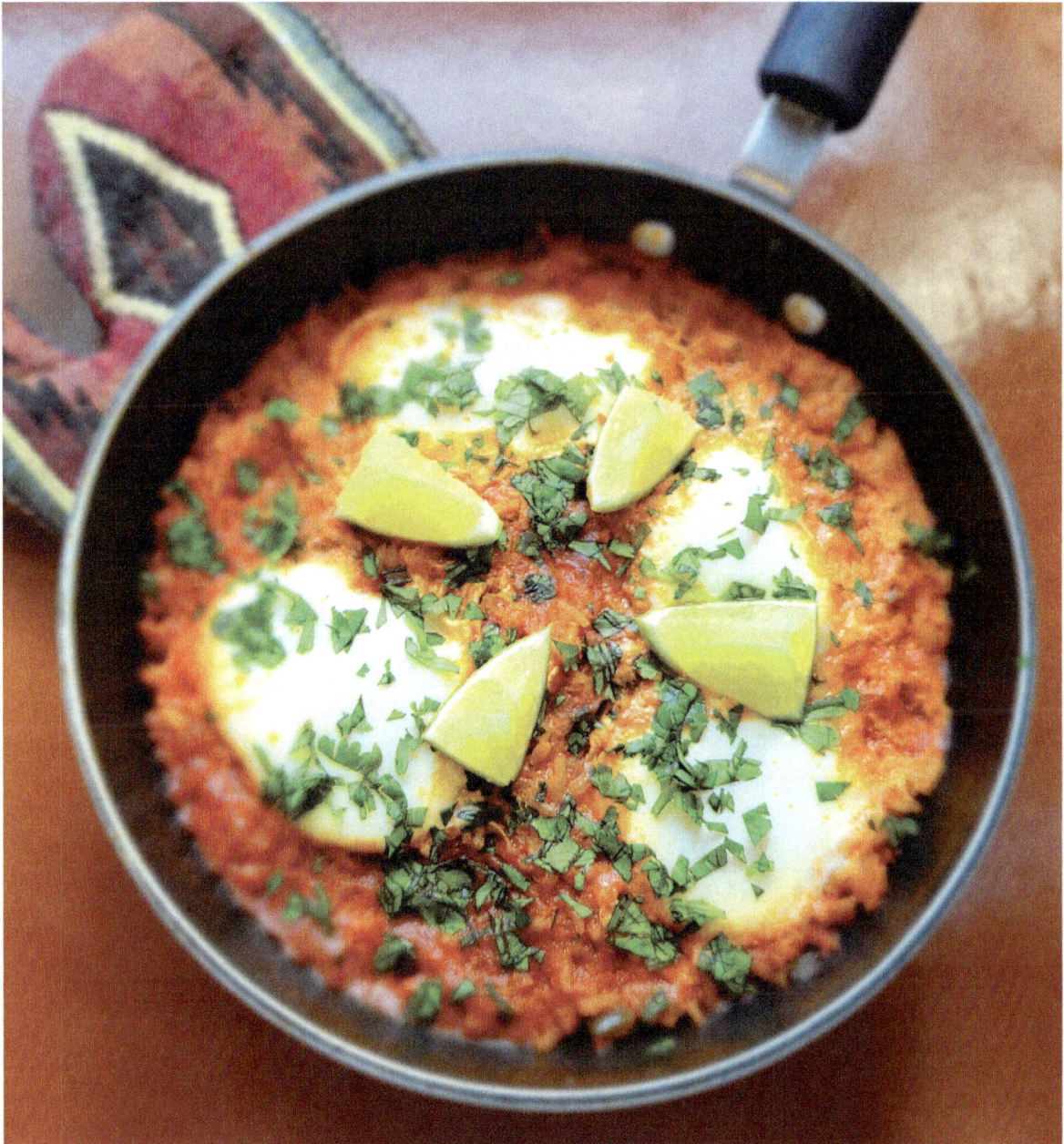

Chorizo Frittata

LOW FODMAP ❤ IBS FRIENDLY ❤ GLUTEN-FREE ❤ DAIRY-FREE

Frittata is like a no-crust quiche that is cooked in a skillet and often finished in the oven, like this version. It's a great dish for using up leftovers, and this chorizo veggie combination is a delicious way to start the day.

If time permits, mix the chorizo ingredients and let marinate in the fridge 4 hours to overnight. When short on time, let it sit for 30 minutes to infuse, then cook.

MAKES 6 SERVINGS

CHORIZO INGREDIENTS

1 tablespoon (15 ml) Low FODMAP Garlic-Infused Oil (page 50), made with extra virgin olive oil, cooled

1/2-pound (227 g) ground pork or ground turkey

2 tablespoons (30 ml) red wine vinegar

1 1/2 teaspoons (2.5 g) smoked paprika

1 teaspoon (2 g) pure mild red chile powder (containing no onion or garlic, the ingredients should list only: red chile. On the Monash App this is called Chilli (chili) red, powdered)

1 teaspoon dried oregano

1/4 teaspoon (.5 g) ground cinnamon

1/4 teaspoon (.5 g) cayenne powder

1/4 teaspoon (1.25 g) fine sea salt

1/4 teaspoon fresh ground black pepper

FRITTATA INGREDIENTS

10 large eggs

2 tablespoons (30 ml) extra virgin olive oil

1 cup (150 g) small diced zucchini

1 large (164 g) red bell pepper, stemmed, seeds and ribs removed, sliced into strips slightly thinner than 1/2-inch (1.25 cm)

1 cup (75 g) rough chopped oyster mushrooms, (you will need to buy 2 cups (150 g) of mushrooms because the heavy stems are cut from the caps and discarded)

1/2 cup (25 g) thin sliced scallions, green parts only

1 teaspoon dried oregano

1/2 teaspoon (2.5 g) fine sea salt

1/4 teaspoon fresh ground black pepper

1 tablespoon (6 g) large flake nutritional yeast, for cheesy flavor

Cilantro leaves for garnish, if desired

Method: Preheat oven to 400 F / 200 C

Chorizo: Mix ingredients including the oil in a medium bowl until fully incorporated. Cover with plastic wrap and marinate in the fridge for at least 30 minutes – 4 hours to overnight, even better.

Frittata: Whisk the eggs in a large mixing bowl until frothy. Set aside.

Brown the chorizo in a 10-inch (25 cm) nonstick ovenproof skillet, stirring with a flat wooden spatula for 4 minutes to really break up the meat. Turn and stir. Cook 4 to 5 minutes longer or until completely cooked through. Spoon the meat onto a plate and set aside.

Bring 2 tablespoons (30 ml) extra virgin olive oil to medium high heat in the same skillet. Add the zucchini, red bell, mushrooms, scallion greens, oregano, salt and pepper. Gently sauté for 4 minutes or until the zucchini and pepper are just becoming tender. Reduce heat to medium. Evenly sprinkle the yeast over the top. Pour in the eggs and gently stir for 3 minutes. Sprinkle the meat evenly on top. Push the meat down to just cover with egg. Bake uncovered for 12 to 15 minutes or until the center is no longer liquid or jiggly. Use an oven mitt to remove from the oven – the handle will be hot!

Slice like a pie to plate. Garnish with cilantro and serve immediately.

Tips: If you are able to tolerate, sprinkle the top with 1/2 cup (50 g) shredded cheddar, Monterey Jack or Manchego cheese before baking.

1/4 cup (40 g) sliced cantaloupe per serving is a sweet side with this dish.

Monash Note: Although chiles (chillies) are generally low in FODMAPs, some people with IBS may be sensitive to the capsaicin they contain. Capsaicin is a natural compound that gives chiles their spicy quality. You may need to limit how much chile you eat if your IBS symptoms are triggered by spicy food.

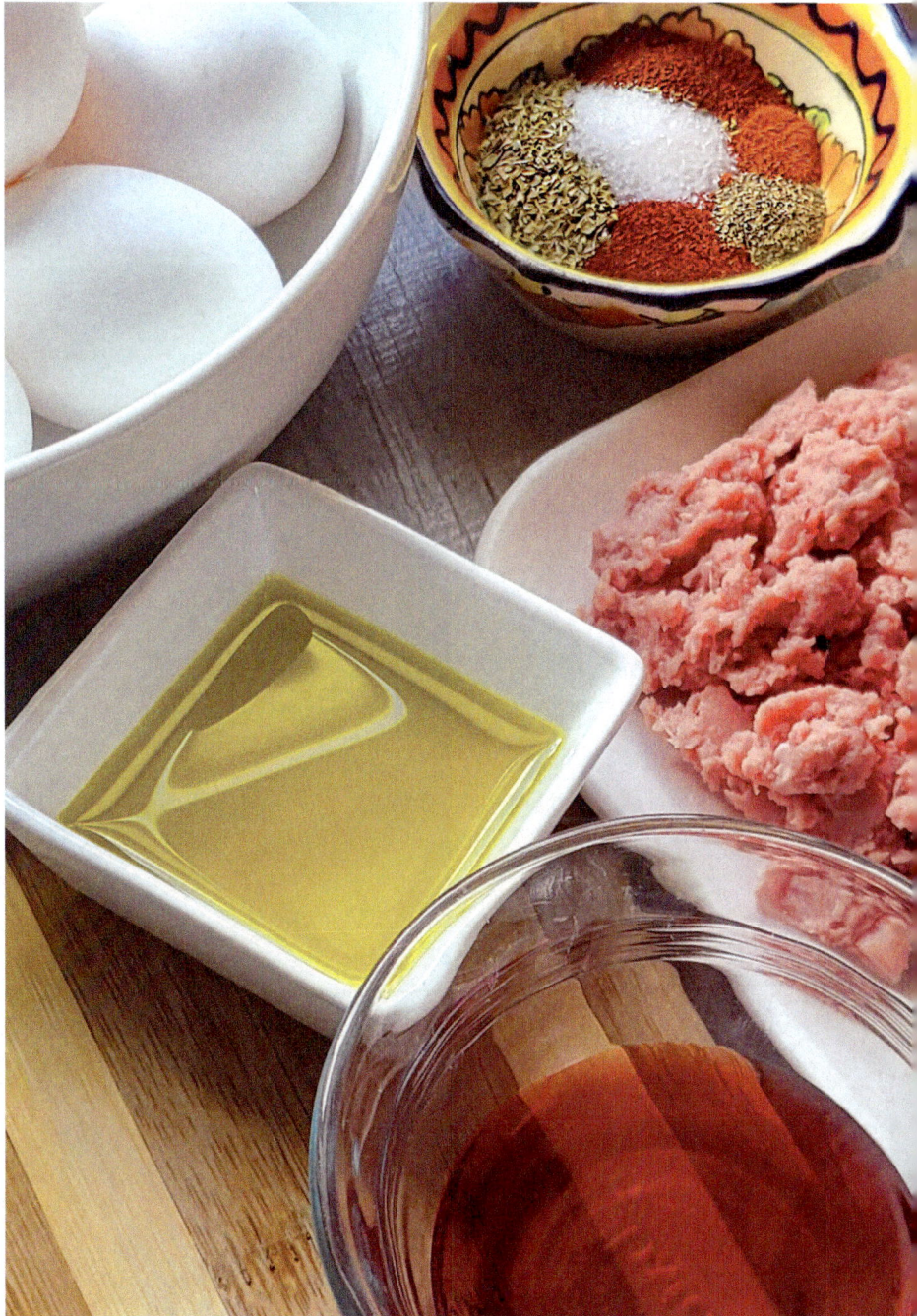

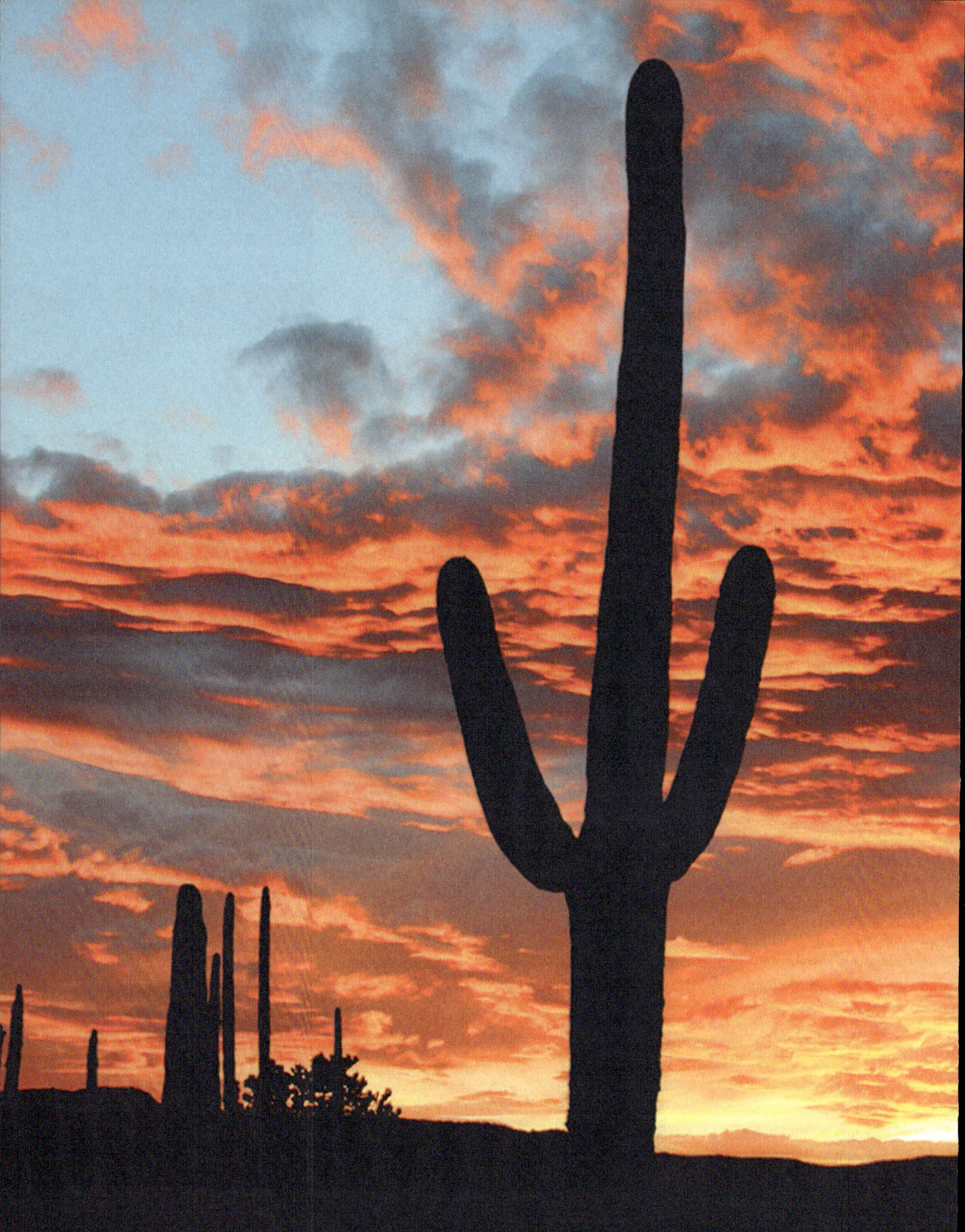

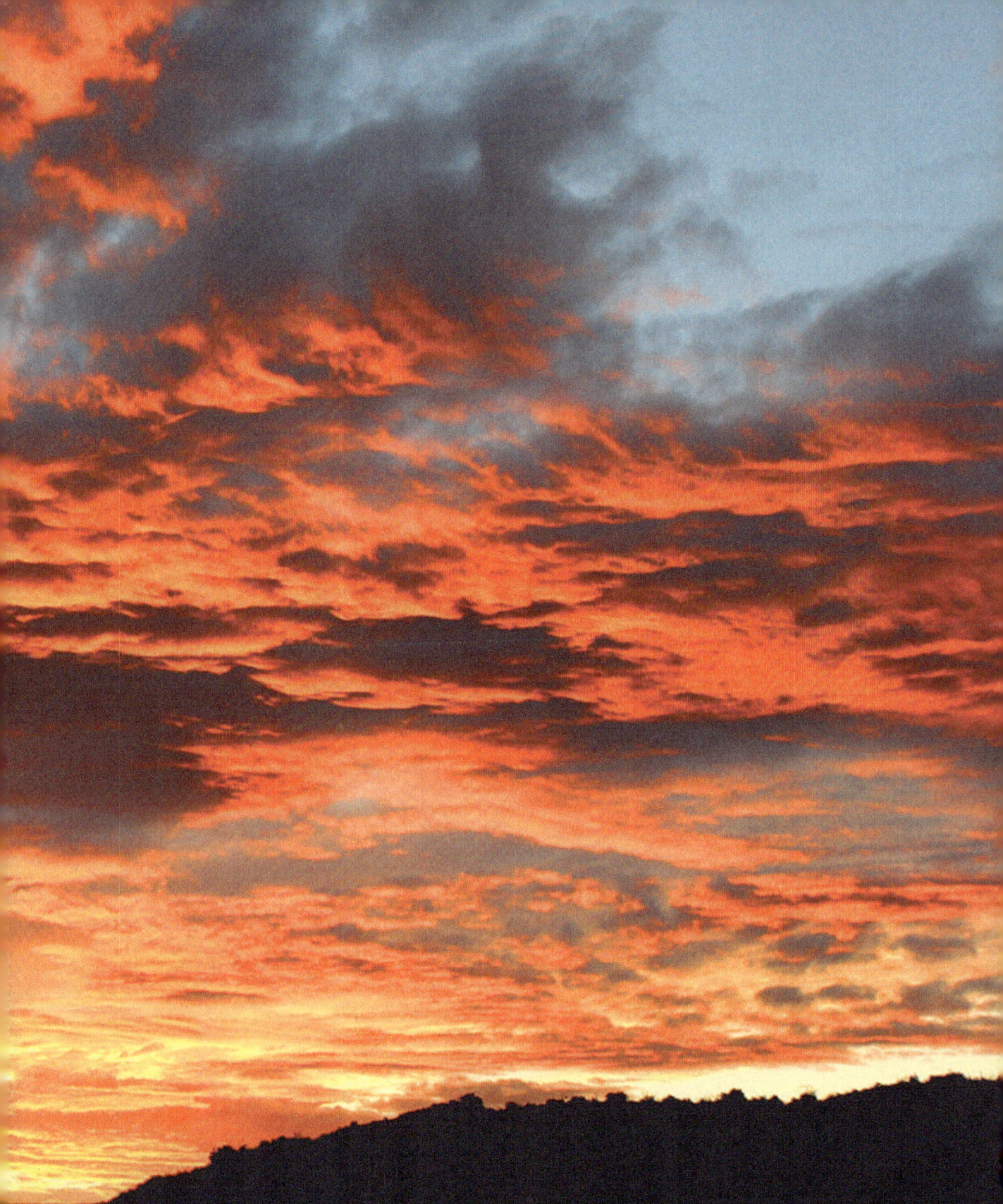

Iconic Southern Arizona

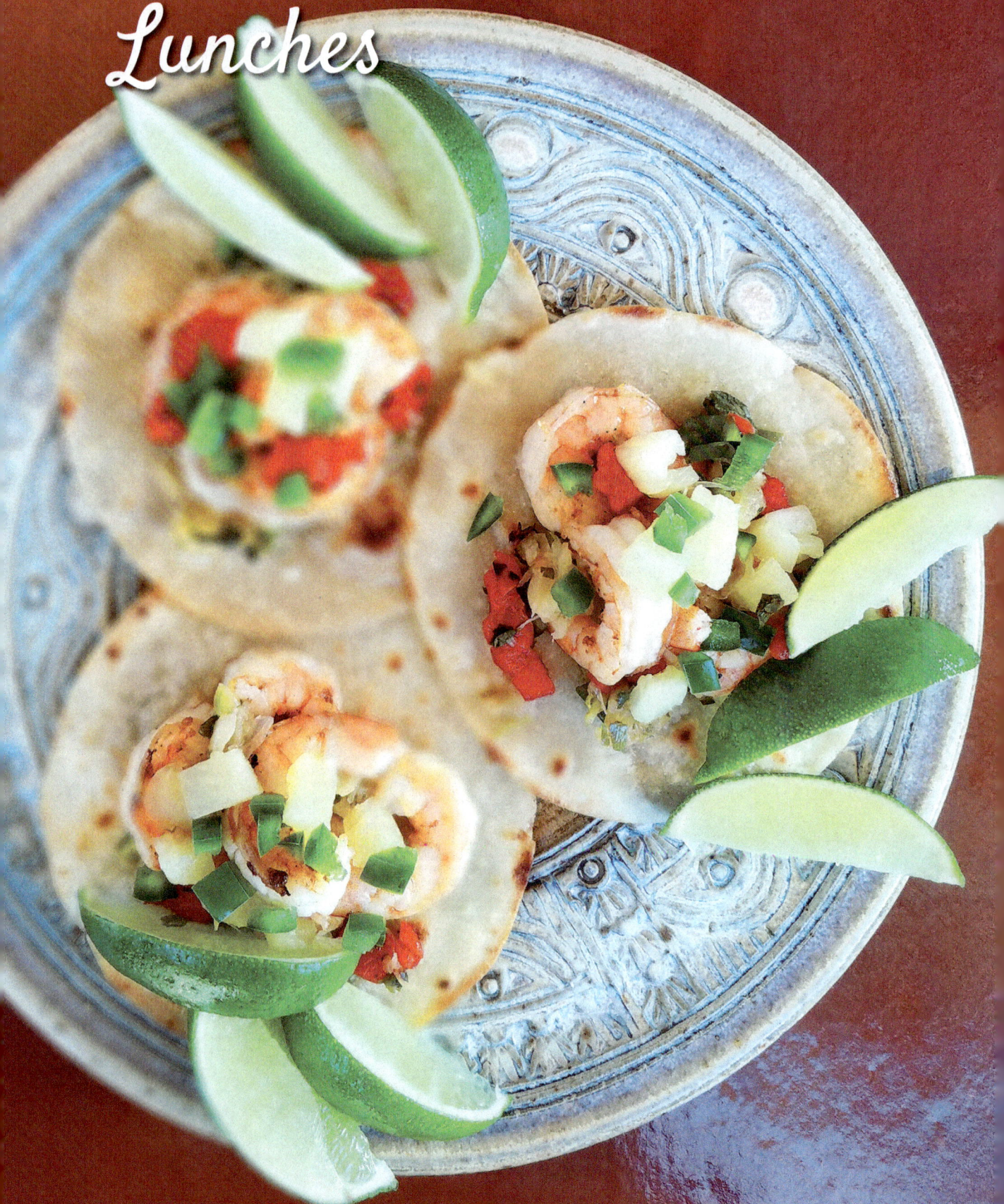

Lunches

- 💜 **Grilled Green Chile Burgers with Bacon**
- 💜 **Burger Patty Tacos**
- 💜 **Shrimp Street Tacos**
- 💜 **Classic Hard Shell Beef Tacos**
- 💜 **Pepper Bellies**
- 💜 **Rayado Ribeye Burritos with Potato & Fiesta Slaw Filling**
- 💜 **Red Bell Pepper Cilantro Burgers with Cumin Lime Mayo**
- 💜 **Pulled Pork Sandwiches with Tangy Sauce & Quick Slaw**
- 💜 **Tofu Tacos With Green Chiles and No Beans Refried "Beans"**

"If I had to live my life over,
I'd live over a Low Fodmap taqueria."
~ Amy Laura

Food brand names are sometimes listed within a recipe, and this means they are Monash Certified. For more brand options we use and love, please visit **FodifyIt.com**

Monash Note: Although chiles (chillies) are generally low in FODMAPs, some people with IBS may be sensitive to the capsaicin they contain. Capsaicin is a natural compound that gives chiles their spicy quality. You may need to limit how much chile you eat if your IBS symptoms are triggered by spicy food.

Grilled Green Chile Burgers with Bacon

LOW FODMAP ❤ IBS FRIENDLY ❤ GLUTEN-FREE ❤ DAIRY-FREE

Most Southwesterners agree that if a burger does not include green chiles it's just not complete. There is an official Green Chile Cheeseburger Trail with map and travel tips that millions of people follow in search of the perfect version. Our fast food burger joints offer green chiles as a topping option. And each year beginning in August, the newly harvested crop is roasted in rolling, flaming chile drums throughout the Southwest, creating an intoxicating, unforgettable aroma that wafts through the air everywhere you go.

As you sink your teeth into this burger, every layer of flavor has all the ingredients for a perfect bite every time, with a hit of those beloved desert emeralds.

If you don't have a bbq grill, pan cook the patties on a stovetop grill or in a nonstick skillet with a bit of extra virgin olive oil. Toast the buns on a stovetop grill or in a toaster.

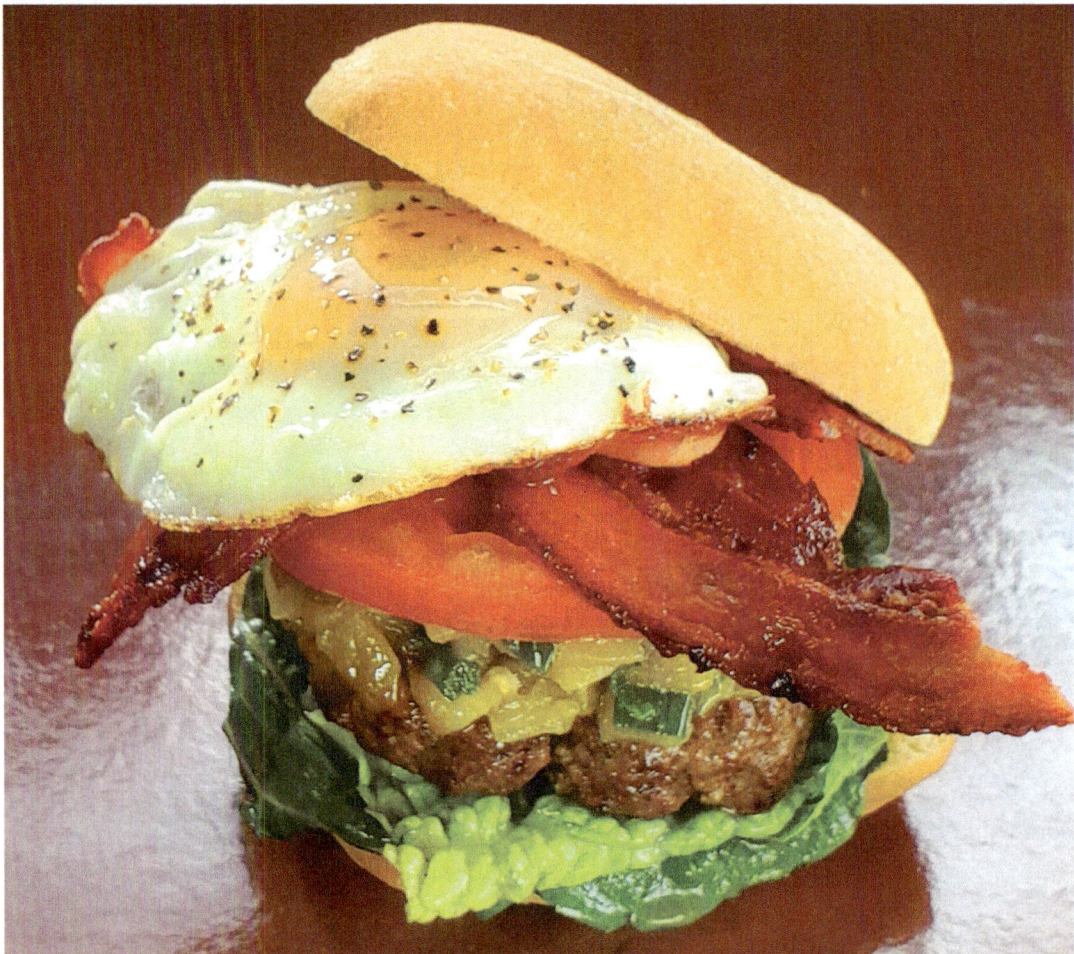

MAKES 2 BURGERS
INGREDIENTS

3 tablespoons (45 g) canned plain chopped green chiles (containing no onion, garlic or other high FODMAP ingredients. On the Monash App they are noted as Chilli (chili) green, mild, chopped, canned)
-OR-
2 medium (61 g each) mild fresh green chiles, roasted and prepped (page 46) will yield approx. 1/4 cup (46 g) diced chile meat (on the Monash App they are noted as: Chile, green, peeled, deseeded)

2 scallions, green parts only, sliced thin

1 tablespoon (14 g) mayonnaise containing no onion or garlic

1/2 teaspoon (1 g) ground cumin

Juice of 1/4 lime

4 - 6-ounces (114 - 170 g) 80/20 ground beef, grass fed if available

1 tablespoon (15 ml) Worcestershire sauce

1/4 teaspoon (1.25 g) fine sea salt

2 low FODMAP gluten-free hamburger buns, or use gluten-free ciabatta rolls such a Schar (Monash Certified)

Lettuce of your choice (crispy Romaine or spring mix is great)

2 slices 1/4-inch (.635 cm) thick common tomato

4 slices thick cut bacon, cooked crispy

2 fried sunny side up large eggs, if you want to be decadent!

Method: Mix the chopped green chiles with the sliced scallion greens in a small bowl and set aside.

Mix the mayo, cumin and lime juice in a separate small bowl and set aside.

Mix the beef with the Worcestershire and salt in a medium bowl using your hands. Careful not to over mix as this will result in a tough texture. Divide into two portions and press gently into patties. Press your thumb into the center to make an indentation so they will grill evenly. Set aside.

Heat your grill to medium high. Using metal tongs and a paper towel doused with a bit of canola oil, grease the grates. Place the patties on the grill and cook for 4 minutes. Flip, top each patty with the green chile and scallion greens and cook 4 to 5 minutes longer, or to desired doneness. Also, when you flip the burgers to finish, place the buns cut side down on the grill to toast until golden brown. Keep an eye on them, they will char quickly.

Assembly: Spread the bottom buns with cumin lime mayo. Top with lettuce, then the chile covered burgers, tomato slices, crisped bacon, fried egg and place the bun top slightly to the side so as not to break the yolks. Serve right away, and give yourself a pat on the back now that you have achieved LoFO green chile burger perfection!

Tips: Fresh green chiles go by names such as New Mexican, Hatch and Anaheim to name a few. If you are not familiar with green chiles, see page 44 for taste and shape descriptions.

If you are able to tolerate dairy, place a slice of cheddar or Monterey Jack cheese (20 g each) over the green chile for the last minute of grilling to melt.

Although Worcestershire sauce contains molasses, garlic and onion, they are in minimal amounts and have been tested by Monash as LoFO in 2 tablespoons (42 g) servings. The amount required to season the burgers is far below the LoFO serving size.

Monash Note: Although chiles (chillies) are generally low in FODMAPs, some people with IBS may be sensitive to the capsaicin they contain. Capsaicin is a natural compound that gives chiles their spicy quality. You may need to limit how much chile you eat if your IBS symptoms are triggered by spicy food.

Burger Patty Tacos

LOW FODMAP ❤ IBS FRIENDLY ❤ GLUTEN-FREE ❤ DAIRY-FREE

Tucson, Arizona introduced me to the iconic saguaro cacti, the enchanting DeGrazia Gallery in the Sun, incredible blazing sunsets, and patty tacos where the burger is pressed into a half-moon shape, grilled or pan cooked and tucked into a corn tortilla with all sorts of toppings. And just like Tucson, I can never get enough of them.

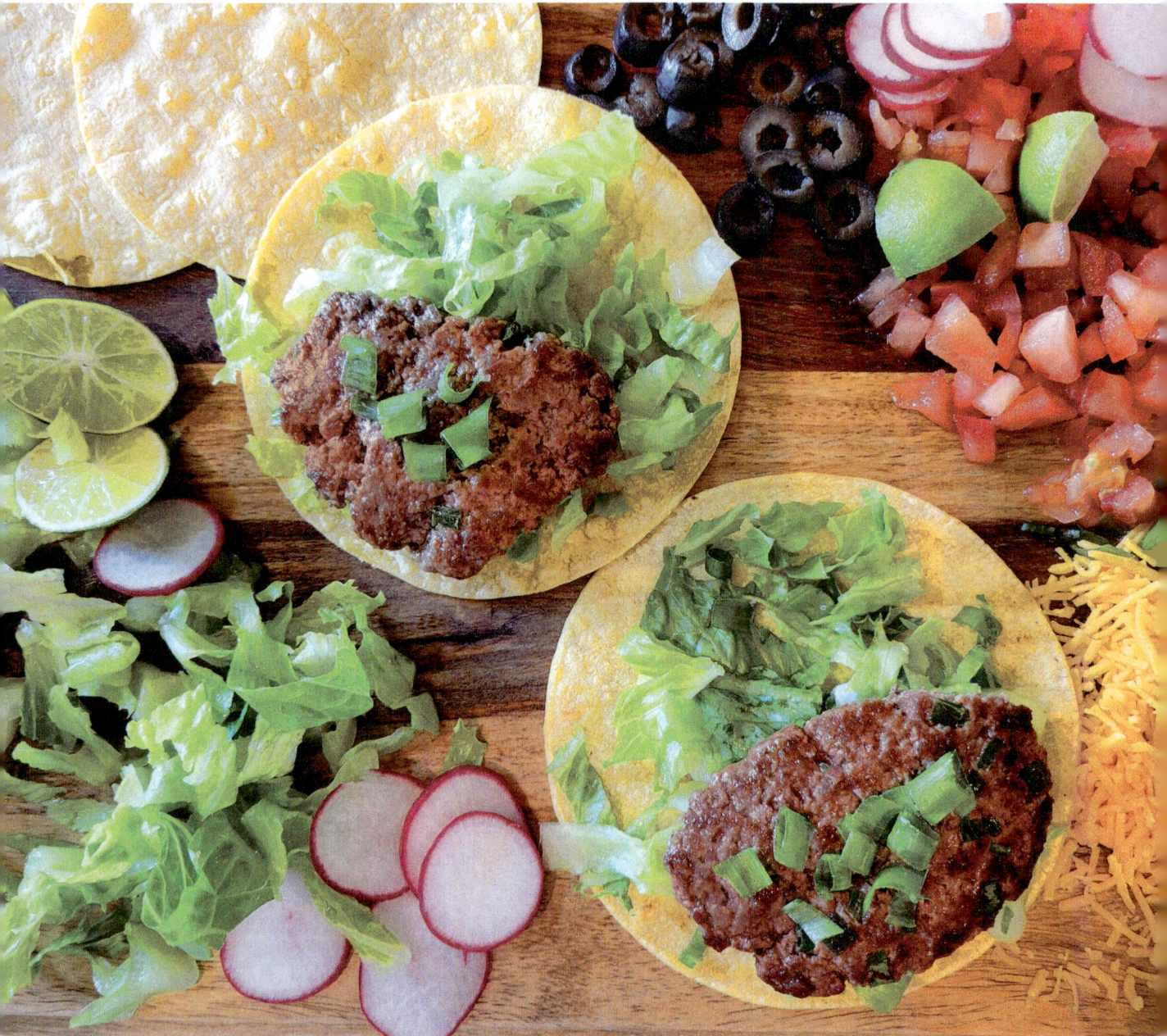

MAKES 4 TACOS – 2 PER SERVING
INGREDIENTS

1/2-pound (227 g) 80/20 ground beef, grass fed if available

1/2 teaspoon (2.5 g) fine sea salt

1/2 teaspoon (1 g) fresh ground black pepper

Canola oil to coat the pan

4 (100 g total) 6-inch (15 cm) low FODMAP gluten-free yellow corn tortillas

1/2 cup (40 g) shredded lettuce (romaine, spring mix and arugula are great)

4 small (40 g total) red radishes, stemmed and diced or sliced

2 scallions, green parts only, sliced thin

1/2 medium (120 g) common tomato, cored and diced

8 large ripe black pitted olives, sliced

1/2 lime, cut into wedges for garnish

Method: Mix the beef, salt and pepper in a medium bowl. Divide into 4 even portions. Take each portion, roll and press with your hands to form a thin half moon shape that will fit inside your tortilla. Set them aside on a plate.

Coat a large nonstick skillet thinly with oil over medium high heat. Place the tortillas in the skillet and warm them to a light toasting, flipping a few times. You want them to be pliable and soft enough to fold around your burgers. Wrap the warm tortillas in a heavy clean kitchen towel, in foil, or place in a tortilla warmer to keep warm.

Lightly coat the pan with oil. Over medium high heat, cook the burgers to your desired doneness. This should take 4 to 5 minutes total, flipping once.

Assembly: Wrap each patty with a warm tortilla. Add the lettuce, radish, scallion greens, tomato and olives inside the tortilla or on top. Garnish with fresh lime wedge. Serve right away. Eat with a fork and knife, or with your hands to get deliciously messy!

Tip: When traveling or cooking at home, a corn tortilla is a great swap for a wheat flour burger bun.

Suggested Dairy Toppings If Tolerated:
1/4 cup (60 g) sour cream or lactose-free sour cream; 1 tablespoon per taco

1/4 cup (28 g) shredded cheddar cheese; 1 tablespoon per taco

Monash Note: Although chiles (chillies) are generally low in FODMAPs, some people with IBS may be sensitive to the capsaicin they contain. Capsaicin is a natural compound that gives chiles their spicy quality. You may need to limit how much chile you eat if your IBS symptoms are triggered by spicy food.

Shrimp Street Tacos

LOW FODMAP ❤ IBS FRIENDLY ❤ GLUTEN-FREE ❤ DAIRY-FREE

Street tacos are made with smaller tortillas making it easier for people buying from street vendors to hold in their hands as they eat and walk. This recipe is a quick and easy light lunch for two with bright, fresh flavors.

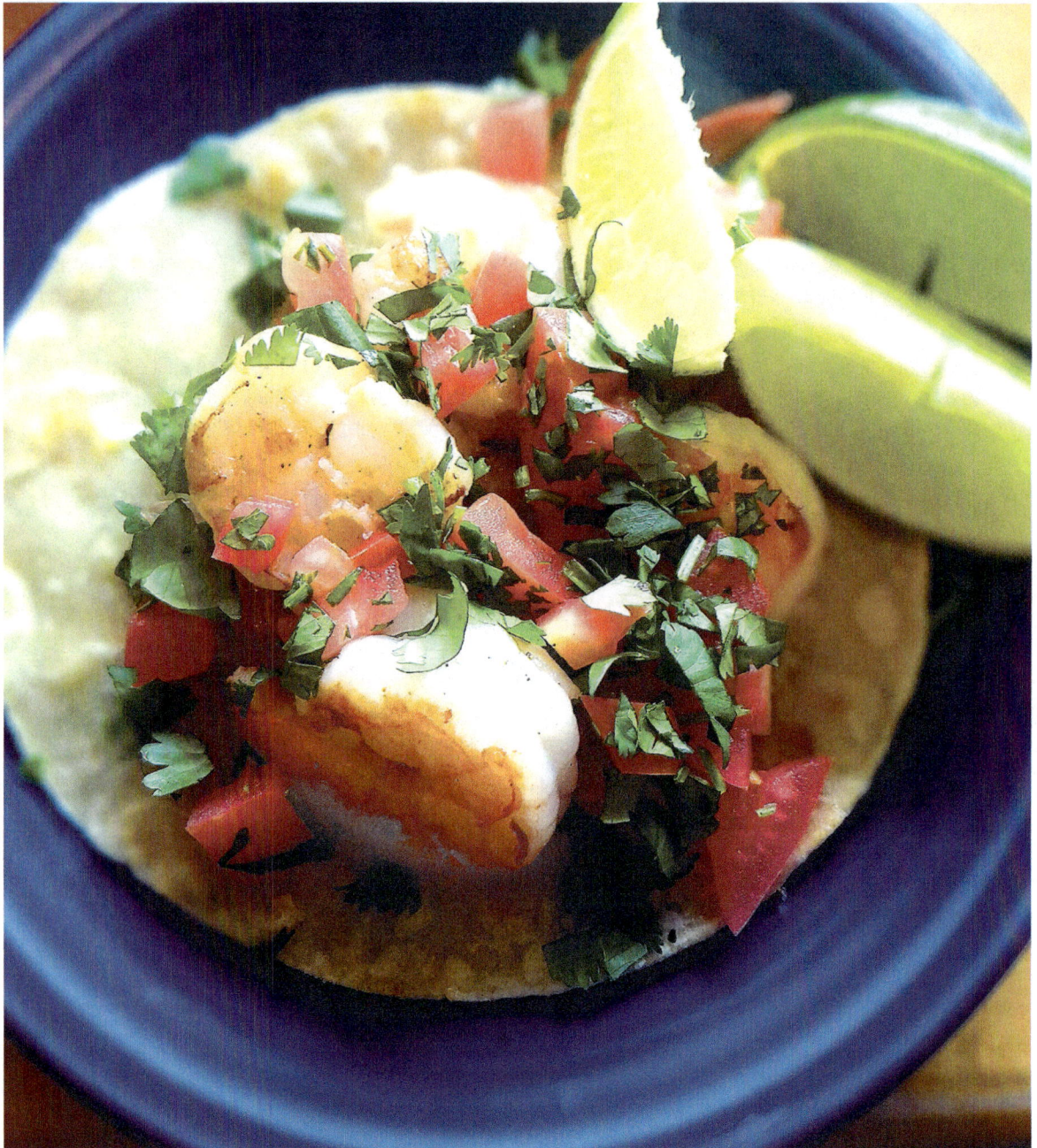

MAKES 2 SERVINGS – 3 TACOS EACH
INGREDIENTS

1 medium (238 g) common tomato, cored, seeded, diced

1/2 (20 g) fresh jalapeño, stem, seeds and ribs removed, diced

Juice of 1/2 lime, plus 1 small sliced lime for garnish

1 tablespoon (15 ml) plus 2 teaspoons (10 ml) canola oil; divided

6, 4 1/2-inch (10 - 11.25 cm) smaller street size LoFO gluten-free corn tortillas, store-bought or homemade (page 104)

18 medium shrimp, shelled, deveined, tails removed

1/4 teaspoon (1 g) fine sea salt, plus more to your taste

1/4 teaspoon fresh ground black pepper

1/4 cup (4 g) fresh medium packed fresh cilantro leaves

Method: Mix the tomato, jalapeño and juice of 1/2 lime in a small bowl. Set aside.

To warm the tortillas, heat 2 teaspoons (10 ml) oil in a large nonstick skillet to medium heat. Place the tortillas in the pan being sure they do not overlap. You may need to do this step in two batches. Move them around to coat with oil. Cook 1 minute and flip. Cook 1 minute and flip until toasted to a light golden brown. This won't take long at all. Wrap tightly in tin foil, a heavy clean kitchen towel, or place in a tortilla warmer.

Add 1 tablespoon (15 ml) oil to the hot skillet. Add the shrimp and lightly dust with salt and pepper. Flip with a spatula for 3 to 4 minutes until the shrimp turns pink, are cooked through and opaque. Remove from the heat.

Assembly: Place 3 tortillas on a plate. Add 3 shrimp to each, then top with the tomato jalapeño lime mix. Garnish with lime slices and cilantro. Repeat for the second plate and serve immediately.

Tip: If you are able to tolerate dairy, 1 teaspoon (3 g) fresh crumbled Queso Fresco per taco adds flavor and a nice creamy texture. If Queso Fresco is not available, feta cheese is fine.

Monash Note: Although chiles (chillies) are generally low in FODMAPs, some people with IBS may be sensitive to the capsaicin they contain. Capsaicin is a natural compound that gives chiles their spicy quality. You may need to limit how much chile you eat if your IBS symptoms are triggered by spicy food.

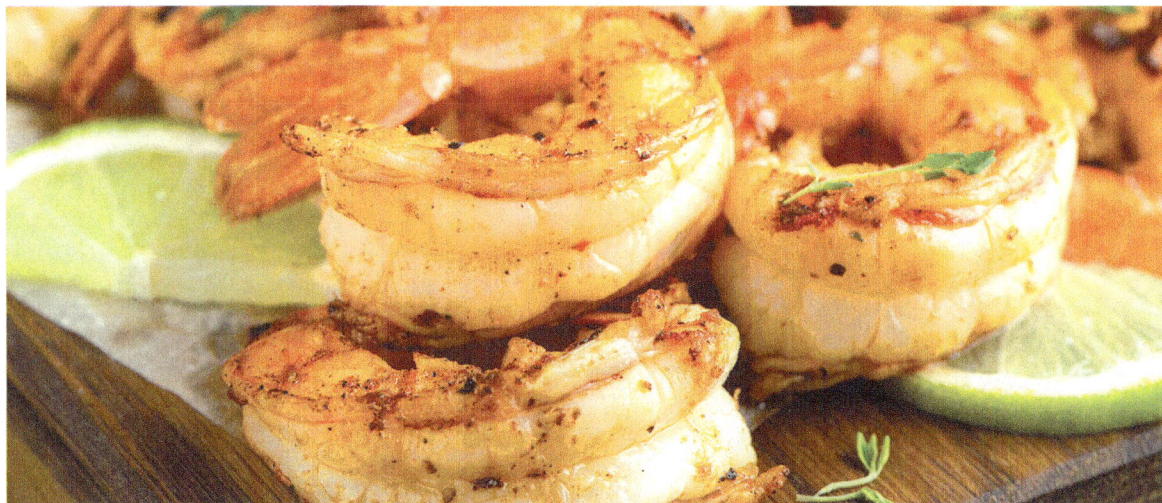

Classic Hard Shell Beef Tacos

LOW FODMAP ❤ IBS FRIENDLY ❤ GLUTEN-FREE ❤ DAIRY-FREE

The classic ground beef taco is one you can count on making an appearance on pretty much any Southwestern menu. Your server will ask if you want a soft or hard (crunchy) tortilla. My family always opted for hard shells and I'm carrying on that tradition.

For a complete LoFO taco plate you need two sides. One option is No Beans Refried "Beans" (page 114) one serving per plate. This is a faux refried recipe I've tested more times than I can count to get it just right. Serve this with one serving of LoFO Mexican Restaurant Style Rice (page 111) — a tasty rice with tiny cubed carrots and spices.

Another sides combo is; 1 taco with 1 serving of Mexican Restaurant Style Rice and 1 serving of Chips and Salsa (page 88) so be sure to plan accordingly.

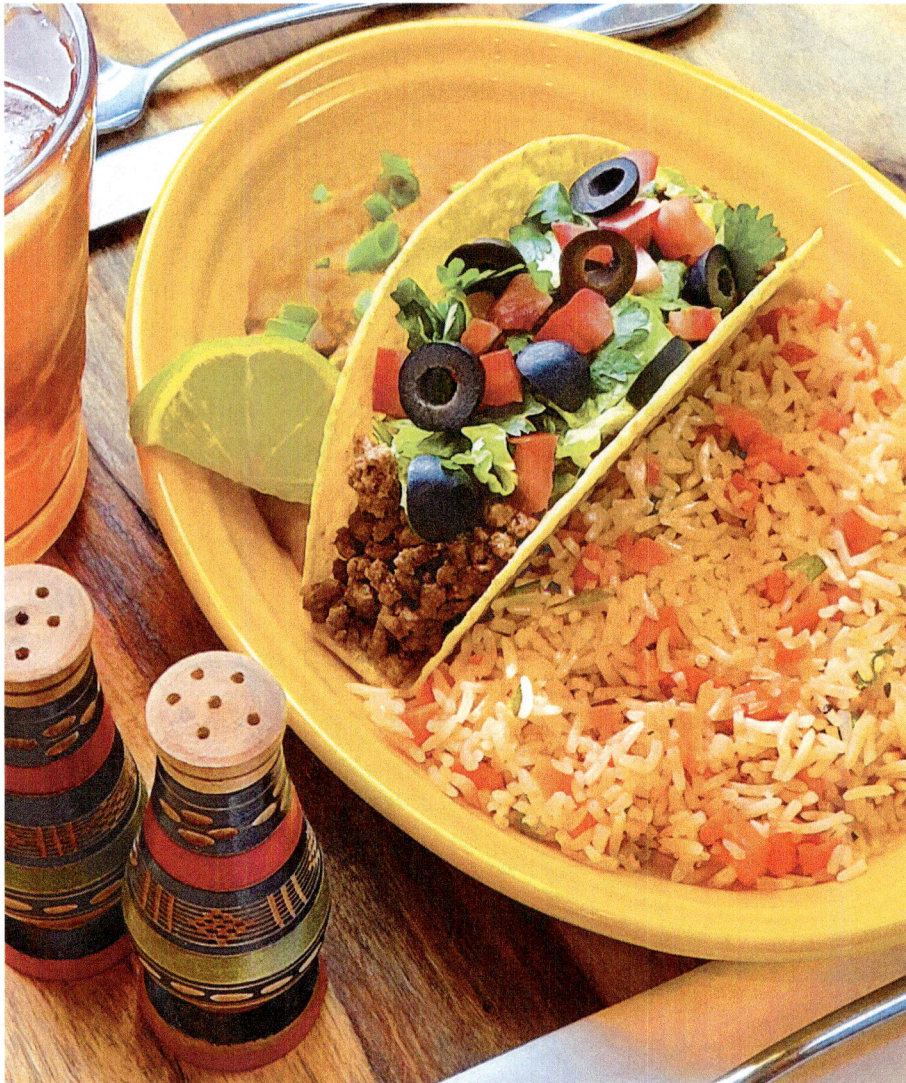

MAKES 4 SERVINGS
TACO SEASONING INGREDIENTS

1 teaspoon (2 g) ground cumin

1 teaspoon (2 g) pure mild red chile powder (containing no onion or garlic, the ingredients should list only: red chile. On the Monash App this is called Chilli (chili) red, powdered)

1/2 teaspoon (1 g) smoked paprika

1/4 teaspoon dried oregano

1/4 teaspoon (1.25 g) fine sea salt

1/4 teaspoon fresh ground black pepper

BEEF INGREDIENTS

2 teaspoons (10 ml) Low FODMAP Garlic-Infused Oil (page 50), made with canola oil

9-ounces (255 g) 80/20 ground beef, grass fed if available

1 tablespoon (3 g) thin sliced scallions, green parts only

1 teaspoons (2 g) masa harina

1/4 cup (60 ml) water

SHELLS

4 (14 g each) gluten-free hard taco shells (I use the crisp flat bottom shells that are more sturdy)

TOPPING INGREDIENTS

3/4 cup (58 g) shredded lettuce, iceberg, Romaine, arugula, spring mix or other lettuce is fine

1 small (75 g) fresh Roma tomato, cored and diced

1/4 cup (4 g) medium packed fresh cilantro, mostly leaves, rough chopped

12 (48 g) canned, pitted ripe black olives, sliced

3 scallions, sliced thin, green parts only

4 lime wedges

Method

Seasoning Mix: Mix the taco seasoning spices in a small bowl and set aside.

Beef: Add the garlic oil to a large nonstick skillet. Heat over medium high heat until it shimmers. Add the beef and scallion greens and cook until the meat is browned, stirring often with a wooden spoon or spatula, breaking up the meat into small pieces as you cook. Drain and return to the skillet.

Add the taco seasoning mix, masa harina and water. Cook over medium heat until bubbling, stirring often. Continue to stir for 3 to 4 minutes. Taste and adjust for salt. Remove from heat and cover to keep warm.

Shells: Heat the hard shells as instructed on the package.

Assembly: Fill the taco shells with equal portions of: beef, lettuce, tomato, cilantro, black olives, scallion greens, with a lime wedge on the side. Serve with your choice of the 2 suggested sides combinations.

Tip: If you are able to tolerate, add a dollop (15 g each) of conventional or lactose-free sour cream, or plain dairy-free, unsweetened coconut yogurt to each taco, and 1/2 cup (50 g) shredded Monterey Jack or cheddar cheese, divided to top each.

Monash Note: Although chiles (chillies) are generally low in FODMAPs, some people with IBS may be sensitive to the capsaicin they contain. Capsaicin is a natural compound that gives chiles their spicy quality. You may need to limit how much chile you eat if your IBS symptoms are triggered by spicy food.

Pepper Bellies

LOW FODMAP ❤ IBS FRIENDLY ❤ GLUTEN-FREE ❤ DAIRY-FREE

My husband grew up in the Mojave Desert of California where vibrant poppy fields blanketed the hillsides, test pilots from Edward's Air Force Base zoomed across the skies, and fabulous, authentic Southwestern food was (and remains) plentiful. When he was in grade school his favorite lunch was Pepper Belly day – small bags of Fritos corn chips filled with beef chili, topped with cheddar cheese and diced onions.

The great thing about Pepper Bellies is that you cut open the tops of the bags, fill them up with chili and kiddos can easily hold and carry them around while scooping with a spoon. This is why they're also called Walking Tacos. A fun, filling lunch for young'uns and the young at heart.

This recipe starts with 1 batch of Mesa Verde Masa Beef Chile (page 136), so be sure to plan accordingly.

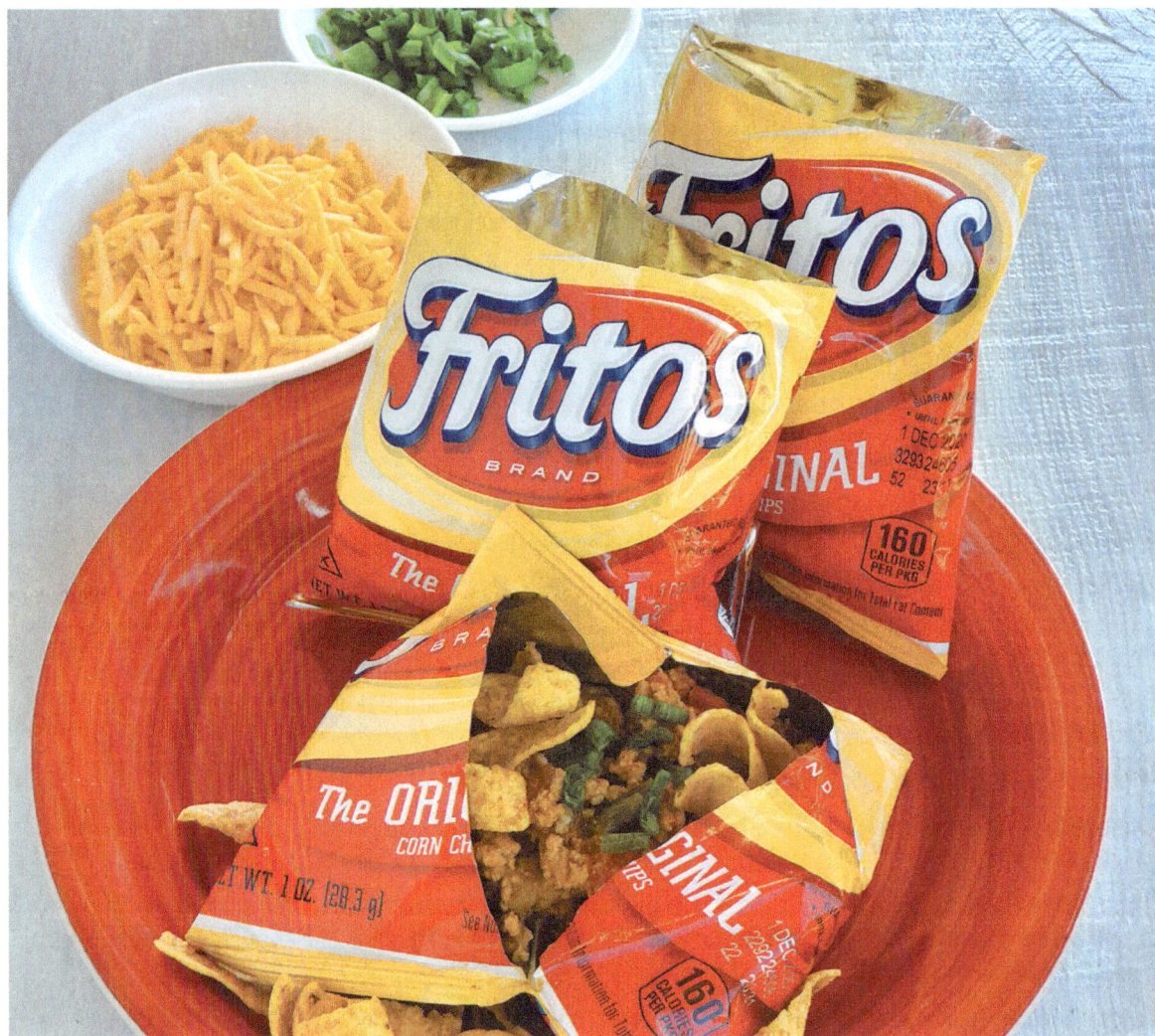

MAKES 8 SERVINGS
INGREDIENTS

1 batch of Mesa Verde Masa Beef Chili (page 136), ready to use and hot

8, 1-ounce (28.3 g) bags Fritos Original corn chips

4 scallions, green parts only, sliced thin

1/2 cup (8 g) medium packed fresh cilantro, mostly leaves, rough chopped

Shredded iceberg or Romaine lettuce, chilled

Method: Cut the tops off the Fritos bags. Spoon in a little chili at a time until each bag is equally filled. Choose desired toppings or place bowls of toppings out for everyone to make their own selections.
Now get ready for a pack of grinning, bright-eyed kids to light up like puppies with a new toy. Actually, expect that reaction from anyone and everyone! Dive right in while the chile is still hot!

Tips: Pictured is one bag cut in the middle and filled, and two upright bags cut at the top. The better method for less spillage is top filled.

If tolerated, offer 3/4 cup (70 g) shredded cheddar cheese to divide and top the bags.

Also if tolerated, add 3/4 cup (180 g) lactose-free or conventional sour cream, divided per taco.

The small 1-ounce (28.3 g) chip bags for this recipe are within the proper LoFO portion amount.

Monash Note: Although chiles (chillies) are generally low in FODMAPs, some people with IBS may be sensitive to the capsaicin they contain. Capsaicin is a natural compound that gives chiles their spicy quality. You may need to limit how much chile you eat if your IBS symptoms are triggered by spicy food.

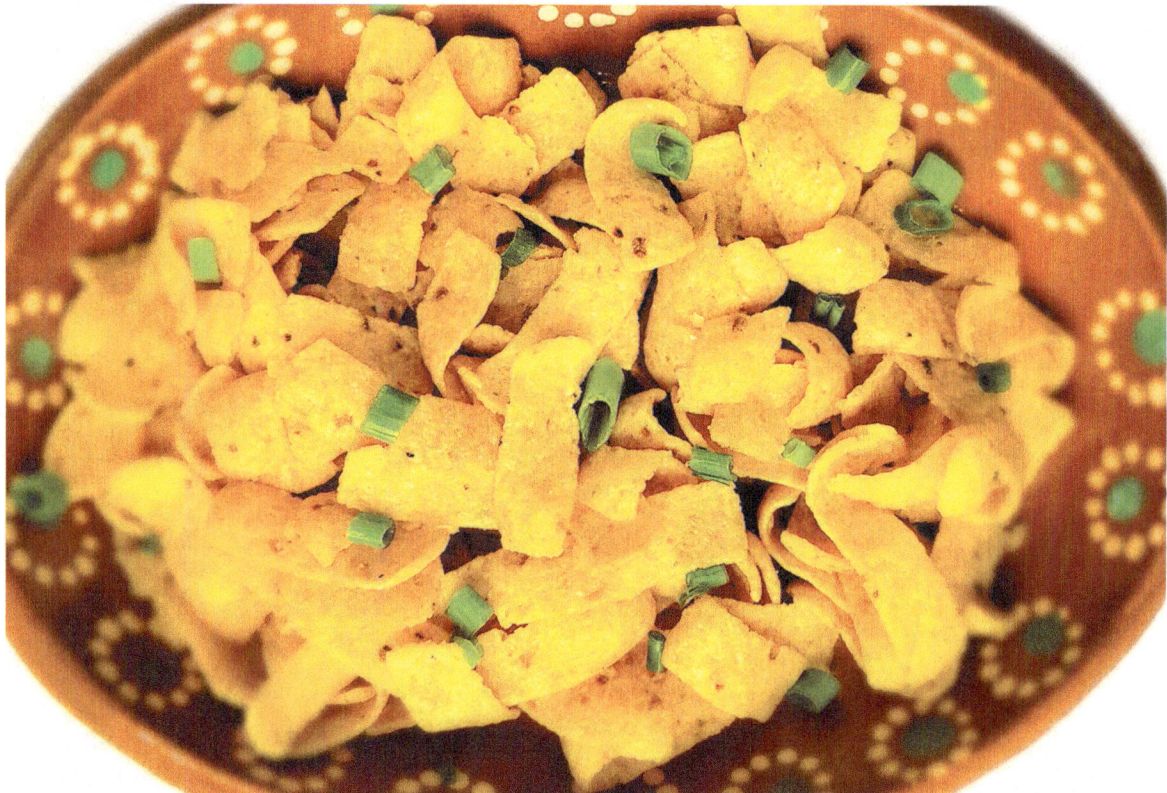

Rayado Ribeye Burritos with Potato & Fiesta Slaw Filling

LOW FODMAP ❤ IBS FRIENDLY ❤ GLUTEN-FREE ❤ DAIRY-FREE

The beauty of this burrito is that it's packed with flavor from the pan-seared ribeye, then the warmth of the steak steams the tangy slaw filling once everything is all rolled up in the tortilla. Serve right away for the best texture and temperature experience.

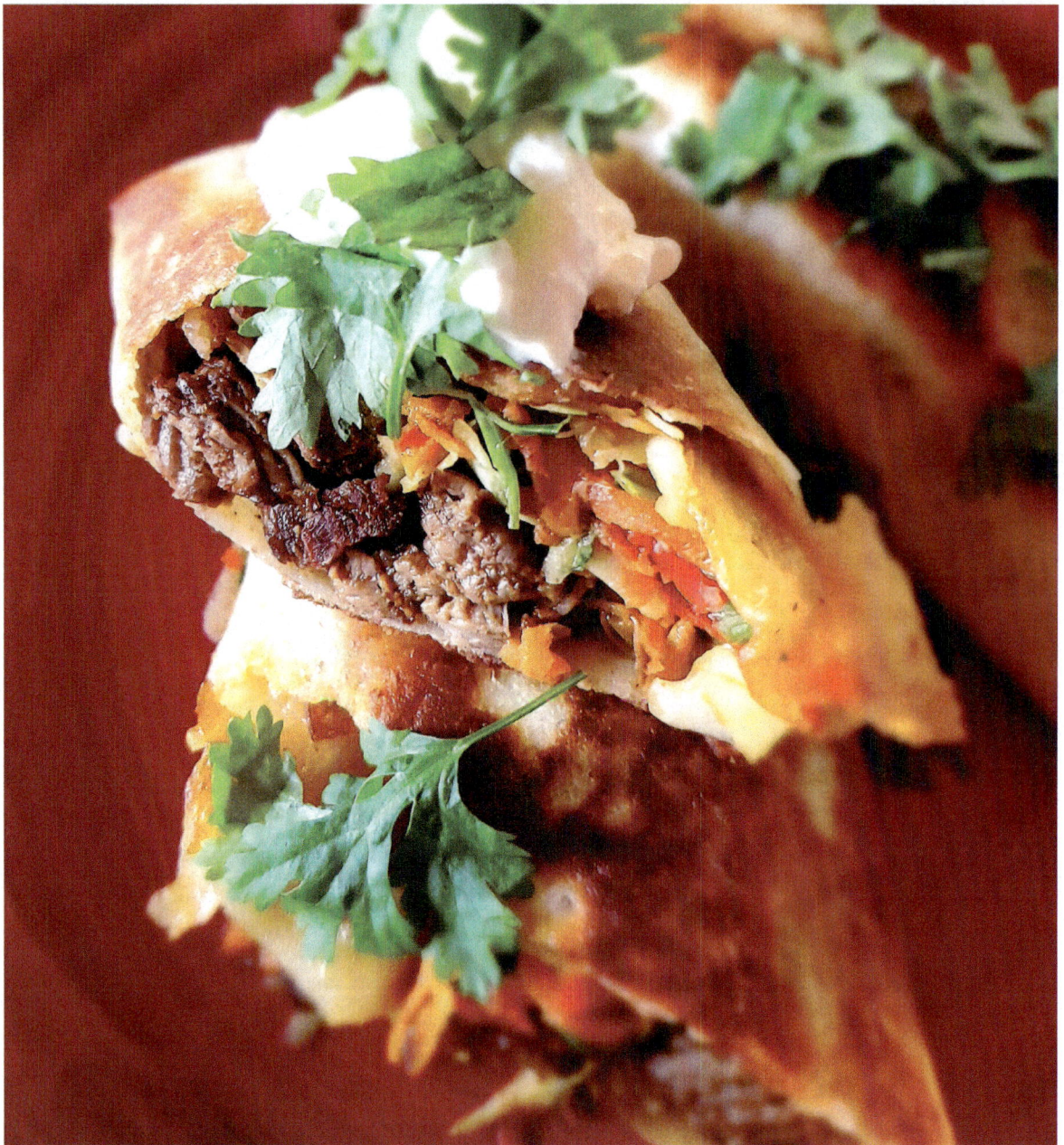

MAKES 2 SERVINGS
SLAW INGREDIENTS

1 large handful (40 g) shredded green cabbage

1/4 (50 g) fresh red bell pepper, stemmed and seeds removed

1/2 carrot (35 g) peeled

1/4 cup (4 g) medium packed fresh cilantro, mostly leaves, minced, plus more leaves for garnish

3 scallions, green parts only, sliced thin

Juice of 1/2 lime

2 teaspoons (9 g) mayonnaise containing no onion or garlic

2 teaspoons (10 ml) red wine vinegar

1/2 teaspoon maple syrup

1/4 teaspoon (1.25 g) fine sea salt

RIBEYE & POTATO INGREDIENTS

1/2 teaspoon (1 g) pure chipotle powder

1/2 teaspoon (1 g) pure mild red chile powder (containing no onion or garlic, the ingredients should list only: red chile. On the Monash App this is called Chilli (chili) red, powdered)

1/2 teaspoon (1 g) ground cumin

1/2 teaspoon (2.5 g) fine sea salt

1/4 teaspoon (.5 g) fresh ground black pepper

1 medium to large ribeye steak (365 g) with nice marbling and not too many large fat pockets, room temperature

3 tablespoon (45 ml) Low FODMAP Garlic-Infused Oil (page 50), made with extra virgin olive oil, or plain olive oil, divided

1 small (140 g) russet potato, peeled, quartered and small diced

2, 9-inch (23 cm) (50 g each) low FODMAP gluten-free burrito tortilla wraps (see Tips)

Method

Slaw: Fit your food processor with the shredding/grating disk. Cut the cabbage, bell pepper and carrot into pieces that will fit through the top feed tube. Turn the processor on and feed the cabbage, pepper and carrot through with the food pusher to shred. Use a spatula to scrape the vegetables into a mixing bowl. Add the remaining slaw ingredients, mix well and set aside.

Ribeye: Mix the chipotle powder, red chile powder, cumin, salt and pepper in a small bowl. Place the ribeye on a plate or cutting board and sprinkle both sides to coat evenly with the rub.

Pour the garlic oil into a medium nonstick skillet over medium high heat. Add the steak and cook to desired doneness. I prefer medium well for burritos, cooking each side for 6 minutes, adding a bit more oil if needed, tented with foil to avoid splatters. Move the steak to a plate and cover with foil to rest.

Reserve the pan drippings to cook the diced potato.

(continued on next page)

(continued from previous page)

Potato: Although you've reserved the pan drippings, the skillet may be coated with charred bits that are too blackened, in which case wipe out the pan and add 1 tablespoon (15 ml) oil.

Bring the drippings/oil to medium high heat. Spoon the diced potato into the pan. Cook, covered loosely with foil for 2 minutes. Flip with a spatula and cook another minute or until the potatoes are tender. Remove from heat.

Assembly: Now that the ribeye has rested, chop it into small pieces, removing and discarding any large bits of fat.

Store-bought low FODMAP gluten-free burrito wraps can be a little dry and may crack when you roll them. By slightly heating them just before you assemble they should roll nice and tight without breaking.

Wipe the cooled medium saucepan with a paper towel to clean. Bring to medium heat. Add one of the wraps to the dry non-oiled pan and let it toast for 1 minute. Flip and toast for 30 seconds to 1 minute or until it feels pliable to the touch.

Place the wrap on a cutting board or plate. Spoon half of the steak bits onto one edge of the wrap closest to you. Spoon half of the slaw over the steak, then half of the potatoes and get ready to roll! Firmly and carefully roll the wrap away from you, about half way. Tuck in the sides and continue to roll into a burrito. Place it seam side down on the work surface; repeat with the second burrito.

Increase the pan heat to medium high. Add 1 tablespoon (15 ml) oil. Lay both burritos in the pan seam side down and immediately roll them all the way around to coat all sides with the oil. Cook for 1 minute seam side down and check for a deep golden brown sear. Flip and cook the other side for 1 minute to golden brown.

To Plate: Cut in half on the diagonal. Top with fresh cilantro and chow down!

Tips: LoFO gluten-free burrito wraps are improving, with more options all the time. I prefer a brown rice flour wrap with tapioca flour, safflower oil, rice bran,xanthan gum and sea salt. Ingredients to avoid; wheat flour or HiFO flours, inulin, honey and any HiFO spices.

If you are able to tolerate dairy, layer in 2 tablespoons (14 g) shredded Monterey Jack or cheddar cheese to each burrito as you assemble. Per your tolerance, top with a dollop (15 g each) of conventional or lactose-free sour cream, or plain dairy-free, unsweetened coconut yogurt.

Pure chipotle powder brands vary in heat. Best to taste test before adding. If you are sensitive to heat, swap it with smoked paprika.

Monash Note: Although chiles (chillies) are generally low in FODMAPs, some people with IBS may be sensitive to the capsaicin they contain. Capsaicin is a natural compound that gives chiles their spicy quality. You may need to limit how much chile you eat if your IBS symptoms are triggered by spicy food.

Red Bell Pepper Cilantro Burgers with Cumin Lime Mayo

LOW FODMAP ❤ IBS FRIENDLY ❤ GLUTEN-FREE ❤ DAIRY-FREE

Biting into a nicely seasoned burger is such a delight. This recipe takes it a step further by mixing fresh red bell peppers, cilantro and scallion greens into the ground beef. And if that's not enough fresh flavor, the cumin lime mayo adds a dollop of earthy, bright creaminess.

MAKES 2 BURGERS
INGREDIENTS

1/2-pound (227 g) 80/20 ground beef, grass fed if available

1/2 medium (60 g) fresh red bell pepper, stemmed, seeds and ribs removed, diced (if your digestion is sensitive to the skins see page 46 for steps on roasting and removing the skins first)

2 tablespoons (2 g) finely chopped cilantro leaves, plus extra cilantro leaves for topping the burgers

2 scallions, green parts only, sliced thin

1/2 teaspoon (2.5 g) fine sea salt

1/4 teaspoon fresh ground black pepper

Canola oil; optional for greasing the skillet

2 tablespoons (28 g) mayonnaise, containing no onion, garlic or other high FODMAP ingredients

Juice of 1/2 lime

1/2 teaspoon (1 g) ground cumin

2 low FODMAP gluten-free buns; Schar brand ciabatta and hamburger rolls are Monash certified

1/2 cup (40 g) lettuce, Romaine, spring mix or arugula

2, 1/4-inch (.63 cm) thick sliced (50 g total) common tomato

Method: Using your hands, gently mix the beef with the red bell, cilantro, scallion greens, salt and pepper until fully incorporated. Don't over mix, as this will make for a tough burger. Form into two burger patties. Press your thumb into the center of the patties to create an indentation, as this will help the burgers to cook evenly.

Grill on medium high heat, use a stovetop griddle, or pan cook with a bit of canola oil to desired doneness. Place on a plate and cover with foil to rest.

Mix the mayo, lime and cumin in a small bowl.

Lightly grill or toast the buns.

Assembly: Spread the seasoned mayo on the bottom and top underside of the buns. Begin assembling with the lettuce, then burger patty, tomato slice, fresh cilantro leaves and bun tops.

Tip: If you are able to tolerate dairy, top each burger patty with 1(20 g) slice of Manchego cheese or cheddar. Add the cheese 1 minute before the burgers are done cooking allowing it to melt.

Pulled Pork Sandwiches with Tangy Sauce & Quick Slaw

LOW FODMAP ❤ IBS FRIENDLY ❤ GLUTEN-FREE ❤ DAIRY-FREE

This recipe is based upon my Slow Oven-Roasted Pulled Pork (page 80), so be sure to read that first and plan your timing accordingly. These sandwiches combine tender pork with a ketchup, cider vinegar, brown sugar-based bbq sauce, crunchy quick slaw and jarred pickled jalapeños for a zingy scrumptious lunch or dinner.

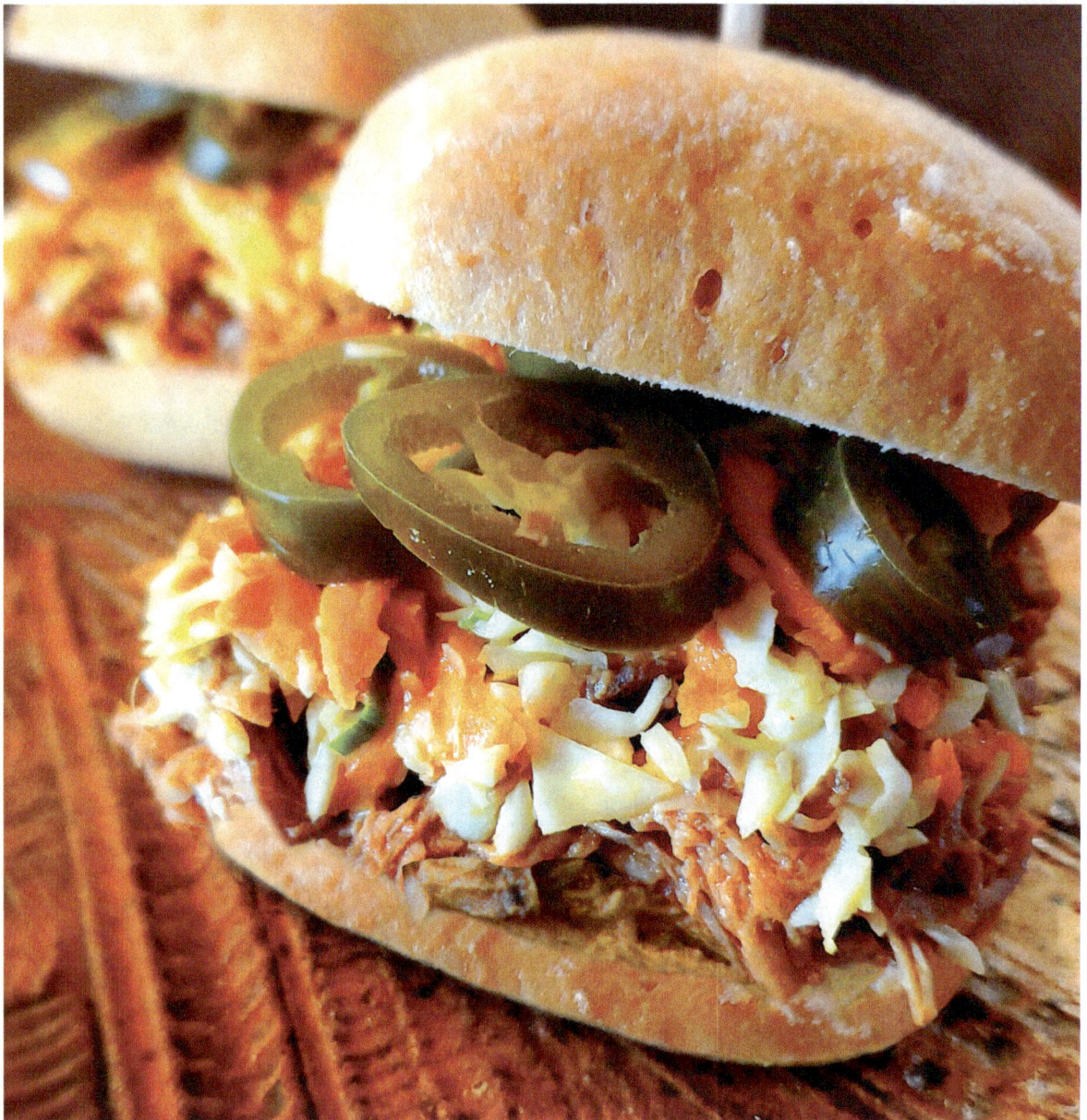

MAKES 2 SERVINGS
QUICK SLAW INGREDIENTS

1/2 (35 g) carrot, grated

2-ounces (55 g) shredded green cabbage

2 scallions, green parts only, sliced thin

1 tablespoon (14 g) mayonnaise containing no onion or garlic

2 teaspoons (10 ml) apple cider vinegar

TANGY BBQ SAUCE INGREDIENTS

2 tablespoons (30 ml) low FODMAP prepared ketchup, containing no onion, garlic or other high FODMAP ingredients. See page 71 for homemade.

2 tablespoons (30 ml) pan drippings from the pulled pork, Low FODMAP Chicken Stock (page 135), or water

1 tablespoon (15 ml) plus 1 teaspoon (5 ml) apple cider vinegar

1 teaspoon (3 g) medium packed light brown sugar

1/2 teaspoon plain, prepared yellow mustard, containing no onion or garlic

1/2 teaspoon Worcestershire sauce

1/2 teaspoon pure chipotle powder containing no onion, garlic or other high FODMAP ingredients

PORK INGREDIENTS

6-ounces (171 g) Slow Oven-Roasted Pulled Pork (page 80), ready to use and hot

BUNS & TOPPING INGREDIENTS

2 low FODMAP gluten-free sandwich rolls; Schar ciabatta and burger buns are Monash certified

2 tablespoons (30 g) drained jarred pickled jalapeños, containing no onion, garlic or other high FODMAP ingredients

Method

Slaw: combine the slaw ingredients in a small bowl. Mix and set aside.

Sauce: Add all of the sauce ingredients to a small saucepan. Bring to a low boil over medium high heat.

Pork: Add the pork to the sauce and gently stir to heat and coat the meat, about 3 minutes.

Buns: Place the buns on a plate and microwave for 10 seconds to soften.

Assembly: Plate with the bottom bun, then the pork, topped with the slaw, pickled jalapeños and top bun. Serve immediately.

Monash Note: Although chiles (chillies) are generally low in FODMAPs, some people with IBS may be sensitive to the capsaicin they contain. Capsaicin is a natural compound that gives chiles their spicy quality. You may need to limit how much chile you eat if your IBS symptoms are triggered by spicy food.

Tofu Tacos With Green Chiles and No Beans Refried "Beans"

LOW FODMAP ❤ IBS FRIENDLY ❤ GLUTEN-FREE ❤ DAIRY-FREE

FODMAP amounts differ with tofu. While firm plain tofu is LoFO at 2/3 cup (160 g) per serving, silken plain tofu is HiFO. Taking the time to press the liquids out of firm tofu makes for a good sear and texture.

These tacos are a delicious Meatless Monday lunch or dinner, and the crisp lettuce, radishes and tortilla shells add lots of crunch.

For No Beans Refried "Beans" see page 114. The recipe yields 6 servings. You will only need 2 servings and the remaining may be used for tomorrow's Huevos Rancheros (page 155), with Classic Beef Tacos (page 178), or dipped with corn tortilla chips.

MAKES 2 SERVINGS – 2 TACOS EACH
FOR PRESSING THE TOFU

10.6-ounces (300 g) block of firm plain tofu

2 medium rimmed sheet pans

2 clean kitchen tea towels

Large cans of veggies or a few heavy books to help press the liquid out of the tofu

TACO INGREDIENTS

2 tablespoons (30 ml) Low FODMAP Garlic-Infused Oil (page 50), made with extra virgin olive oil

2 tablespoons (30 ml) soy sauce, gluten-free if you are following a gluten-free diet

1/2 teaspoon (1 g) ground cumin

1/2 teaspoon (1 g) smoked paprika

1/4 teaspoon (1.25 g) fine sea salt

1/2 lime for spritzing the tofu

2 servings No Beans Refried "Beans"(page 114), ready to serve and hot

4 gluten-free hard taco shells (I use crisp flat bottom shells (13 g each) that are more sturdy)

1/2 cup (40 g) shredded iceberg lettuce, chilled

1/4 cup (45 g) canned mild chopped green chiles, containing no onion, garlic or other high FODMAP ingredients (on the Monash App they are noted as Chilli (chili) green, mild, chopped, canned)
-OR-
2 medium (61 g each) mild fresh green chiles, roasted and prepped (page 46) will yield approx. 1/4 cup (46 g) diced chile meat (on the Monash App they are noted as: Chile, green, peeled, deseeded)

1/2 small (60 g) common tomato, small diced

3 scallions, green parts only, sliced thin

2 (40 g total) red radishes, sliced thin

1/4 cup (25 g) fresh grated carrot

Cilantro, a small handful of mostly leaves, rough chopped

Method: To press the tofu, fold and place one towel on a rimmed baking sheet. Cut the tofu block lengthwise in half and place onto the towel. Cover with the second towel and position the other baking pan on top. Weigh it down with cans of veggies or books to press for 30 minutes. Place the tofu on a cutting board and cut into 1/2-inch (.63 cm) cubes.

Pour the garlic oil in a medium saucepan over medium high heat. Toss in the tofu and stir with a spatula to sear all sides. Add the soy sauce and cook 2 minutes. Remove from heat and sprinkle evenly with the cumin, paprika and salt. Toss to coat. Spritz with lime juice.

Assembly: Place 2 hard taco shells on each plate. Evenly distribute the refried "beans" into the shells, then the lettuce, tofu, chopped green chiles, tomatoes, sliced scallions, radishes and top with carrot and cilantro.

Tips: For vegetarian No Beans Refried "Beans" substitute the bacon drippings for Low FODMAP Garlic-Infused Oil (page 50) made with extra virgin olive oil, and swap water in place of the chicken stock.

If tolerated, evenly divide 1/4 cup (25 g) shredded cheddar, Manchego or Monterey Jack cheese to top the 4 tacos.

Monash Note: Although chiles (chillies) are generally low in FODMAPs, some people with IBS may be sensitive to the capsaicin they contain. Capsaicin is a natural compound that gives chiles their spicy quality. You may need to limit how much chile you eat if your IBS symptoms are triggered by spicy food.

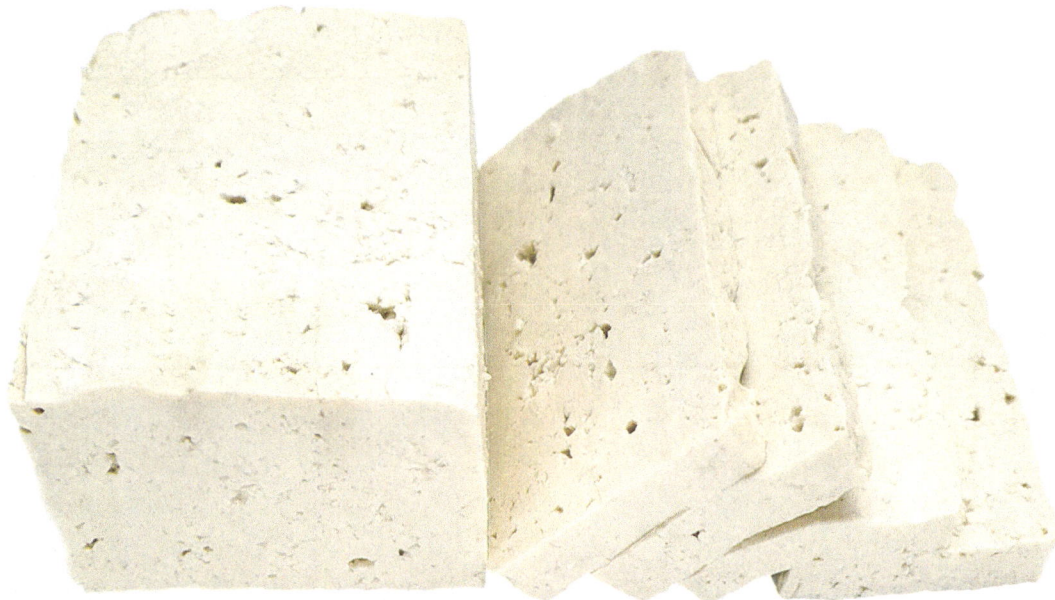

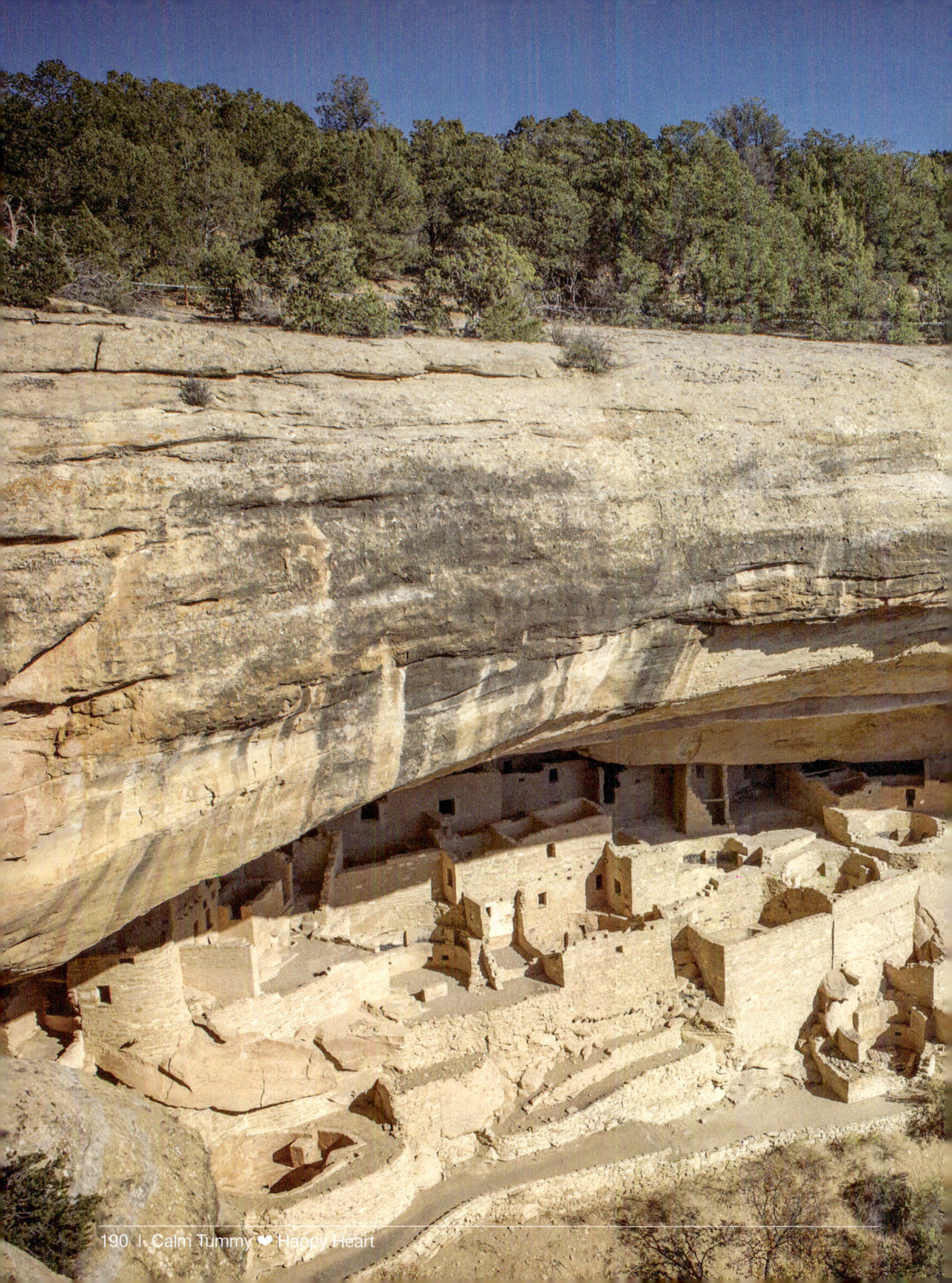

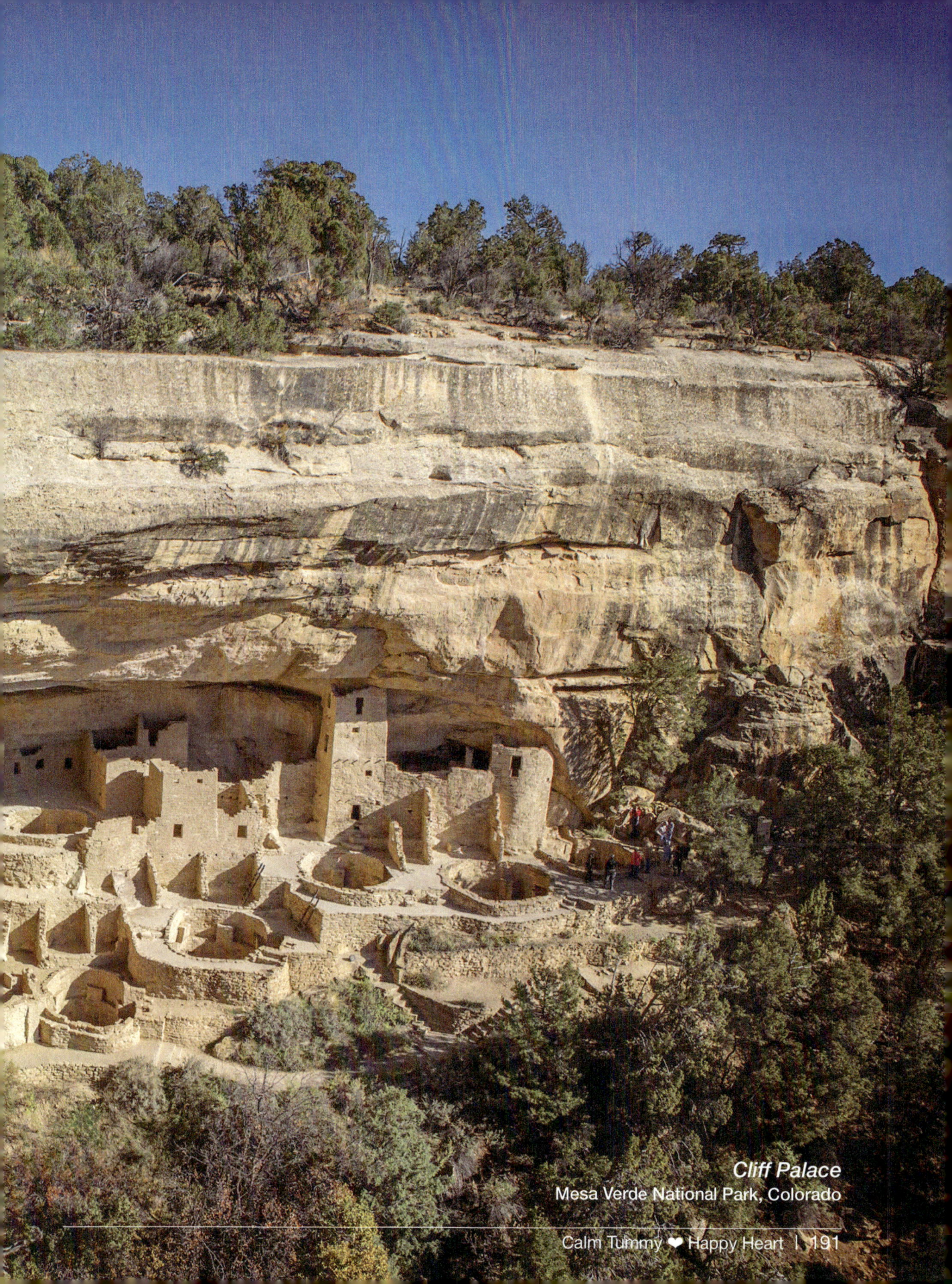

Cliff Palace
Mesa Verde National Park, Colorado

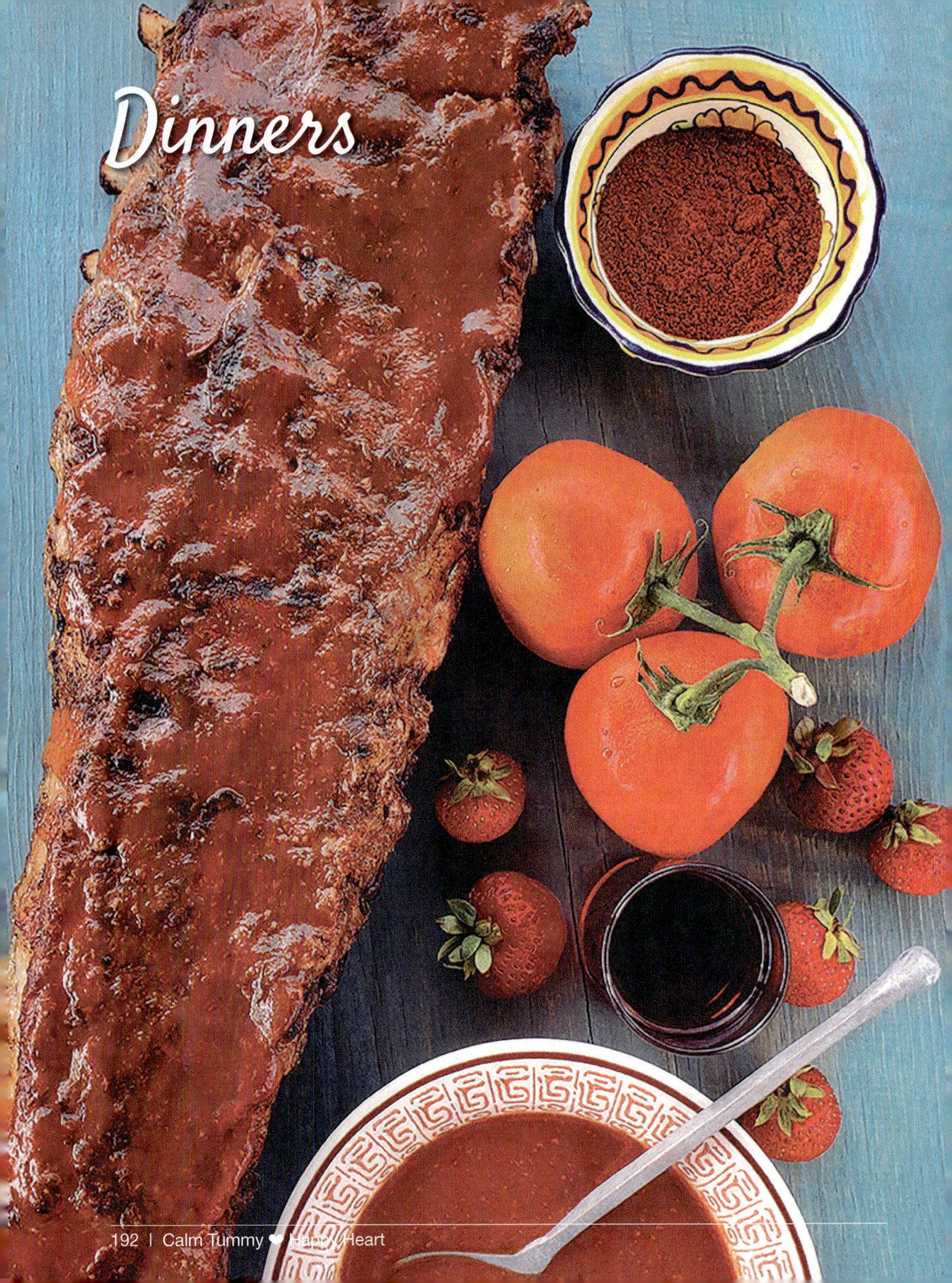

Dinners

- Grilled Rack of Ribs with Strawberry BBQ Sauce

- Steak Tampiquena

- Vegetarian Ranch House Pie

- Pollo Dorado with Lemon Poblano Sauce

- Mexican Lasagna

- Seafood Enchiladas

- Chicken Poblano Enchiladas

- Fajitas - Chicken, Beef or Shrimp

- Meatloaves with Cornmeal & Brown Sugar Glaze

- Pork Loin Medallions with Tornado Juice BBQ Sauce

- Chicken Tamales with Carrot Chive Dough & Green Chile Sauce

- Crispy Chicken Poblano Chiles Rellenos

Food brand names are sometimes listed within a recipe, and this means they are Monash Certified. For more brand options we use and love, please visit **FodifyIt.com**

Monash Note: Although chiles (chillies) are generally low in FODMAPs, some people with IBS may be sensitive to the capsaicin they contain. Capsaicin is a natural compound that gives chiles their spicy quality. You may need to limit how much chile you eat if your IBS symptoms are triggered by spicy food.

Grilled Rack of Ribs with Strawberry BBQ Sauce

LOW FODMAP ❤ IBS FRIENDLY ❤ GLUTEN-FREE ❤ DAIRY-FREE

When I was growing up, if anyone walked anywhere near our outdoor grill, my Pa would magically appear out of nowhere and ask "What's up? What are we grilling?" For years I watched him meticulously marinate, sear, char, smoke, rotate and sauce meats and vegetables. So it's no surprise that when I was sixteen years old, the first recipe I developed on my own was for bbq ribs.

This recipe is different from the honey-onion-garlic based sauce I first made, but it's equally flavorful. Shout out to Pa – he cleaned the grill after each gooey charred bbq test and I'll always be eternally grateful for that. Not to mention, that's why his grill is always spotless!

This recipe uses strawberries for fresh sweetness, with tangy red wine vinegar and mustard balanced by brown sugar and a kick of cayenne heat. By baking the ribs in the oven for 2 hours, tightly wrapped in foil, they become tender. A 10 minute finish on the grill, then dunked in sauce and you're ready for a sticky, delicious chow down!

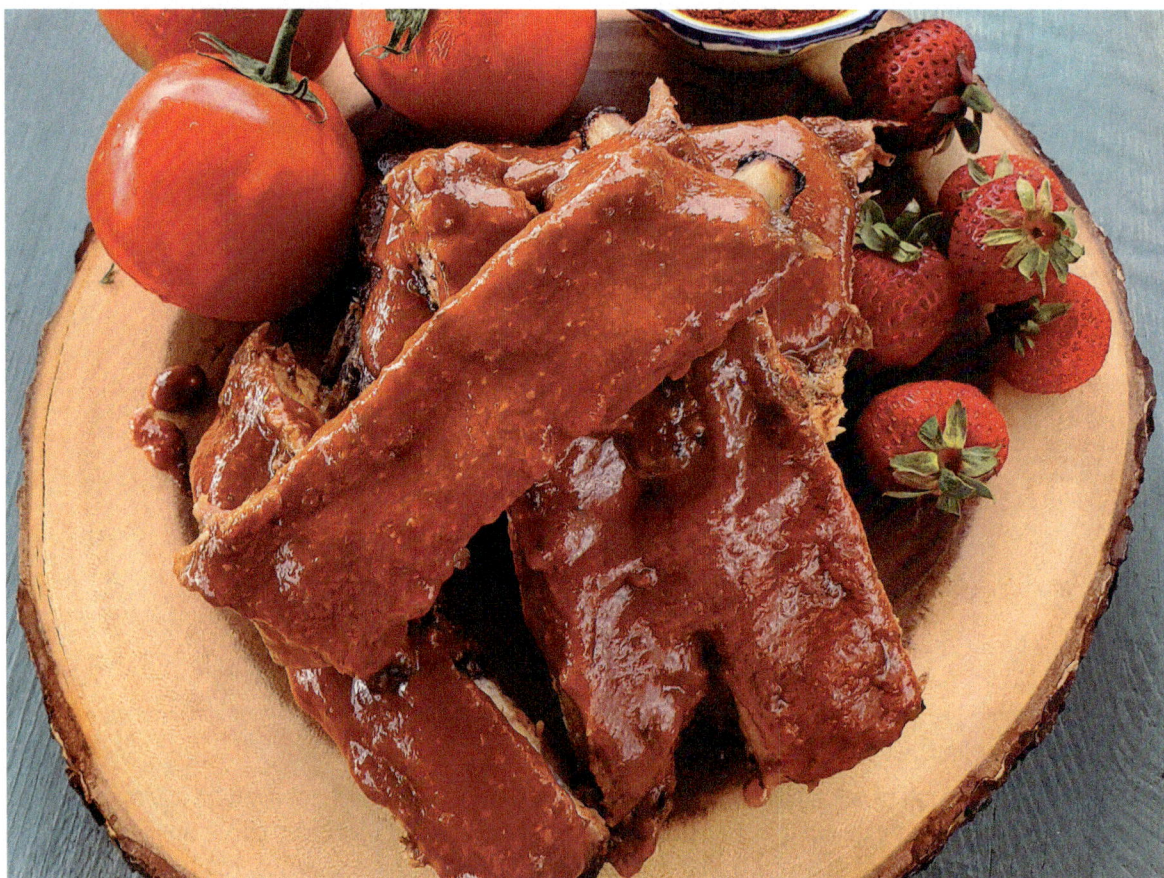

MAKES 4 SERVINGS
BBQ SAUCE INGREDIENTS (MAKES 2 CUPS 475 ML)

10 strawberries, sweet and ripe, hulled

1 cup (240 ml) canned plain tomato sauce

1/2 cup (80 g) medium packed light brown sugar

1/2 cup (120 ml) red wine vinegar

1/4 cup (55 g) plain, prepared yellow mustard, containing no onion or garlic

2 tablespoons (30 ml) Worcestershire sauce

2 tablespoons (30 g) tomato paste, containing no high fructose corn syrup or other high FODMAP ingredients

3 teaspoons (15 ml) unsulphured molasses

2 teaspoons (2 g) minced chives

1 teaspoon (2 g) smoked paprika

1 teaspoon (2 g) pure mild red chile powder (containing no onion or garlic, the ingredients should list only: red chile. On the Monash App this is called Chilli (chili) red, powdered)

1/2 teaspoon (1 g) cayenne, optional

RIBS INGREDIENTS

2 full racks (2 - 2.5-pounds each rack) (907 g – 1.14 kg each rack) pork ribs, silverskin removed (St. Louis cut are a favorite)

2 teaspoons (10 g) fine sea salt

2 teaspoons (4 g) fresh ground black pepper

Canola oil for greasing the grill grates

Method: Preheat oven to 350 F / 177 C

BBQ Sauce: Place all sauce ingredients in a blender and purée for 1 minute. Pour into a medium saucepan and bring to a low boil. Reduce to simmer, covered for 10 minutes. Stir occasionally. When the sauce thickens to coat the back of a spoon, remove from heat, cover and set aside.

Ribs: Place the racks meat side up on 2 foil-covered rimmed baking sheets. Sprinkle each rack with salt and pepper. Massage into the meat with your fingers. Spoon 2 tablespoons (30 ml) sauce on each rack and smooth evenly over the top of the ribs.

Cover tightly with foil and bake for 2 hours.

Heat your bbq grill to medium high. Using metal tongs and a paper towel doused with a bit of canola oil, grease the grates. Remove the ribs from the foil and place on the grates. Close the lid and grill for 5 minutes. Turn them over, close the lid and grill another 5 minutes. Place on a cutting board and using a sharp knife, slice into individual ribs for serving. Heat the bbq sauce over medium high heat. Dunk the ribs in the warm sauce. Serve immediately.

Tips: Baked potatoes and a nice leafy green salad with cucumber, grated carrot, and a splash of red wine vinegar and olive oil are perfect sides.

If you do not have a bbq grill, after baking the ribs for 2 hours remove the top foil wrap and use the broiler in your oven to hit them with a good brown char, about 2 -3 minutes per side. Then slice and dunk with warm sauce.

Monash Note: Although chiles (chillies) are generally low in FODMAPs, some people with IBS may be sensitive to the capsaicin they contain. Capsaicin is a natural compound that gives chiles their spicy quality. You may need to limit how much chile you eat if your IBS symptoms are triggered by spicy food.

Steak Tampiquena

LOW FODMAP ❤ IBS FRIENDLY ❤ GLUTEN-FREE ❤ DAIRY-FREE

Tampiquena recipes vary from region to region and this version is a favorite preparation inspired by an authentic Mexican restaurant we discovered in a tiny Southwestern Colorado town. It begins with marinating thin cut ribeye steaks, stuffing them with ham, Serrano chile and scallion greens, rolling them into logs and wrapping in bacon to grill. But it doesn't stop there. You then sauté plump shrimps to place on top of the stuffed steaks, along with Pico de Gallo and a Red Chile Sauce.

You will need to make New Mexican Red Chile sauce (page 62) for topping the steaks, so be sure to plan accordingly. Any remaining sauce may be served over plain scrambled eggs, salt and pepper grilled chicken grilled, or shrimp sautéed in olive oil with a dusting of salt and pepper.

MAKES 2 SERVINGS
PICO DE GALLO INGREDIENTS

1/2 medium (100 g) common tomato, diced

1 heaping tablespoon (2 g) fine chopped fresh cilantro leaves

2 scallions, green parts only, sliced thin

2 red radishes (20 g) diced

Juice of 1/4 lime

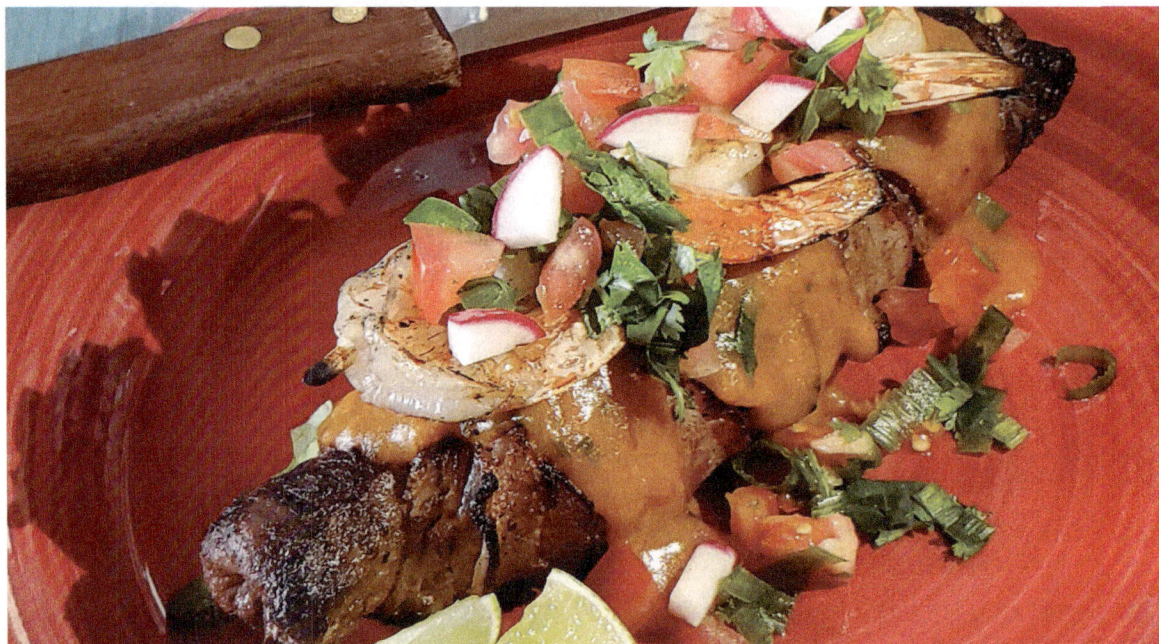

Monash Note: Although chiles (chillies) are generally low in FODMAPs, some people with IBS may be sensitive to the capsaicin they contain. Capsaicin is a natural compound that gives chiles their spicy quality. You may need to limit how much chile you eat if your IBS symptoms are triggered by spicy food.

SAUCE INGREDIENTS

See page 62 for Red Chile Sauce. You will need two servings.

STEAK INGREDIENTS

3 tablespoons (44 ml) Low FODMAP Garlic-Infused Oil (page 50), made with canola oil, divided

Juice of 1 lime

1 teaspoon (2 g) pure mild red chile powder (containing no onion or garlic, the ingredients should list only: red chile. On the Monash App this is called Chilli (chili) red, powdered)

1 teaspoon (5 g) fine sea salt

1/2 teaspoon fresh ground black pepper

2 thin cut boneless ribeye steaks (approx. 265 g each) wide cut to 6 x 9-inches (15 x 23 cm), or 2 boneless thick ribeyes pounded thin with a meat mallet to 6 x 9-inches (15 x 23 cm)

ROLL & GRILL INGREDIENTS

6 toothpicks, soaked in water for at least 10 minutes

6 thin slices (90 g total) low FODMAP ham, fresh deli sliced

1 fresh (28 g) Serrano chile; stem, seeds and ribs removed, cut into long matchsticks

2 scallions, green parts only, thin sliced

4 pieces bacon

SHRIMP INGREDIENTS

6 medium or jumbo shrimp, shelled and deveined, tails removed

A very light dusting of salt and fresh ground black pepper, 1/8 teaspoon each

Method

Pico de Gallo: Mix the ingredients in a small bowl and set aside.

Sauce: Make the Red Chile Sauce as instructed on page 62; 2 servings required.

Steaks: Mix 2 tablespoons oil, lime juice, chile powder, salt and pepper in a small bowl. Coat the steaks with the marinade and let infuse in a sealed plastic baggie for 30 minutes while also bringing the meat to room temperature. Dab off excess oil with a paper towel and place the steaks on a cutting board or work surface. Get ready to roll!

Roll and Grill: Place three slices of ham on each steak to cover as best you can. Divide the Serrano sticks and scallion greens into two portions and sprinkle evenly over the ham. Roll each steak into a log lengthwise. Using 2 pieces of bacon per, wrap them around the log to cover. Use toothpicks to secure the bacon.

Bring your bbq grill to medium high heat. Sear the logs 8 to 10 minutes, turning with metal tongs 1/4 of a turn each time to sear evenly. Reduce the heat to medium, close the grill lid and cook to desired doneness. Remove the toothpicks. Let rest on a plate tented with foil to keep warm.

Shrimp: Bring 1 tablespoon oil to medium heat in a small saucepan. Add the shrimp and lightly dust with salt and pepper. Stir with a spatula until they turn pink and are opaque and done inside.

Assembly: Place the rolled steaks on 2 plates. Top with 1 serving each of Red Chile Sauce. Place 3 shrimps on top of each, then sprinkle with the Pico de Gallo. Serve immediately with big steak knives.

Tips: If you do not have a bbq grill, the steak rolls can be pan cooked in canola oil.
If you are able to tolerate, roll 2 slices (40 g) Monterey Jack cheese with the steak fillings.

Suggested Sides: Cilantro Green Rice with Spinach & Lime (page 110), or a small salad of arugula or Romaine lettuce, common cucumber, shredded carrot and sliced radish with a dash of red wine vinegar and extra virgin olive oil.

Vegetarian Ranch House Pie

LOW FODMAP ❤ IBS FRIENDLY ❤ GLUTEN-FREE ❤ DAIRY-FREE

Ranch House Pie, also called shepherd's pie, is a favorite dish for folks who are up before dark, work outdoors tending chores for most of the day, and want a hearty meal to keep their energy up. I've revised my original beef recipe to a LoFO Meatless Monday version that is so flavorful, no one will miss the meat!

My original recipe contained lots of onion, garlic, green peas, beans, sweet corn, and the potato topping was blended with cheeses and heavy cream. This LoFO version replaces scallion greens for the onion, properly garlic-infused oil for chopped garlic cloves, tiny sliced green beans to resemble peas, lentils for the beans, and it's dairy-free.

Please note that 6 tablespoons (90 ml) Low FODMAP Garlic-Infused Oil (page 50) is required for this recipe, made with extra virgin olive oil and ready to use.

MAKES 8 SERVINGS
WHIPPED POTATO TOPPING INGREDIENTS

3 large (1140 g total) russet potatoes, peeled and 1/2-inch (1.25 cm) cubed

1 teaspoon (5 g) fine sea salt

3 tablespoons (45 ml) Low FODMAP Garlic-Infused Oil

1/2 cup (120 ml) plain, unsweetened almond milk

1/4 cup (60 ml) canned full-fat coconut milk for cooking, containing no inulin, well-stirred, plus up to 1/4 cup more if needed for a creamy smooth consistency

2 teaspoon (2 g) minced chives

1/2 teaspoon fresh ground black pepper

FILLING INGREDIENTS

2 tablespoons (30 ml) Low FODMAP Garlic-Infused Oil

5 (375 g total) carrots, peeled and cut into pea-sized cubes

2 medium (300 g total) parsnips, peeled and small diced

15 (75 g) fresh, trimmed green beans, cut into tiny pea-sized pieces

1/2 cup (25 g) thin sliced scallions, green parts only

1 cup (150 g) 1/2-inch(1.25 cm) diced, peeled zucchini

10-ounces (283 g) canned brown lentils, drained

8-ounces (227 g) canned plum tomatoes, drained and crushed, containing no garlic onion or other high FODMAP ingredients

1 cup (75 g) rough chopped oyster mushrooms (you will need to buy 2 cups (150 g) of mushrooms because the heavy stems are cut from the caps and discarded)

1 cup (240 ml) water

(continued on next page)

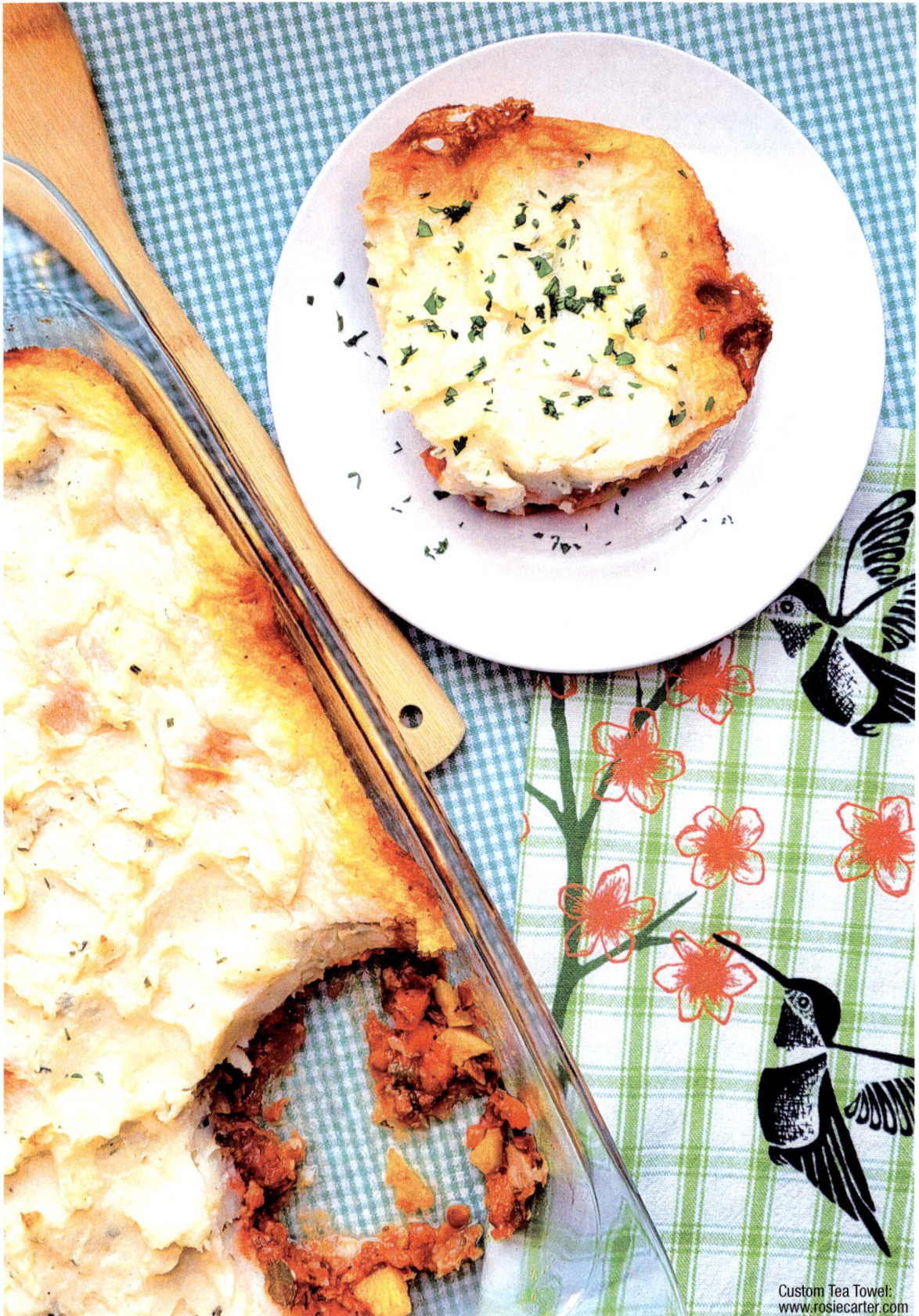

(continued from previous page)

2 tablespoons (30 ml) Worcestershire sauce

2 teaspoons (4 g) large flake nutritional yeast

2 teaspoons (4 g) pure mild red chile powder (containing no onion or garlic, the ingredients should list only: red chile. On the Monash App this is called Chilli (chili) red, powdered)

1 teaspoon (2 g) ground cumin

1/2 teaspoon (2.5 g) fine sea salt

1/2 teaspoon dried oregano

1/2 teaspoon fresh ground black pepper

3 tablespoons (45 ml) cold water

3 tablespoons (24 g) cornstarch, gluten-free if you are following a gluten-free diet

Method: Preheat the oven to 400 F / 200 C

Potato Topping: Bring 7 to 8 cups (1.7 - 2 L) of water to a rolling boil in a soup pot. Add the potatoes and 1 teaspoon salt. Reduce heat to medium high and boil for 15 minutes or until they are very tender. Drain well and spoon into a mixing bowl. Add 3 tablespoons (45 ml) garlic oil, the milks, chives, and pepper. Use a hand blender to whip until smooth. Taste to adjust for salt. Set aside.

Filling: Pour 2 tablespoons (30 ml) garlic oil into a large nonstick skillet over medium high heat. Add the parsnips, carrots, green beans and scallion greens. Cook for 4 to 6 minutes or until the carrots and parsnips are just tender, stirring often. Add the zucchini, lentils, tomatoes, mushrooms, water, Worcestershire, yeast and spices. Stir and cook at a low boil for 5 minutes until hot and bubbly. Mix the water and cornstarch to create a slurry in a small bowl, and add to the skillet. Stir for 2 minutes or until the filling is bubbly and thickened.

Assembly: Pour the filling into a greased 9 x 13-inch (23 x 33 cm) casserole dish. Spoon large scoops of the mashed potatoes over the filling and use the backside of a spoon to gently spread evenly to cover. Bake for 15 to 20 minutes or until it bubbles up around the edges and the potato topping just begins to brown. Serve immediately.

Tips: Adding 2-ounces (60 ml) of red wine to the filling offers an aromatic layer of flavor. A robust, Spanish Tempranillo made from black grapes goes very nicely with this dish.

A simple salad of shredded Romaine lettuce, sliced radishes and cucumber, and grated carrot with a splash of red wine vinegar and olive oil is a fresh side for this dish.

If you are able to tolerate, conventional or lactose-free whole milk may be used in place of the almond and coconut milks for the potato topping.

Just in case the filling should bubble over while baking, place a rimmed sheet pan covered with foil on the oven rack below the pie.

Monash Note: Although chiles (chillies) are generally low in FODMAPs, some people with IBS may be sensitive to the capsaicin they contain. Capsaicin is a natural compound that gives chiles their spicy quality. You may need to limit how much chile you eat if your IBS symptoms are triggered by spicy food.

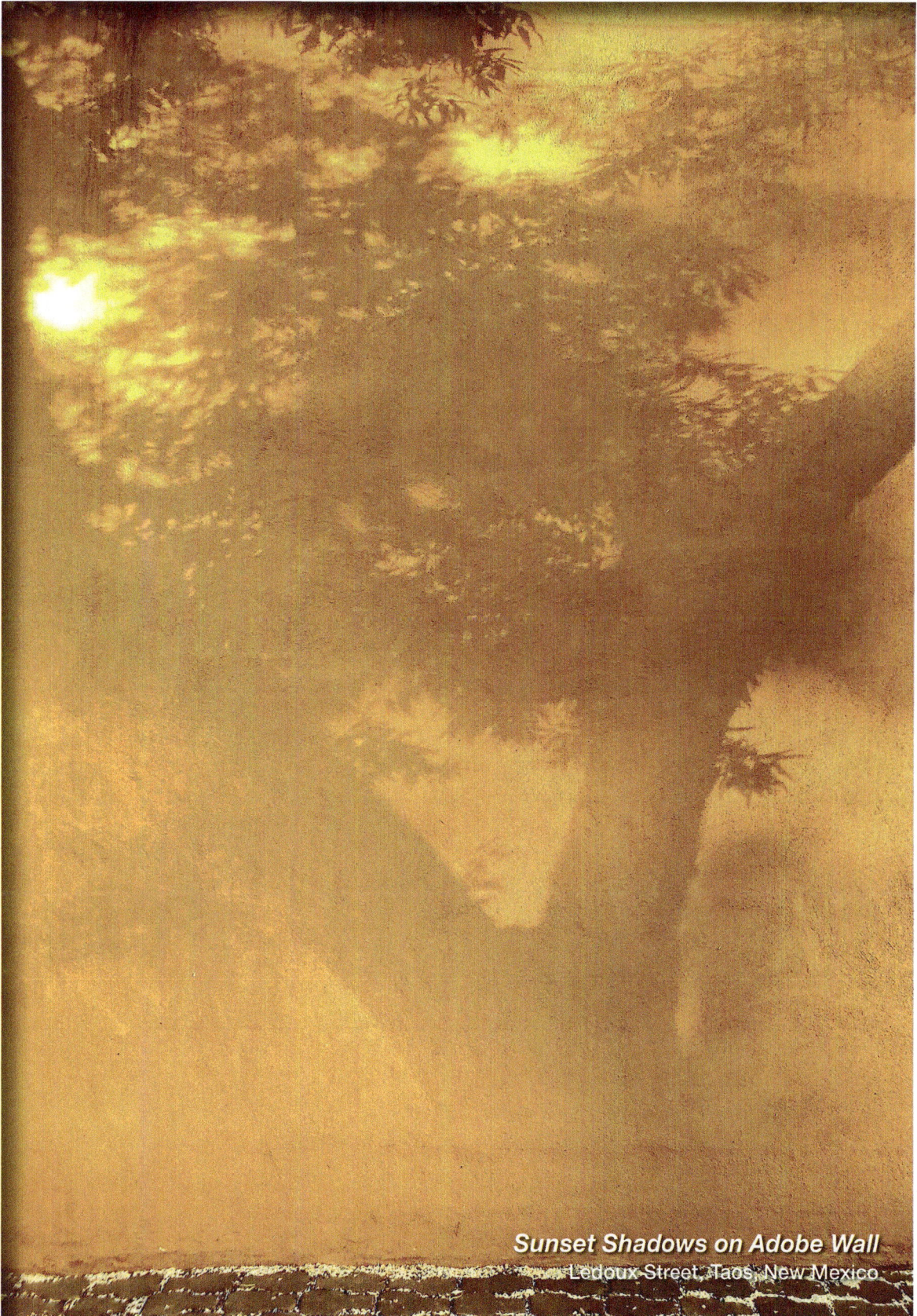

Sunset Shadows on Adobe Wall
Ledoux Street, Taos, New Mexico

Pollo Dorado
with Lemon Poblano Sauce

LOW FODMAP ❤ IBS FRIENDLY ❤ GLUTEN-FREE ❤ DAIRY-FREE

How do you make the ultimate golden not-fried fried chicken fillets ever? By coating them in corn tortilla chips! Not only do they serve up a gorgeous warm color, the flavor is delicious earthy maize (corn) with crunch!

Spooning Lemon Poblano Sauce onto a plate and topping it with a crispy chicken fillet is a fantastic pairing with the herb-y chile pepper, citrus and little hit of heat (depending on your poblanos). This dish is a perfect dinner for two.

The poblanos will need roasting and prepping to remove the skins, stems and seeds so be sure to plan accordingly.

MAKES 2 SERVINGS

LEMON POBLANO SAUCE INGREDIENTS

2 tablespoons (27 g) Low FODMAP Garlic-Infused Oil (page 50), made with canola oil

2 medium (97 g each) fresh poblano peppers, roasted and prepped as instructed on page 46, will yield approx. 1/2 cup (90 g) of chile meat, rough chopped

1/3 cup (6 g) fresh, medium packed cilantro leaves, some stems are okay

4 scallions, green parts only, rough chopped

1/4 cup (59 ml) unsweetened, plain almond milk

2 tablespoons (36 g) plain dairy-free, unsweetened coconut yogurt

Juice of 1 lemon

1/2 teaspoon (1 g) ground cumin

1/4 scant teaspoon (1 g) fine sea salt

1/4 scant teaspoon fresh ground black pepper

CHICKEN INGREDIENTS

2 chicken breasts (550 g total), boneless skinless

1/2 cup (74 g) low FODMAP gluten-free all-purpose baking flour, containing xanthan gum (page 55 for description)

1 teaspoon (5 g) fine sea salt

1/2 teaspoon fresh ground black pepper

1 large egg

25 (75 g) regular style corn tortilla chips, gluten-free, blended into coarse crumbs in a food processor (makes approx. 1-cup)

3 tablespoons (45 ml) canola oil

Cooking spray oil

Fresh cilantro, finely chopped for garnish

Method

Sauce: Use a medium nonstick skillet to make the garlic infused oil as instructed on page 50. Once the garlic bits are removed, leave the oil in the pan off heat.

Place the poblano meat, cilantro, scallion greens, almond milk, yogurt, lemon juice, cumin, salt and pepper into a blender. Purée for 1 minute until smooth with tiny bits of herbs showing. Place the skillet with oil over medium heat. Pour in the sauce and stir until warm and just bubbly. Remove from heat and cover with a lid to keep warm.

Chicken: Preheat oven to 425 F / 220 C

Butterfly the chicken by placing your hand flat on top of one breast and cut into the side lengthwise to divide in half, stopping at 1-inch (2.5 cm) before slicing all the way through. Open the fillet flat and it will be heart-shaped. Repeat for the second breast. Cut away any fatty pieces. Make sure your knife is nice and sharp, otherwise the meat will shred as you slice into it (speaking from experience here).

Set up your dredging station in 3 shallow bowls or pie pans as follows:

1 – Mix the flour with salt and pepper in the first pan and whisk to mix.

2 – Beat the egg in the second pan.

3 – Pour the tortilla chip crumbs into the last pan.

First, dredge the breast in the flour to coat completely. Shake off any excess. Then dredge in the beaten egg, again covering completely. Finally, coat in the chip crumbs using your hands to push the crumbs into the breast for maximum coverage. Repeat for second breast.

Grease a small, rimmed baking sheet with canola oil. Place the chicken on the pan and coat the tops lightly with cooking spray oil.

Bake for 10 minutes. Flip with a spatula. Bake 10 minutes longer until golden crisp and done, showing no pink in the centers. Timing will vary according to the thickness and temperature of your chicken.

If the sauce has cooled, place it over medium high heat until it's just bubbly and warmed through.

Assembly: Pour half of the sauce onto a dinner plate. Top with a golden chicken breast. Sprinkle with cilantro. Repeat for the second plate. Serve immediately.

A tasty side for this dish is a serving of Cilantro Green Rice with Spinach & Lime (page 110).

Tips: These golden chicken fillets also make great sandwiches. Or, slice them into strips to serve over a salad.

For the sauce, the dairy-free yogurt I prefer has a creamy coconut base that gives only the slightest hint of coconut flavor. If you are able to tolerate, use a lactose-free or conventional cow's milk plain yogurt.

Monash Note: Although chiles (chillies) are generally low in FODMAPs, some people with IBS may be sensitive to the capsaicin they contain. Capsaicin is a natural compound that gives chiles their spicy quality. You may need to limit how much chile you eat if your IBS symptoms are triggered by spicy food.

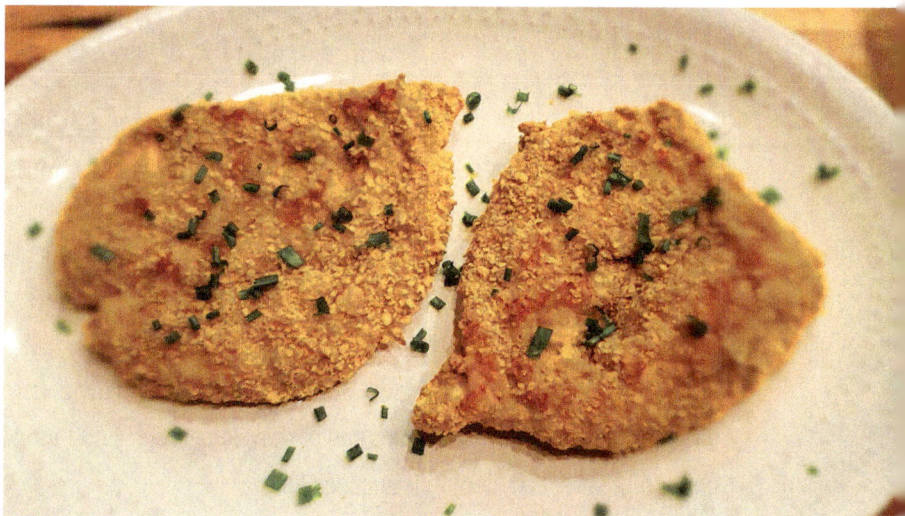

Mexican Lasagna

LOW FODMAP ❤ IBS FRIENDLY ❤ GLUTEN-FREE ❤ DAIRY-FREE

Also known as taco casserole because it incorporates taco ingredients into layers of perfect bites, this recipe offers robust flavors for lunch, dinner or for a bring-a-dish event.

Lasagna noodles are swapped out with yellow corn tortillas, white onion is subbed with scallion greens, and a silky LoFO Béchamel Sauce (page 65) with chopped green chiles and large flake nutritional yeast replaces the cheese. The grated carrot and fresh toppings add a cool salad to balance this hot, savory dish.

You will need to make the Béchamel Sauce first - the full recipe amount.

This lasagne has been known to instantaneously disappear so be sure to get your serving!

MAKES 8 SERVINGS
BÉCHAMEL LAYER INGREDIENTS

Béchamel Sauce, ready to use, hot

2, 4-ounce cans (226 g) mild chopped green chiles (containing no onion, garlic or other high FODMAP ingredients. On the Monash App they are noted as Chilli (chili) green, mild, chopped, canned)

BEEF LAYER INGREDIENTS

2-pounds (907 g) 80/20 ground beef, grass fed if available

3 teaspoons (6 g) ground cumin

1 1/2 teaspoons (7 g) fine sea salt

1 teaspoon (2 g) pure mild red chile powder (containing no onion or garlic, the ingredients should list only: red chile. On the Monash App this is called Chilli (chili) red, powdered)

1 teaspoon (2 g) smoked paprika, optional

1 teaspoon dried oregano

1/2 teaspoon fresh ground black pepper

1/2 teaspoon cayenne, optional

PEPPER & TOMATO LAYER INGREDIENTS

2 tablespoons (30 ml) Low FODMAP Garlic-Infused Oil (page 50), made with extra virgin olive oil

1 large (164 g) fresh red bell pepper, stemmed, seeds and ribs removed, diced

1/2 cup (25 g) thin sliced scallions, green parts only

1 can (14.5-ounce / 411 g) whole peeled Roma tomatoes, chopped small, plus 1/4 cup (60 ml) of the can juices

ADDITIONAL INGREDIENTS

18 (450 g total) 6-inch (15 cm) low FODMAP gluten-free yellow corn tortillas

2 large (200 g total) carrots, peeled and grated, (reserve 1/4 cup for garnish topping)

1 cup (75 g) shredded iceberg lettuce, chilled

1/2 cup (90 g) canned, pitted ripe black olives, sliced

1/4 cup (4 g) medium packed fresh cilantro, mostly leaves, rough chopped

Method: Heat the oven to 350 F / 177 C

Béchamel Sauce: Stir the chiles into Béchamel Sauce; set aside, covered; keep warm.

Beef Layer: Place the beef in a large nonstick skillet over medium high heat. Use a wooden spatula to brown and break up the beef into crumbles as best you can. Drain. Return the beef to the pan. Add the cumin, salt, red chile powder, paprika, oregano, pepper and cayenne. Sauté on medium high for 1 minute to fully incorporate the spices. Spoon the beef into a bowl and set aside.

Pepper & Tomato: In the same skillet, pour in 2 tablespoons (30 ml) of oil over medium high heat. Add the red bell, scallion greens, chopped tomatoes and tomato juices. Cook uncovered at medium high heat until the liquids evaporate and the pepper is tender, stirring often; set aside.

Assembly: Coat a 9 x 13 inch (23 x 33 cm) casserole with cooking spray oil. Line the bottom with 6 tortillas, overlapping as needed. Evenly spread 1/2 of the beef over the tortillas. Spoon 1/2 of the pepper & tomato mixture over the beef, then 1/3 of the green chile béchamel. Spread each layer evenly with a spatula as best you can. Sprinkle with half of the grated carrots. Repeat for the next layering.

Place the remaining 6 tortillas over the top and spread the remaining 1/3 béchamel over them to completely coat.

Cover with foil and bake 25 minutes until bubbly and warmed through. Remove from the oven and let rest for 10 minutes, covered.

Top with lettuce, black olives, cilantro and remaining grated carrot.

Tip: If you are able to tolerate, layer in and top with 2 cups (200 g) shredded cheddar or Monterey Jack cheese.

Monash Note: Although chiles (chillies) are generally low in FODMAPs, some people with IBS may be sensitive to the capsaicin they contain. Capsaicin is a natural compound that gives chiles their spicy quality. You may need to limit how much chile you eat if your IBS symptoms are triggered by spicy food.

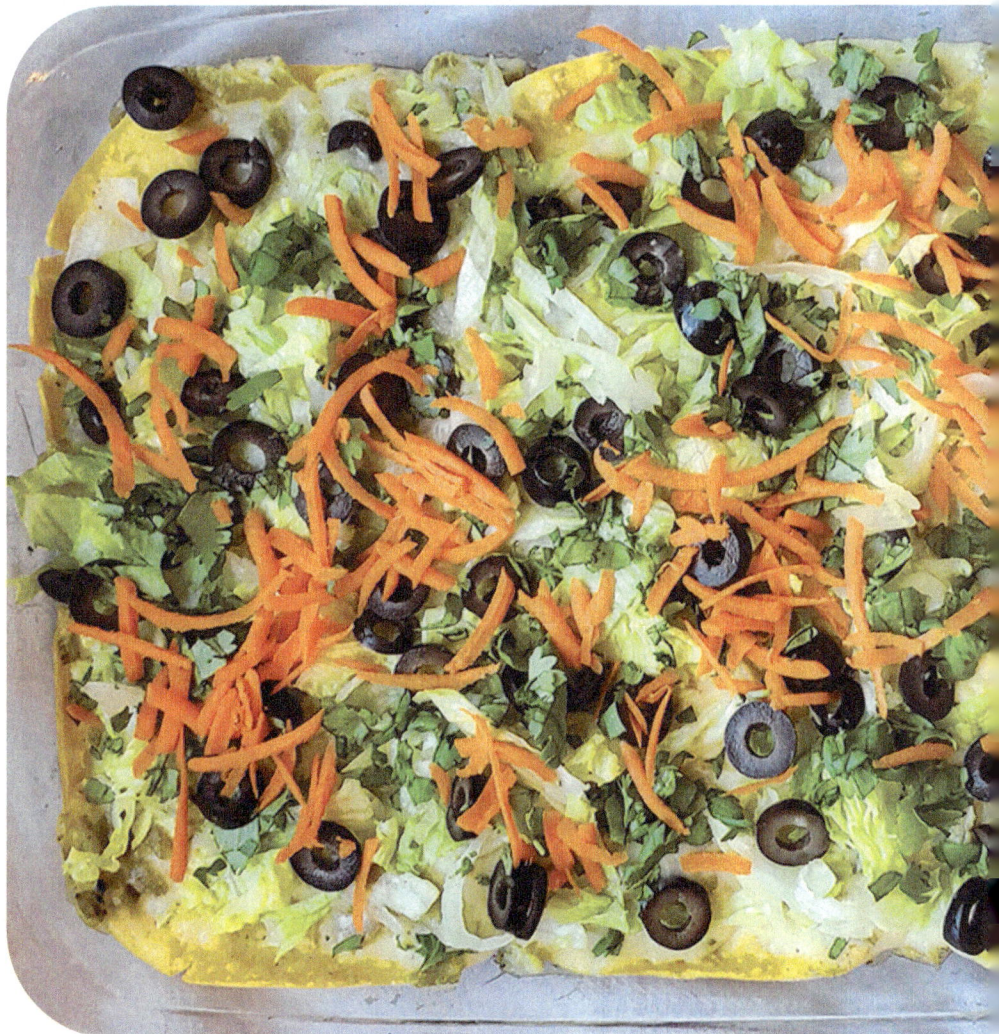

Seafood Enchiladas

LOW FODMAP ❤ IBS FRIENDLY ❤ GLUTEN-FREE ❤ DAIRY-FREE

What's not to love about corn tortillas rolled with a creamy seafood filling and topped with an enhanced, silky Béchamel Sauce? You will need to make a full batch of the Béchamel Sauce first (page 65). And keep in mind that while enchiladas require several steps to prepare, once you start assembling it's actually a simple dish to make.

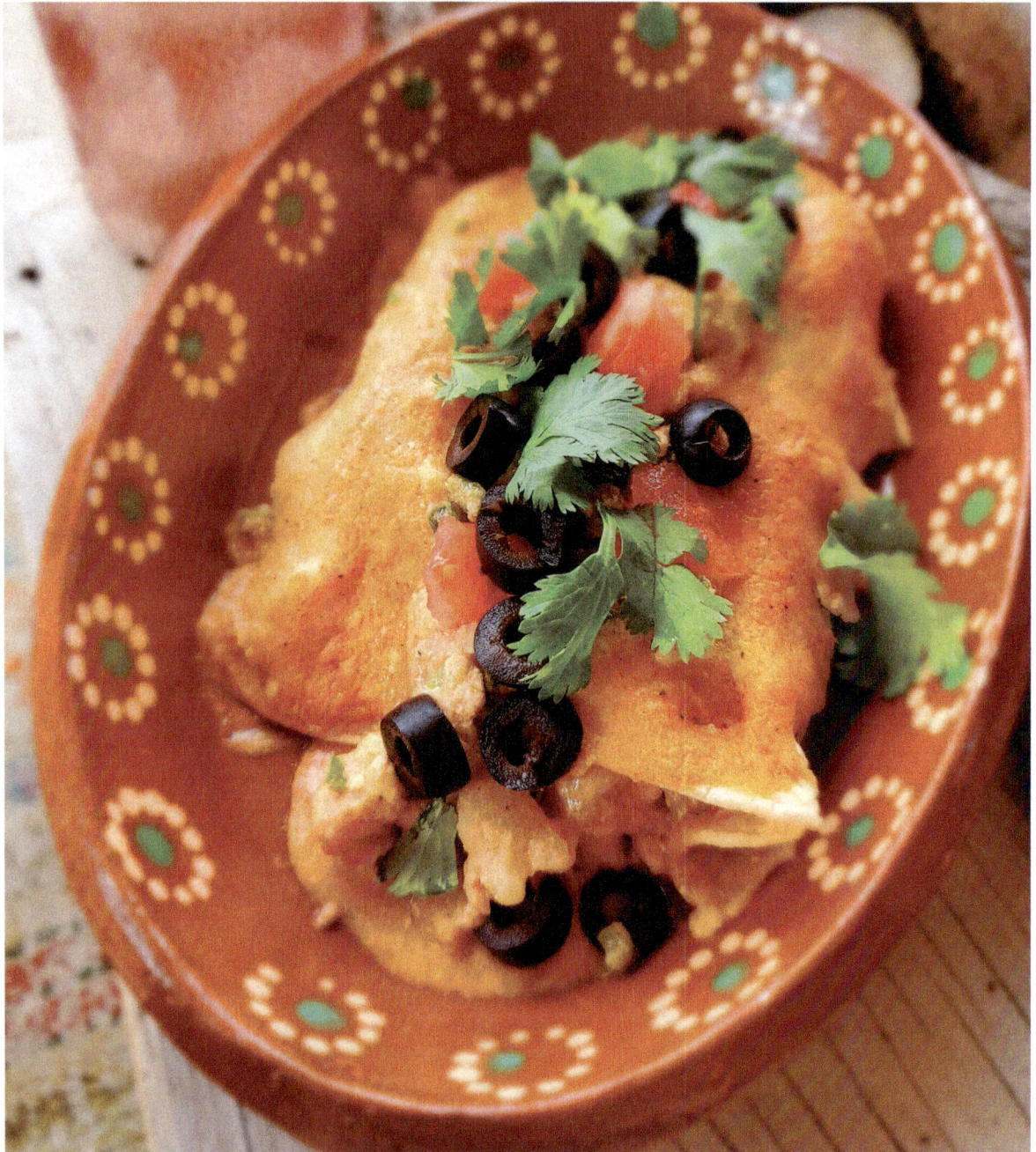

MAKES 6 SERVINGS
BÉCHAMEL SAUCE INGREDIENTS

1 batch Béchamel Sauce With Gluten-Free Roux (page 65)

1/4 cup (72 g) plain dairy-free, unsweetened coconut yogurt

1 small (28 g) Serrano pepper, stemmed seeded and minced

2 tablespoons (30 g) tomato paste, containing no high fructose corn syrup or other high FODMAP ingredients

1/2 teaspoon (1 g) pure mild red chile powder (containing no onion or garlic, the ingredients should list only: red chile. On the Monash App this is called Chilli (chili) red, powdered)

2 tablespoons (30 ml) dry white wine

FILLING INGREDIENTS

2 tablespoons (30 ml) Low FODMAP Garlic-Infused Oil (page 50), made with extra virgin olive oil

1/4 cup (13 g) thin sliced scallions, green parts only, minced

3 small (75 g total) Serrano peppers, stemmed seeded and minced

1/2-pound (227 g) raw medium shrimp, shelled deveined and tails removed, rough chopped

2 skinless salmon fillets (8-ounces / 227 g total) checked for bones and cut into 1/2–inch (1.25 cm) cubes

8-ounces (227 g) large sea scallops, rinsed under cool water and patted dry, sliced into 1/2-inch (1.25 cm) pieces

1/2 teaspoon (1 g) ground cumin

1/2 teaspoon(1 g) pure mild red chile powder (containing no onion or garlic, the ingredients should list only: red chile. On the Monash App this is called Chilli (chili) red, powdered)

1/2 teaspoon (2.5 g) fine sea salt

1/4 teaspoon fresh ground black pepper

1/4 cup (72 g) plain dairy-free, unsweetened coconut yogurt

1 medium (238 g) common tomato, cored and diced

1 cup (16 g) medium packed fresh cilantro, mostly leaves, rough chopped, divided

Juice of 1 lime

ADDITIONAL INGREDIENTS

12, 6-inch (15 cm) (25 g each) low FODMAP gluten-free white or yellow corn tortillas

2 tablespoons (30 ml) canola oil, plus more as needed

1/2 medium (120 g) common tomato, diced

15 (60 g) canned, pitted ripe black olives, sliced

Shredded Romaine lettuce

(continued on the next page)

(continued from previous page)

Method:

Béchamel: Prepare the sauce and stir in the yogurt, Serrano, tomato paste, chile powder and wine. Set aside, covered.

Filling: Pour 2 tablespoons (30 ml) oil into a large nonstick skillet over medium high heat. Add the scallion greens, minced Serrano and sauté for 2 minutes. Reduce heat to medium.

Add the shrimp and gently stir for 3 minutes. Add the salmon and stir for 3 minutes. Gently fold in the scallops. Add the cumin, chile powder, salt, pepper, yogurt, diced tomato and 1/2 cup (8 g) cilantro. Fold and cook for 2 minutes. The seafood should be par-cooked, as it will finish in the final baking step. Remove from heat and stir in the lime juice. Set aside.

Tortillas: To warm the tortillas, pour 2 teaspoons (30 ml) canola oil into a large nonstick skillet over medium high heat. Add the tortillas to the pan (as many that will fit without overlapping) and cook them for 5 seconds. Flip and cook 5 seconds more. Warm them in batches, adding more oil as needed. Stack them in a tortilla warmer or wrapped foil as you go.

Preheat oven to 400 F / 200 C

Generously grease a 9 x 13 inch (23 x 33 cm) baking dish with cooking spray oil.

Assembly: Divide the seafood filling into 12 portions by creating 6 sections in the bowl and scooping one half of that section for each tortilla. Lay one tortilla flat on a work surface and place the filling down the center. Roll the enchilada and place seam side down in the baking dish. Repeat for the remaining. If you have leftover filling, spoon it on top of the enchiladas. Pour the Béchamel Sauce over to fully cover all 12 from end to end. Use the back of a spoon to evenly spread.

Bake for 10 to 15 minutes or until heated through.

Garnish the top with diced tomato, black olives, 1/2 cup (8 g) cilantro, and lettuce. Serve immediately, 2 enchiladas per person.

Tip: If you are able to tolerate dairy, evenly distribute 1 1/2 cups (150 g) shredded Monterey Jack cheese on top of the enchiladas before baking. Per your tolerance, the plain, dairy-free, unsweetened coconut yogurt may be subbed with lactose-free or conventional yogurt or sour cream.

Monash Note: Although chiles (chillies) are generally low in FODMAPs, some people with IBS may be sensitive to the capsaicin they contain. Capsaicin is a natural compound that gives chiles their spicy quality. You may need to limit how much chile you eat if your IBS symptoms are triggered by spicy food.

Chicken Poblano Enchiladas

LOW FODMAP ♥ IBS FRIENDLY ♥ GLUTEN-FREE ♥ DAIRY-FREE

Succulent chicken mixed with spices and a creamy Béchamel Sauce, rolled in corn tortillas and covered in a luscious green poblano chile sauce with garden fresh toppings - this is comfort food to the max!

For this recipe, I suggest that you make a Whole Poached Chicken (page 82) that takes a little over an hour to cook, cool and shred. The chicken will also yield a delicious, robust stock for freezing in portions to thaw as needed. When short on time, use a plain store-bought rotisserie chicken to shred and use the meat.

For the Poblano Sauce, the peppers will need roasting and steaming to remove the skins, stem and seeds, in which case plan ahead for cooking that component.

MAKES 6 SERVINGS
BÉCHAMEL SAUCE INGREDIENTS

2 cups (475 ml) Béchamel Sauce With Gluten-Free Roux (page 65), ready to use and hot

CHICKEN INGREDIENTS

2 1/2 cups (375 g) cooked chicken, shredded, ready to use

1 cup (50 g) thin sliced scallions, green parts only

2 teaspoons (4 g) ground cumin

1/2 teaspoon (2.5 g) fine sea salt, or none if your rotisserie chicken is salted

1/2 teaspoon fresh ground black pepper

POBLANO SAUCE INGREDIENTS

2 tablespoons (30 ml) Low FODMAP Garlic-Infused Oil (page 50), made with extra virgin olive oil, or plain olive oil is also fine

4 medium (97 g each) fresh poblano peppers, roasted and prepped (page 46), chopped fine, to yield approx 1 cup (180 g) of chile meat

1 small (119 g) common tomato, diced

1/2 cup (25 g) thin sliced scallions, green parts only

1 teaspoon (2 g) ground cumin

1 teaspoon (2 g) pure mild red chile powder (containing no onion or garlic, the ingredients should list only: red chile. On the Monash App this is called Chilli (chili) red, powdered)

3/4 cup (180 ml) LoFO chicken stock (page 135), or use the stock from the poached chicken recipe

1/2 cup (8 g) medium packed fresh cilantro, mostly leaves, finely chopped

1/4 teaspoon fine sea salt

1/4 teaspoon fresh ground back pepper

(continued on next page)

(continued from previous page)

ADDITIONAL INGREDIENTS

12, 6-inch (15 cm) (25 g each) low FODMAP gluten-free white or yellow corn tortillas (yellow are more sturdy)

1 cup (75 g) shredded lettuce, chilled

1/2 cup (8 g) medium packed fresh cilantro leaves

1/2 cup (60 g) common tomato, diced

5 (50 g total) red radishes, sliced thin

15 (60 g) canned, pitted ripe black olives, sliced

Method

Chicken: In a bowl, sprinkle the shredded chicken evenly with the scallions greens, cumin, salt, and pepper. Stir and toss to coat. Add the béchamel and gently stir to combine. Cover and set aside.

Poblano Sauce: Pour the oil into a medium nonstick skillet over medium high heat. Add the chopped poblano chile meat, diced tomato, and scallion greens. Sauté for 2 minutes. Add the cumin, red chile powder, stock, cilantro, salt and pepper. Stir and cook 2 minutes. Remove from heat. Carefully spoon or pour into a blender. Cover the lid with a clean, heavy kitchen towel to avoid splatters. Purée until smooth. Set aside, covered to keep warm.

Tortillas: To warm the tortillas, heat 2 teaspoons (10 ml) canola oil in a large nonstick skillet to medium high. Add the tortillas to the pan (as many that will fit without overlapping) and cook them for 5 seconds. Flip and cook 5 seconds more. This step is for just warming them enough to roll the enchiladas without breaking. Warm them in batches, adding more oil as needed. Stack them in a tortilla warmer or wrapped in foil as you go.

Generously grease a 9 x 13-inch (23 x 33 cm) baking dish with cooking spray oil.

Preheat oven to 375 F / 190 C

Assembly: Spread 3 tablespoons (45 ml) poblano sauce on the bottom of the dish.

Scoop the chicken filling into 12 equal sized portions (approx. 1/4 cup each) on a cutting board or work surface. Lay one tortilla flat and spoon 1 portion of the filling down the center. Roll the enchilada and place seam side down in the baking dish. Repeat for the remaining enchiladas. Pour the poblano sauce over to fully cover all 12 from end to end, using the back of a spoon to evenly spread.

Bake 12 to 15 minutes or until warmed through.

Garnish the top with lettuce, cilantro, diced tomato, radishes and black olives. Serve immediately, 2 enchiladas per person.

Tip: If you are able to tolerate, add 1 cup (100 g) shredded cheddar or Monterey Jack cheese to the chicken filling, and sprinkle the top of the enchiladas with 1/2 cup more (50 g) before baking.

Monash Note: Although chiles (chillies) are generally low in FODMAPs, some people with IBS may be sensitive to the capsaicin they contain. Capsaicin is a natural compound that gives chiles their spicy quality. You may need to limit how much chile you eat if your IBS symptoms are triggered by spicy food.

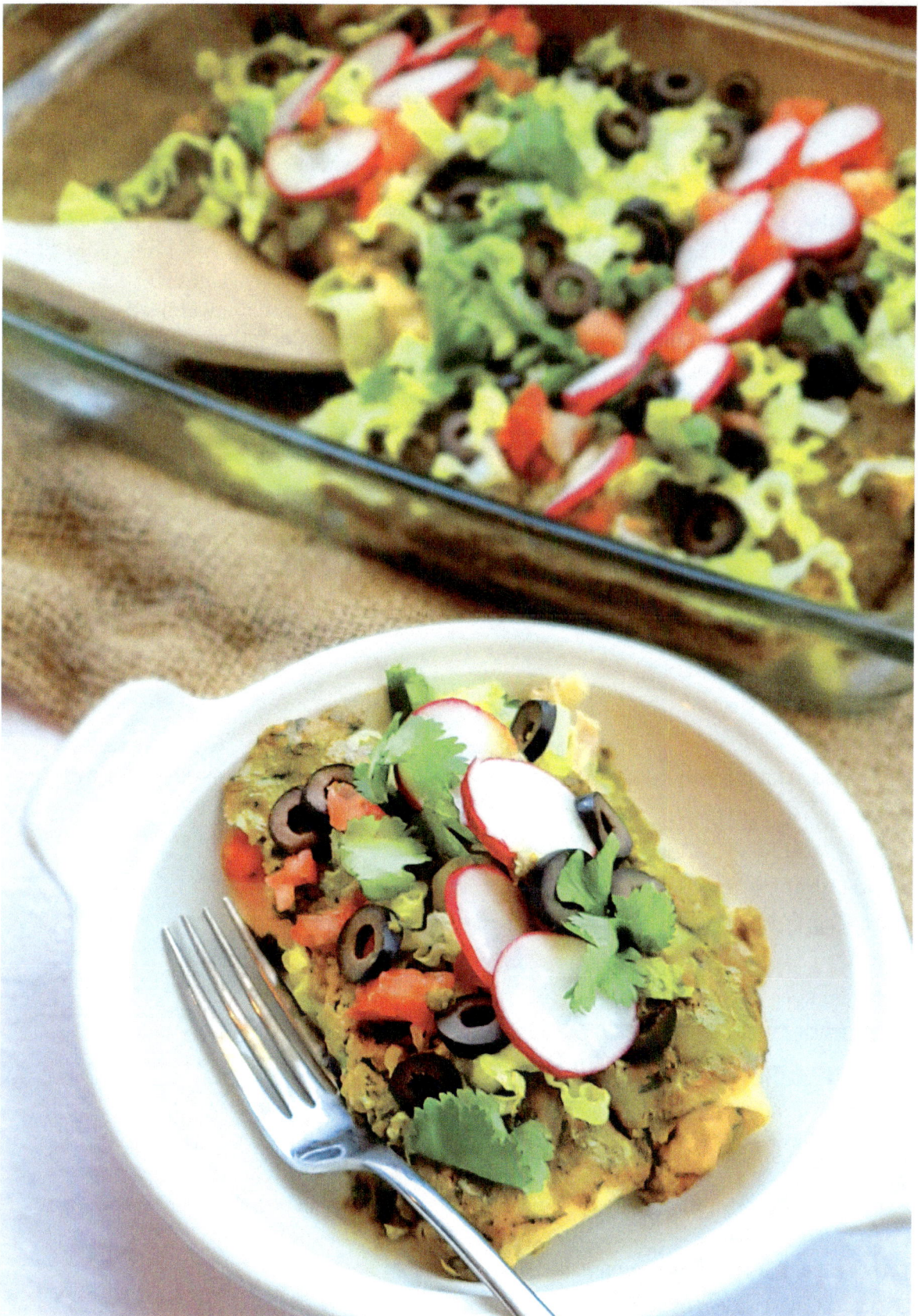

Fajitas - Chicken, Beef or Shrimp

LOW FODMAP ♥ IBS FRIENDLY ♥ GLUTEN-FREE ♥ DAIRY-FREE

Fajitas are fun because everyone gets to choose their fillings and assemble them as they like! This recipe of citrus and spice marinated chicken with thin sliced peppers (rajas) is easy to convert into LoFO. The main swaps are to use scallion greens in place of white onions, white corn tortillas instead of flour tortillas, and proper amounts of peppers. Marinating your protein of choice is also a cinch, as the ingredients are the same for beef, chicken and shrimp (see the Tips section). Cilantro Green Rice with Spinach & Lime (page 110) is a nice side dish for fajitas.

Please note that you will need approx. 6 tablespoons (90 ml) of Low FODMAP Garlic-Infused Oil for this recipe (page 50), made with canola oil and ready to use.

MAKES 8 SERVINGS
MARINADE & CHICKEN INGREDIENTS

3 tablespoons (45 ml) Low FODMAP Garlic-Infused Oil

Juice of 2 limes

1 teaspoon (2 g) ground cumin

1 teaspoon (2 g) pure chipotle powder

1 teaspoon (5 g) fine sea salt

1/2 teaspoon fresh ground

black pepper

2 1/2-pounds (1134 g) boneless skinless chicken breasts, sliced lengthwise into scant 1/2-inch (1.25 cm) thin strips

TOPPING INGREDIENTS

Juice of 1 lime

3 small (225 g total) fresh plum tomatoes, cored and diced

1/2 cup (8 g) fresh medium packed cilantro, rough chopped

TORTILLA INGREDIENTS

Cooking spray oil

16 (25 g each) 6-inch (15 cm) low FODMAP gluten-free white corn tortillas

PEPPER INGREDIENTS

2 tablespoons (30 ml) Low FODMAP Garlic-Infused Oil (page 50), plus a bit more if needed

2 large (325 g total) fresh green bell peppers, stemmed, seeds and ribs removed, sliced into scant 1/2-inch (1.25 cm) strips

2 medium (235 g total) fresh red bell peppers, stemmed, core and ribs removed, sliced into scant 1/2-inch (1.25 cm) strips

1/4 cup (13 g) thin sliced scallions, green parts only

2 limes, cut into 8 wedges each

(continued on the next page)

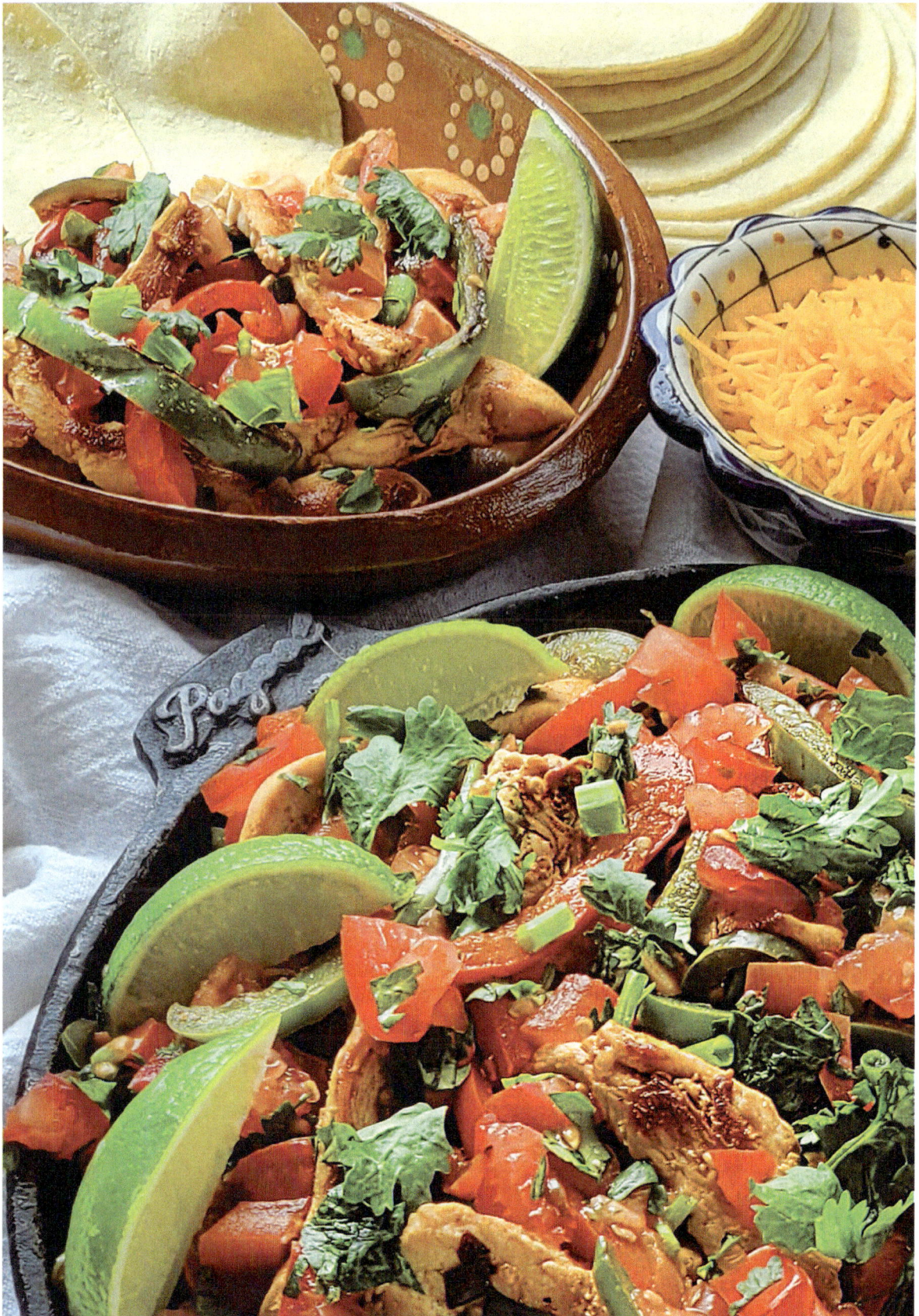

(continued from previous page)

Method

Chicken: Mix the marinade ingredients in a large plastic baggie and add the chicken strips. Seal the baggie and move the chicken around with your hands to massage and coat. Allow to infuse for 20 minutes.

Topping: Mix the topping ingredients in a small bowl and chill in the fridge until ready to plate.

Tortillas: Coat a large nonstick skillet lightly with cooking oil spray. Over medium high heat, and add 3 to 4 tortillas (or as many that will fit into the pan). Warm them for 30 seconds, flip and warm another 30 seconds. Wrap them in a heavy clean kitchen towel, in foil or place in a tortilla warmer as you go. Repeat for the remaining tortillas. Set aside.

Cooking the Chicken and Peppers: Pour 2 tablespoon (30 ml) infused oil into a large heavy bottom nonstick skillet over medium high heat. Add the chicken and using a spatula, turn and stir around the pan to fry for 6 to 8 minutes or until they are just caramel brown and no longer pink in the middle. Move the chicken to a plate, cover with foil to keep warm.

Add 2 tablespoons (30 ml) oil to the same pan over medium high heat. Add the sliced peppers. Let them sear undisturbed for 2 minutes. Use a spatula to stir and flip for 6 minutes or until char blistered to your taste. Add the scallion greens.

Add the chicken back into the pan with the peppers and stir to re-heat. Remove from heat and sprinkle with the topping mixture.

Assembly Family Style: Arrange lime wedges around the edge of the pan. Bring to the table and place on a trivet or hot pad, with a large serving spoon for scooping. Pass the warm tortillas around, 2 per serving.

Tips: If tolerated, offer 1 cup (100 g) lactose-free or conventional sour cream, and 1 cup (100 g) shredded cheddar in bowls on the table to pass around.

If you are sensitive to pepper skins, see page 46 for steps on roasting and removing the skins before searing.

BEEF FAJITAS 1, 2 1/2-pounds (1134 g) flank or strip steak. Marinate the steak for 45 minutes using the same ingredients used for the chicken. Pan cook or grill 7 to 8 minutes each side on medium high heat, or to your preferred doneness. Let rest on a cutting board for 10 minutes. Using a sharp knife, cut into thin slices against the grain.

SHRIMP FAJITAS 2 1/2-pounds (1134 g) medium shrimp, shells and tails removed, deveined. Rinse under cool water. Marinate 20 minutes. When cooking, stir them until they turn pink and are opaque in the center.

Monash Note: Although chiles (chillies) are generally low in FODMAPs, some people with IBS may be sensitive to the capsaicin they contain. Capsaicin is a natural compound that gives chiles their spicy quality. You may need to limit how much chile you eat if your IBS symptoms are triggered by spicy food.

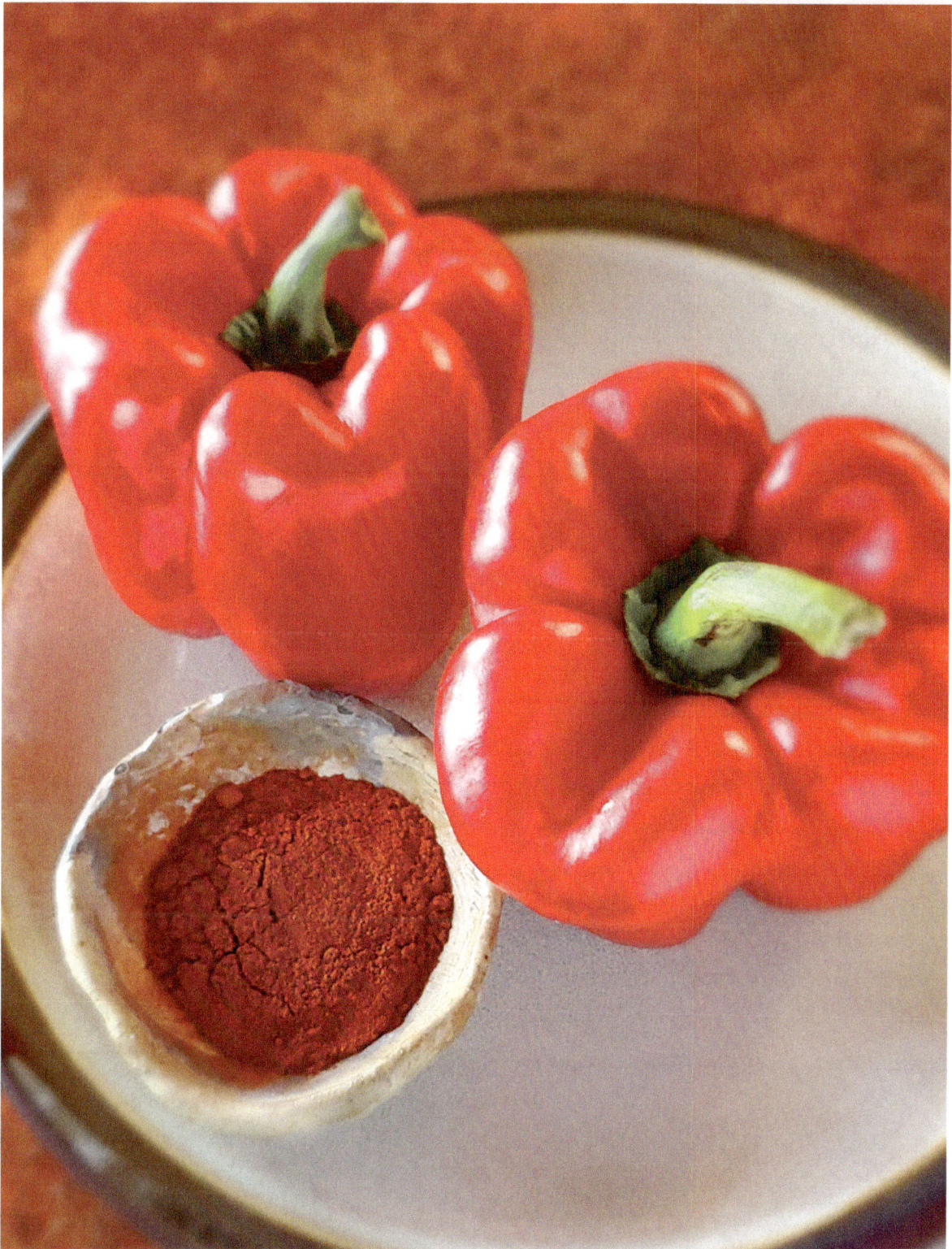

Meatloaves with Cornmeal & Brown Sugar Glaze

LOW FODMAP ❤ IBS FRIENDLY ❤ GLUTEN-FREE ❤ DAIRY-FREE

Who doesn't love the end cut of a meatloaf? The softer, inner slices are tasty and tender, but the end cut has more caramelized flavor with a crusty texture.

These individual loaves are such a treat because everyone gets their own "end cut" with texture, and coating of a tomato, chive, brown sugar and cider vinegar glaze.

MAKES 8 INDIVIDUAL LOAF SERVINGS
MEATLOAVES INGREDIENTS

2 tablespoons (30 ml) Low FODMAP Garlic-Infused Oil (page 50), made with extra virgin olive oil

3/4 cup (56 g) finely chopped bok choy

3/4 cup (38 g) thin sliced scallions, green parts only

2 medium (238 g total) fresh red bell peppers, stemmed, seeds and ribs removed, minced (if your digestion is sensitive to the skins see page 46 for steps on roasting and removing the skins first)

1/2 cup (120 ml) plain, unsweetened almond milk or canned full-fat coconut milk for cooking, containing no inulin, well-stirred

3 large eggs, beaten

1/2 cup (120 ml) Low FODMAP Chicken Stock (page 135)

3 tablespoons (45 g) tomato paste, containing no high fructose corn syrup or other high FODMAP ingredients

2 teaspoons (10 g) fine sea salt

2 teaspoons (4 g) cumin

1 teaspoon fresh ground black pepper

1/2 teaspoon cayenne

2-pounds (907 g) 80/20 ground beef, grass fed if available

1 cup plus 2 tablespoons (172 g) low FODMAP medium grind whole grain yellow cornmeal

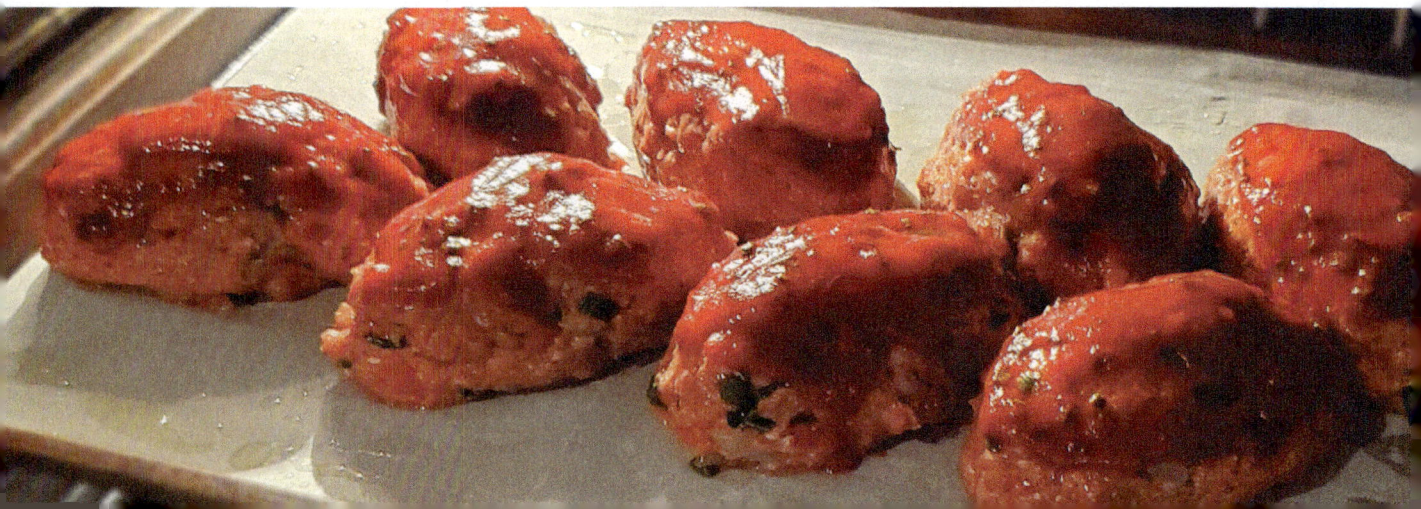

GLAZE INGREDIENTS

1/3 cup (80 ml) water

1/4 cup (60 g) tomato paste, containing no high fructose corn syrup or other high FODMAP ingredients

1/4 cup (60 ml) apple cider vinegar

3 tablespoons (30 g) medium packed light brown sugar

2 tablespoons (30 ml) Worcestershire sauce

2 teaspoons (2 g) minced fresh chives

Method: Preheat the oven to 350 F / 177 C

Cover a large rimmed baking sheet with parchment. Generously coat with cooking spray oil.

Meatloaves: Pour the oil in a large nonstick skillet over medium high heat. Add the bok choy, scallion greens and red bell. Sauté for 10 minutes or until the bok choy is just fork tender. If the pan gets too hot, reduce heat to medium. Set aside to cool for 5 minutes.

Whisk the milk, eggs, stock, 3 tablespoons (45 g) tomato paste, salt, cumin, pepper and cayenne in a large mixing bowl to thoroughly combine. Add the beef, cornmeal and sautéed vegetables. Mix together with your hands.

Divide the mixture into 8 portions. Take one portion and shape it into an oval with pointed ends, or into a rectangular loaf shape. Place on the baking sheet. Repeat for the remaining loaves, arranging them evenly spaced apart on the pan.

Glaze: Whisk the glaze ingredients with 1/4 cup (60 g) tomato paste. If too thick, add 1 teaspoon (5 ml) more water at a time until you have a ketchup consistency. Spoon over the loaves and around the edges to coat.

Bake 30 minutes and check. When the internal temperature has reached 160 F / 71 C remove from the oven, tent with foil and let rest for 10 minutes or until the internal temperature has reached 165 F / 74 C.

When plating, scoop away any gelatinous grey 'stuff' that may have formed around the bottom of the loaves while baking.

Meatloaves will keep up to 3 days in the fridge when stored in an airtight container, and will freeze up to 3 months.

Tip: Fiesta Slaw (page 116) and LoFO Garlic-Infused Mashed Potatoes (page 115) pair nicely with this recipe; one serving per person.

Monash Note: Although chiles (chillies) are generally low in FODMAPs, some people with IBS may be sensitive to the capsaicin they contain. Capsaicin is a natural compound that gives chiles their spicy quality. You may need to limit how much chile you eat if your IBS symptoms are triggered by spicy food.

Pork Loin Medallions with Tornado Juice BBQ Sauce

LOW FODMAP ❤ IBS FRIENDLY ❤ GLUTEN-FREE ❤ DAIRY-FREE

Tornado juice (whiskey) bbq sauce elevates this dish above the usual oven-roasted pork loin. Rather than pouring the sauce over the sliced medallions, they are placed into the warm pan of bbq to coat before plating. This way, every bite is savory bbq bliss.

MAKES 4 SERVINGS

PORK MEDALLION INGREDIENTS

1, 1 1/2-pound (680 g) boneless pork loin, trimmed of most fat

1 teaspoon (5 g) fine sea salt

1/2 teaspoon fresh ground black pepper

2 tablespoons (30 ml) canola oil

1/4 cup (60 ml) water

TORNADO BBQ SAUCE INGREDIENTS

1 cup (240 ml) Low FODMAP Chicken Stock (page 135) or water

1/4 cup (60 ml) canned tomato purée

1.7-ounces (50 ml) whiskey (aka. tornado juice)

1/4 cup (60 ml) soy sauce, gluten-free if you are following a gluten-free diet

1/4 cup (60 ml) red wine vinegar

1 tablespoon (15 ml) Low FODMAP Garlic-Infused Oil (page 50), made with extra virgin olive oil

1/2 cup (100 g) medium packed light brown sugar

1 tablespoon (3 g) fresh minced chives

1 tablespoon (6 g) pure mild red chile powder (containing no onion or garlic, the ingredients should list only: red chile. On the Monash App this is called Chilli (chili) red, powdered)

1 teaspoon (5 g) plain, prepared yellow mustard, containing no onion or garlic

1 teaspoon (2 g) cayenne, optional

1 tablespoon (8 g) cornstarch

1 tablespoon (15 ml) cold water

Method: Preheat oven to 325 F / 165 C

Pork Loin: Dust the pork loin with salt and pepper, rubbing the seasonings well into the meat. Pour the oil into a large ovenproof skillet over medium high heat. Using tongs or a large bbq fork, brown and rotate the loin on all sides. Turn the pork fat side up (if there is a fat cap). Add water to the pan, cover with ovenproof lid and bake for 35 to 40 minutes or until the internal temperature is 145 F / 63 C.

Using oven mitts, remove from the oven and place the loin on a cutting board or plate covered with foil to rest. Reserve 2 tablespoons of the pan drippings.

Sauce: Heat the drippings in the same pan - that may still be hot so again, be sure to use those oven mitts. Over medium heat, add the stock, tomato purée, tornado juice, soy sauce, vinegar, garlic oil, brown sugar, chives, chile powder, mustard and cayenne. Using a spatula, stir gently to mix and also incorporate the tasty roasted bits from the bottom of the pan. Let the sauce reduce at a low boil for 5 minutes, stirring often. Mix the cornstarch and water to create a slurry. Add to the sauce and continue to stir until thickened.

Slice the loin into 1/2-inch (1.25 cm) thick medallions and add to the sauce. Coat the medallions, turning them a few times for 3 to 4 minutes. Serve immediately.

Tips: Baked potatoes and a side salad of arugula, sliced cucumber, grated carrot and splash of red wine vinegar and olive oil pair nicely with this dish.

Tornado BBQ Sauce also goes beautifully with chicken, pork chops, and as a hamburger glaze.

Monash Note: Although chiles (chillies) are generally low in FODMAPs, some people with IBS may be sensitive to the capsaicin they contain. Capsaicin is a natural compound that gives chiles their spicy quality. You may need to limit how much chile you eat if your IBS symptoms are triggered by spicy food.

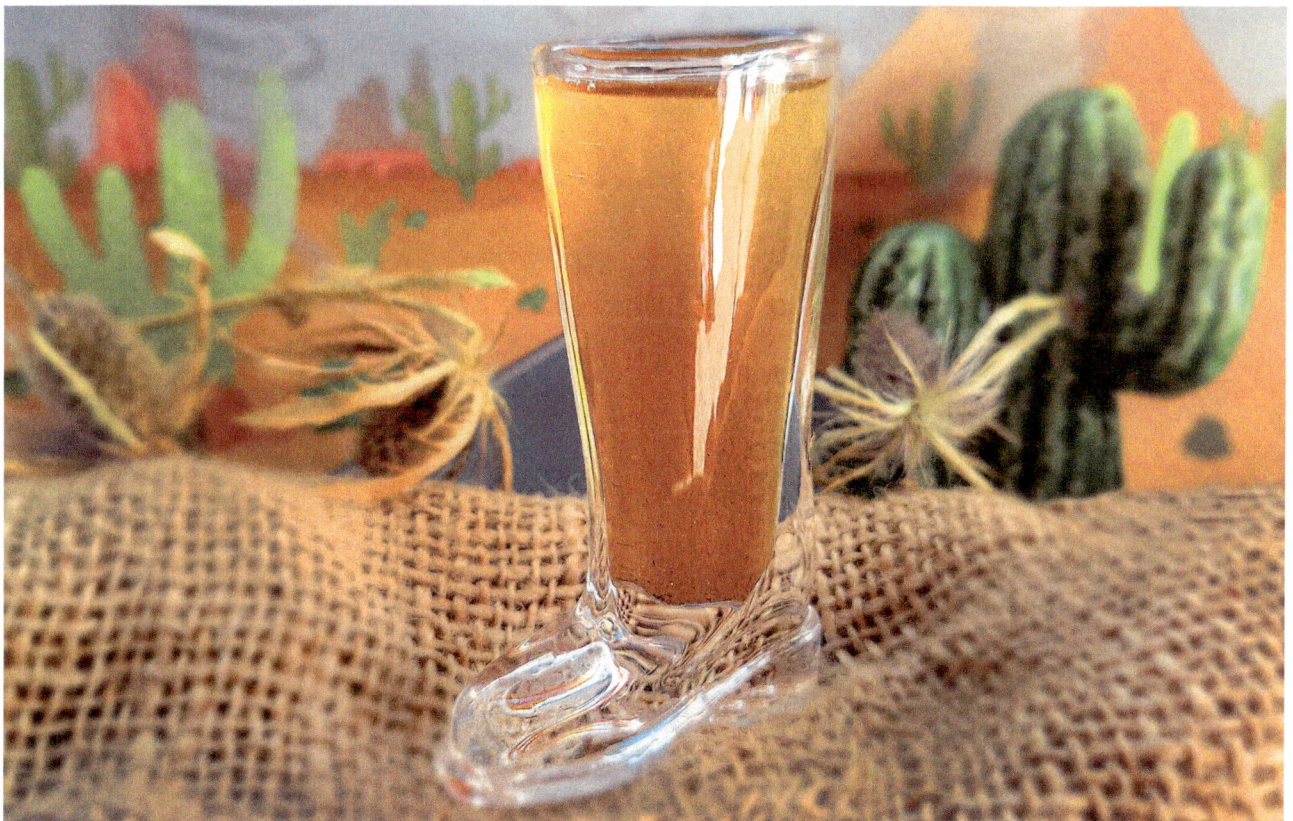

Chicken Tamales with Carrot Chive Dough & Green Chile Sauce

LOW FODMAP ❤ IBS FRIENDLY ❤ GLUTEN-FREE ❤ DAIRY-FREE

Tamales are a holiday tradition, and an afternoon party of assembling and tying them into cornhusk "gifts" is huge fun.

The masa dough is traditionally mixed with lard. This version is low-fat due to chicken stock and fluffy egg whites standing in for lard. I've also added mashed carrots and chives for flavor and a lovely, warm color.

Coating the cornhusks with cooking spray oil before laying in the dough and fillings keeps the tamales from sticking to the husks.

A store-bought, plain rotisserie chicken containing no high FODMAP ingredients works well for the chicken shred, or you can make your own Whole Poached Chicken with Stock (page 82).

2 batches of New Mexican Green Chile Sauce (page 60) are also needed, so be sure to plan accordingly.

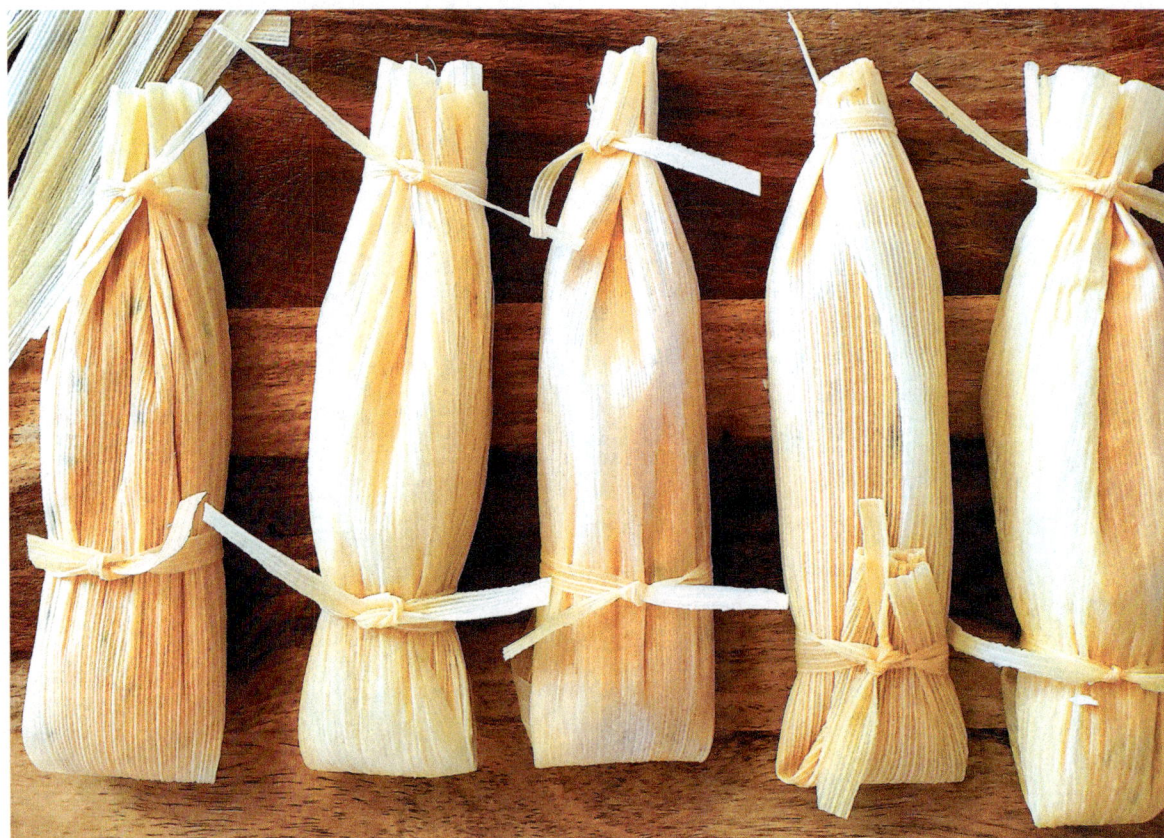

MAKES 10 TAMALES – 2 PER ENTRÉE COURSE – 1 PER APPETIZER

CORNHUSKS

20, 9.5 to 10-inch (24 to 25 cm) cornhusks

SHREDDED CHICKEN

2 1/2 cups (375 g) shredded cooked chicken, from a plain, store-bought rotisserie chicken containing no high FODMAP ingredients, or Whole Poached Chicken with Stock (page 82), ready to use

GREEN CHILE SAUCE

2 batches New Mexican Green Chile Sauce (page 60), ready to use

FILLING INGREDIENTS

5 small (375 g total) Roma tomatoes, cored and small diced

1/2 cup (8 g) fresh medium packed cilantro, mostly leaves, finely chopped

1/2 cup (25 g) thin sliced scallions, green parts only

1/2 teaspoon (2.5 g) fine sea salt

1/2 teaspoon (1 g) ground cumin

Juice of 1/2 lime, plus lime wedges for plating

DOUGH INGREDIENTS

4 cups water

2 large (170 g total) carrots, peeled and small diced

2 large egg whites

1 1/3 cups (165 g) gluten-free masa harina

1 tablespoon (3 g) minced fresh chives

1 teaspoon (5 g) fine sea salt

1 teaspoon (4 g) baking powder, gluten-free if you are following a gluten-free diet

1 1/2 cups (350 ml) low FODMAP Chicken Stock (page 135), or from the Whole Poached Chicken recipe, heated in a pan or microwave to lukewarm

Cooking spray oil for coating the cornhusks

Method

Cornhusks: Place the cornhusks in a large bowl and cover with very warm water, but not boiling. Place a plate over the top to weigh them down. Let soak while you prep the rest of the recipe.

Filling: Place the filling ingredients in a medium bowl. Stir well. Add the shredded chicken, stir to combine and set aside.

Dough: Pour the water into a medium saucepan over high heat. Add the carrots and boil for 10 to 15 minutes or until very tender. Use a slotted spoon to scoop them into a bowl. Mash them into mush with a wooden spatula.

Use a hand mixer to beat the egg whites to stiff peaks. Set aside.

Whisk together the masa, chives, 1 teaspoon (5 g) salt, and the baking powder in a separate medium bowl. Pour in the lukewarm chicken stock and spoon in the carrot mash. Use your hand to blend it into a sticky dough. Gently fold in the egg whites with a spatula. The consistency will be light and very soft. Use a spoon to divide the dough into 10 equal portions in the bowl. (continued on the next page)

(continued from previous page)

Cornhusk Ties: Take 2 cornhusks, shake off excess water and tear long 1/4-inch (.63 cm) thick strips lengthwise. You will need to knot 2 strips together to create a tie long enough to wrap around each tamale. Start with 20 strips to make 10 ties. You will need 10 more ties for securing the tamales tops. If some ties break, you have extra husks if needed.

Call the kids, family and friends. It's time for a tamale wrapping party!

Tamale Wrapping: Take 1 soaked whole cornhusk, shake off any excess water and place it on a work surface.

1 – The husk is shaped like a fan, so you want the wide side toward you and the smaller side facing away. Lightly coat the husk with cooking spray oil.

2 - Scoop 1 portion of the dough (approx. 1/4 cup) into the center of the husk. Use your fingers to spread it into a 4 x 4 inch (10 x 10 cm) square.

3 - Place 2 tablespoons filling down the center of the dough.

4 - Push the husk sides inward to press the filling and dough together.

5– Fold the husk sides inwards to overlap and close the tamale..

6 – Fold the bottom up to enclose the filling.

7 – Tie the bottom flap of the tamale with a long strip of cornhusk. Then tie the narrow top to secure. Repeat for remaining tamales.

Place a steamer basket in the bottom of a large soup pot. Fill with enough water to just touch the bottom of the steamer. Place 4 whole cornhusks to overlap and cover the steamer. Bring the water to a rolling boil. Arrange the tamales upright in the pot with their narrow ends up. Reduce heat to medium high for a low boil, cover with a lid and steam for 20 minutes. Use tongs to lift up one of the bottom cornhusks to see if the water has evaporated. You will most likely need to add more hot water, just to the steamer basket level. Steam for 25 minutes longer, covered.

Assembly: After untying and opening the husk, take the shorter end of the 'fan' and tie it with a string of cornhusk. Trim the sides with scissors for a pretty open fan display. Assemble 2 per plate for an entrée, or 1 per for an appetizer. Top with Green Chile Sauce and cilantro, with a lime wedge to the side if desired.

Tips: If tolerated, add 1 tablespoon (5 g) grated cheddar, Monterey Jack or Manchego cheese to the filling of each tamale before wrapping and steaming.

If you use the Whole Poached Chicken recipe to make your shred, you will also have plenty of stock for mixing the dough.

Just in case there's a question, the cornhusks are inedible.

Monash Note: Although chiles (chillies) are generally low in FODMAPs, some people with IBS may be sensitive to the capsaicin they contain. Capsaicin is a natural compound that gives chiles their spicy quality. You may need to limit how much chile you eat if your IBS symptoms are triggered by spicy food.

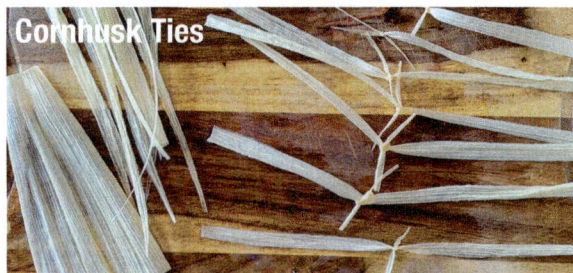

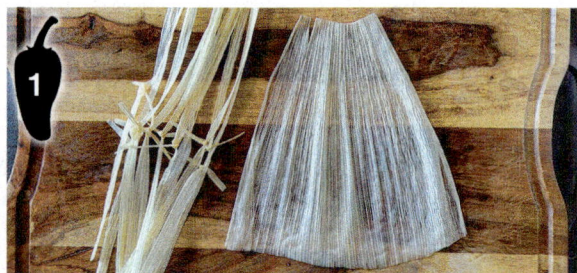

Cornhusk Ties

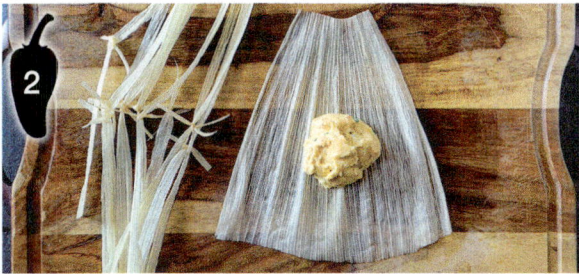

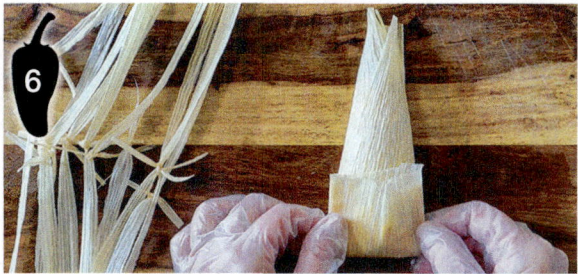

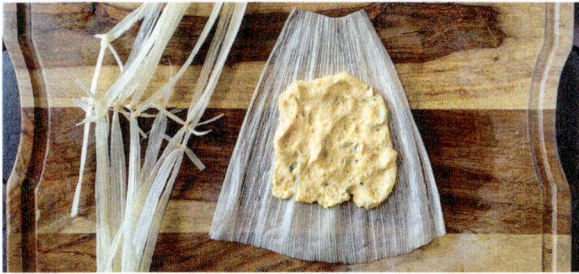

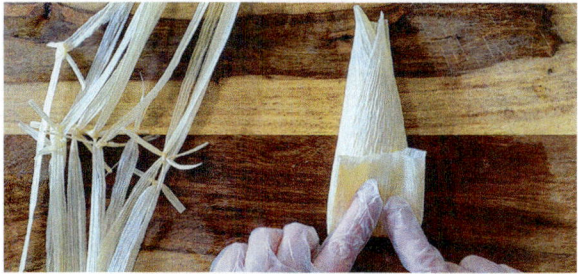

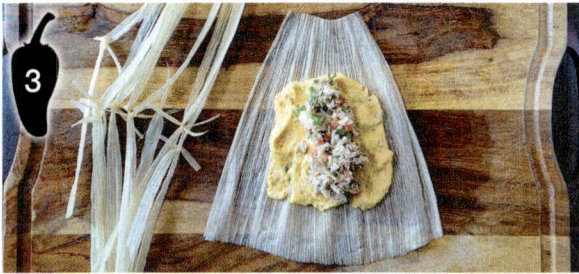

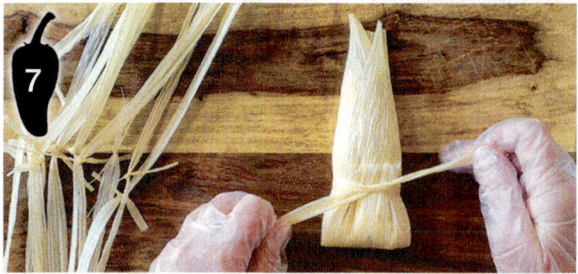

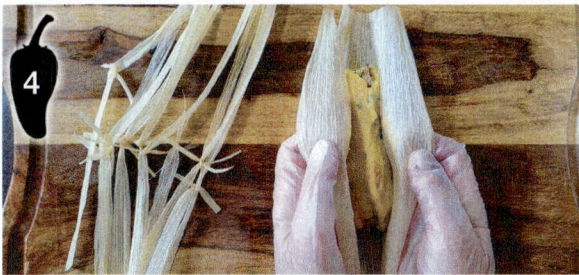

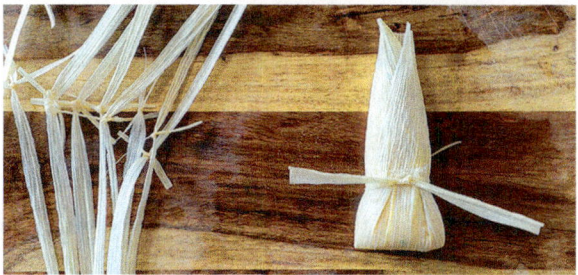

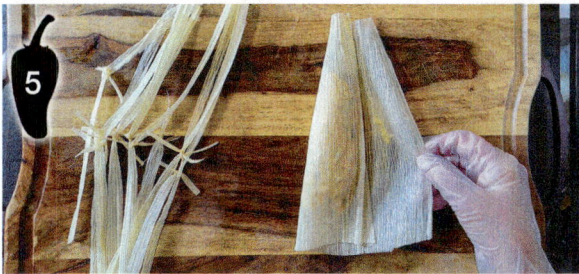

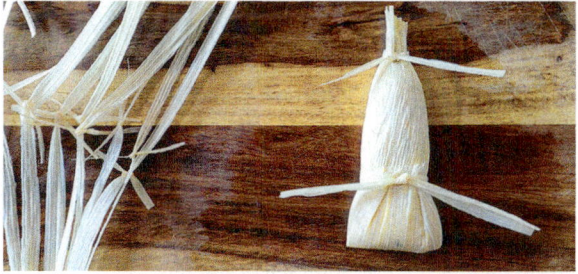

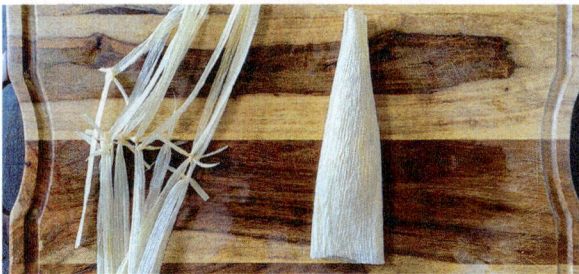

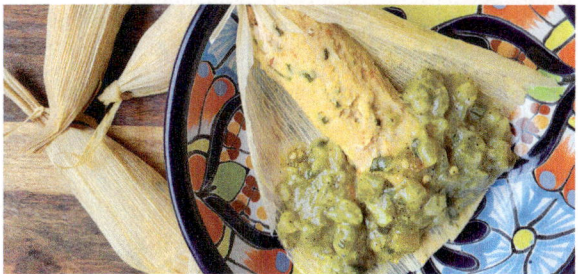

Crispy Chicken Poblano Chiles Rellenos

LOW FODMAP ❤ IBS FRIENDLY ❤ GLUTEN-FREE ❤ DAIRY-FREE

Poblanos are a mild to low-heat pepper and are great for chiles rellenos (stuffed chiles) because of their thick, sturdy chile meat that holds well when filled. They are commonly stuffed with meat and lots of cheese, dipped in a batter of whipped egg whites, flour, baking powder and salt, then pan fried in oil.

This healthier LoFO version is coated in low FODMAP gluten-free panko breadcrumbs and baked for a crispy crunch!

You will need to prepare the Béchamel Sauce, roasted poblano peppers and cooked rice ahead of time, so be sure to plan accordingly

MAKES 4 SERVINGS
INGREDIENTS
8 wooden toothpicks soaked in water

BÉCHAMEL SAUCE
One-half batch Béchamel Sauce (page 65), ready to use

POBLANOS
4 fresh medium (97g each) poblano peppers, roasted and prepped as instructed on page 46, using the sliced pocket relleno method with stem intact, ready to use

CILANTRO RICE INGREDIENTS
1 cup (190 g) cooked white rice

1/4 cup (4 g) medium packed cilantro, mostly leaves, chopped fine

Juice of 1/2 lime

1/4 teaspoon (1.25 g) fine sea salt

1/4 teaspoon fresh ground black pepper

CHICKEN INGREDIENTS
2 medium (550 g total) chicken breasts, boneless, skinless

1 scant teaspoon (4 g) fine sea salt

1/2 teaspoon fresh ground black pepper

2 tablespoons (30 ml) canola oil

1/2 teaspoon (1 g) pure mild red chile powder (containing no onion or garlic, the ingredients should list only: red chile. On the Monash App this is called Chilli (chili) red, powdered)

1/2 teaspoon (1 g) smoked paprika

1/2 teaspoon (1 g) ground cumin

1/2 cup (25 g) thin sliced scallions, green parts only

(continued on next page)

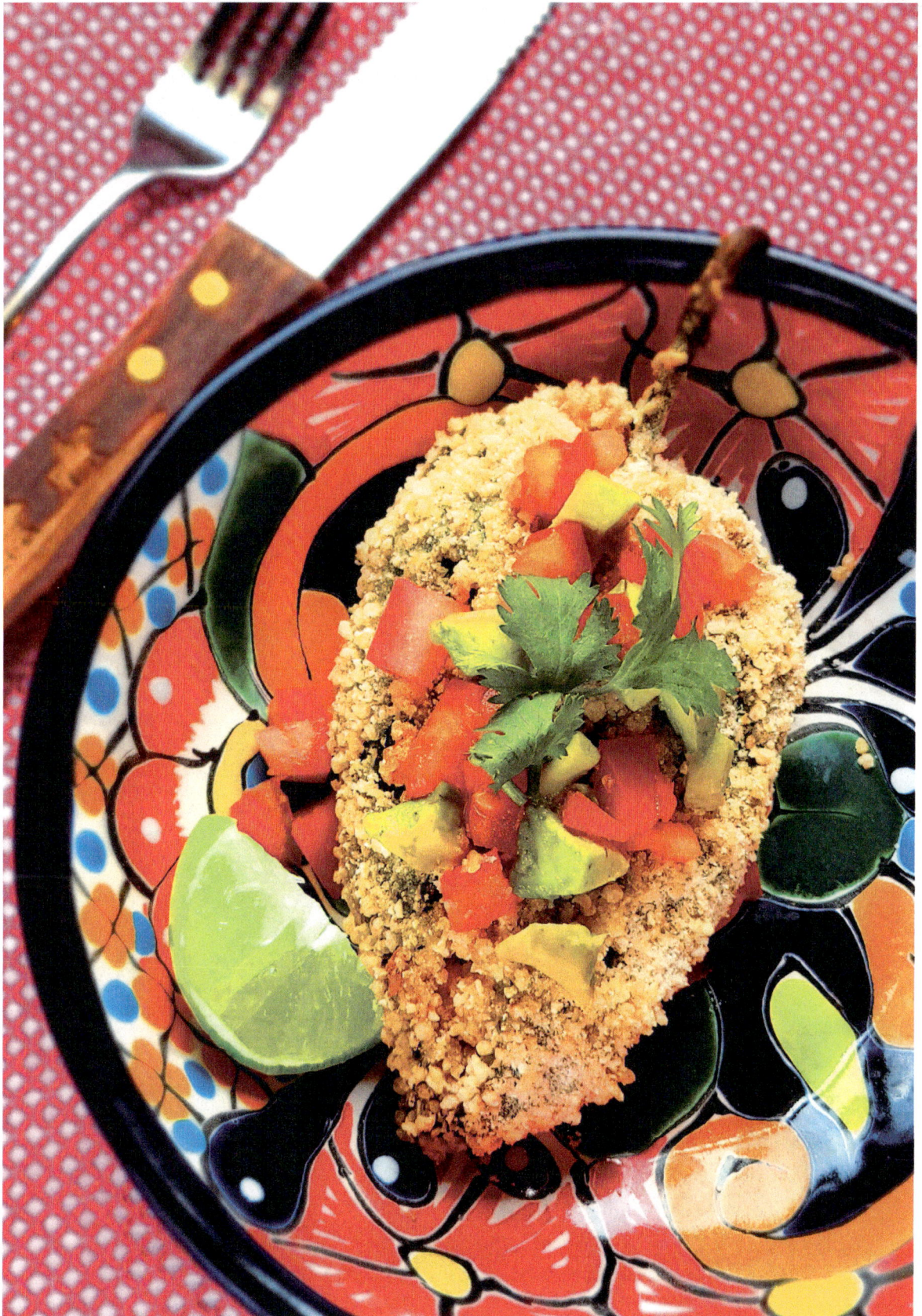

(continued from previous page)

DREDGING STATION

3/4 cup (110 g) low FODMAP gluten-free all-purpose baking flour, containing xanthan gum (see page 55 for LoFO flour descriptions)

1/4 teaspoon (1.25 g) fine sea salt

1/4 teaspoon fresh ground black pepper

2 large eggs

2 tablespoons (30 ml) plain, unsweetened almond milk

1 3/4 cups (175 g) low FODMAP gluten-free plain panko breadcrumbs

TOPPING INGREDIENTS

Cooking spray oil

1/3 (50g) small, fresh Roma tomato, small diced

 2-ounces (60 g) avocado, cubed into small pieces

4 lime wedges

Small bunch of cilantro leaves

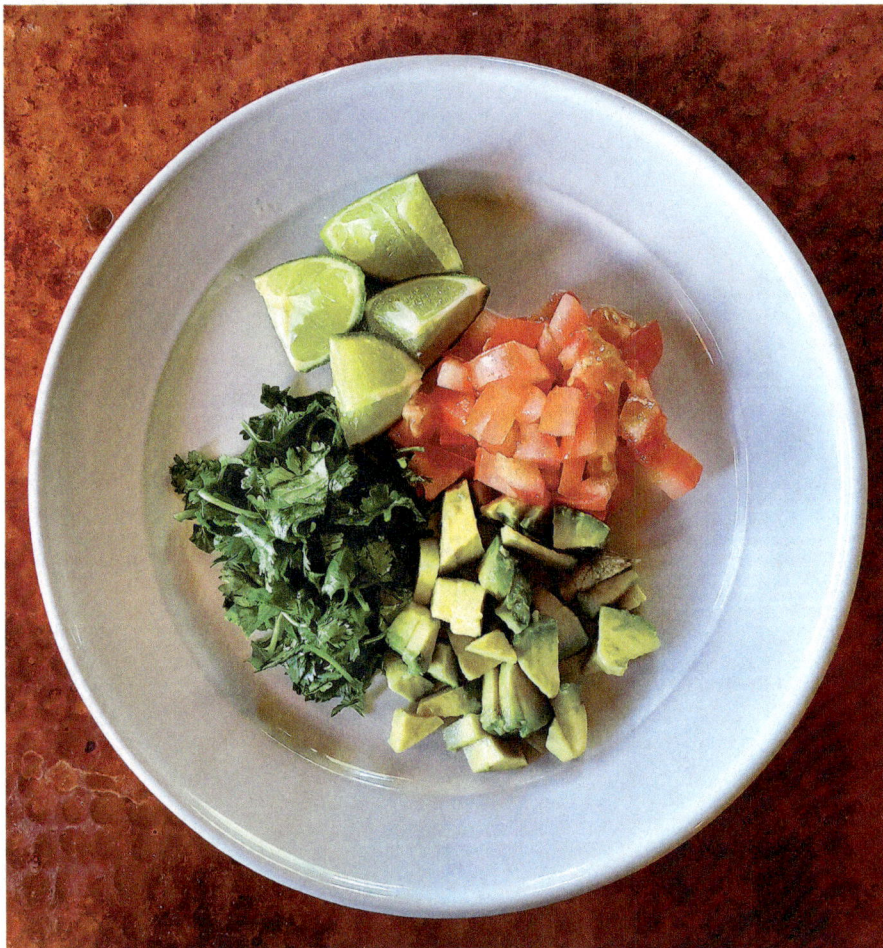

Method: Preheat the oven to 400 F / 200 C.

Rice: Mix the cooked rice, cilantro, lime juice, salt and pepper in a small bowl. Set aside.

Chicken: Butterfly the chicken by placing your hand flat on top of one breast and cut into the side lengthwise to divide in half, stopping at 1-inch (2.5 cm) before slicing all the way through. Open the fillet flat and it will be heart-shaped. Repeat for the second breast. Cut away any fatty pieces. Make sure your knife is nice and sharp, otherwise the meat will shred as you slice into it. Lightly dust them with salt and pepper.

Pour the canola oil into a large nonstick skillet over medium high heat. Place the breasts in the pan and cook for 6 minutes. Flip and cook 5 to 6 minutes or until the centers are no longer pink. If the oil becomes too hot or smoky as you cook, reduce heat to medium. Move the chicken to a cutting board and let rest for 5 minutes. Cut them into 1/2-inch (1.25 cm) cubes and place in a medium mixing bowl. Mix the red chile powder, smoked paprika, and cumin, then lightly dust over the chicken. Use a fork to mix and evenly coat, as the chile powder will turn your fingers red. Add the scallion greens and toss to mix. Set aside.

Dredge & Assembly: To assemble your dredging station, place 3 medium-sized bowls in a row. Fill one with flour, salt and pepper and whisk. Beat the eggs and almond milk until frothy in the second bowl. Place the breadcrumbs in the third.

Fill each poblano 3/4 full with the chicken mixture. Fill almost to the top with cilantro rice. Top with 3 tablespoons (45 ml) béchamel (or however much will fit into each pocket). Gently push the opening together and secure by closing the pocket with 2 toothpicks each.

Take one relleno, place in the flour and carefully turn and dust with your hands to fully coat. Shake away any excess. Next, dredge it in the eggs to completely cover. Roll it in the breadcrumbs, turning it a few times to completely coat. Place on a greased baking sheet and repeat for the remaining rellenos. Lightly coat the tops with cooking spray oil.

Bake for 25 to 30 minutes, uncovered, until the breadcrumbs are golden brown. Remove from the oven. Extract the toothpicks and discard.

To Plate: Place 1 relleno on each plate or serving bowl. Evenly divide the diced tomato and avocado and place on the tops. Garnish with lime wedges and cilantro leaves. Serve immediately.

Tips: 1-pound (454 g) amounts protein options other than chicken: Slow Oven-Roasted Pulled Pork (page 80), pan cooked shrimp in canola oil and a light dusting of salt and pepper, or Plain Shredded Beef (page 79 in the Tips section).

If tolerated, add 1/4 cup (25 g) shredded parmesan cheese to the breadcrumbs for dredging.

Also if tolerated, fill the rellenos with 1 tablespoon (7 g) shredded cheddar or Monterey Jack cheese each.

If you rinse the chiles under water to remove the skins, gently pat them inside and out with paper towels to dry before filling and breading. This will keep them crisp underneath.

Rellenos should be eaten the same day, as they don't refrigerate well and become soft.

Monash Note: Although chiles (chillies) are generally low in FODMAPs, some people with IBS may be sensitive to the capsaicin they contain. Capsaicin is a natural compound that gives chiles their spicy quality. You may need to limit how much chile you eat if your IBS symptoms are triggered by spicy food.

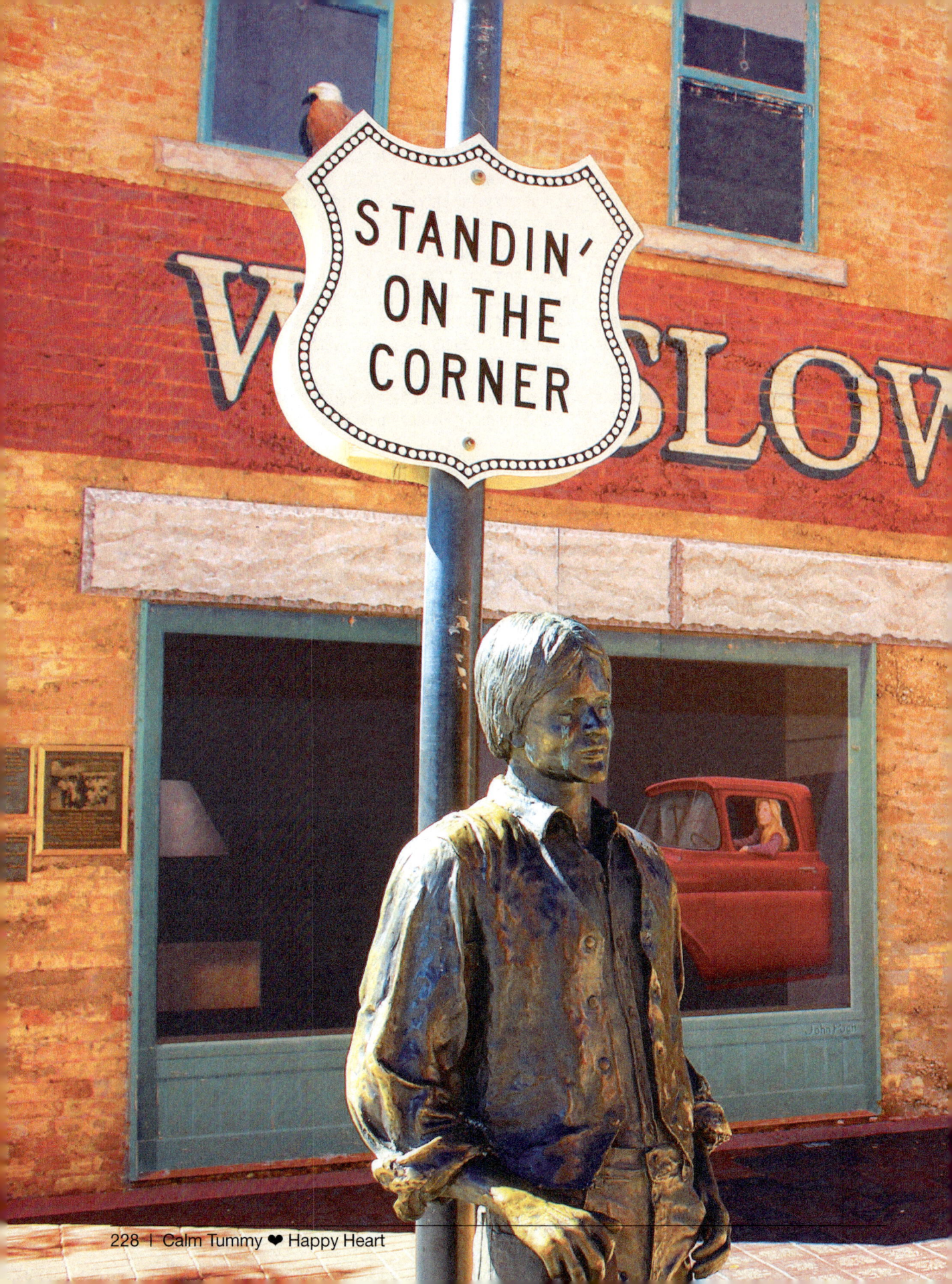

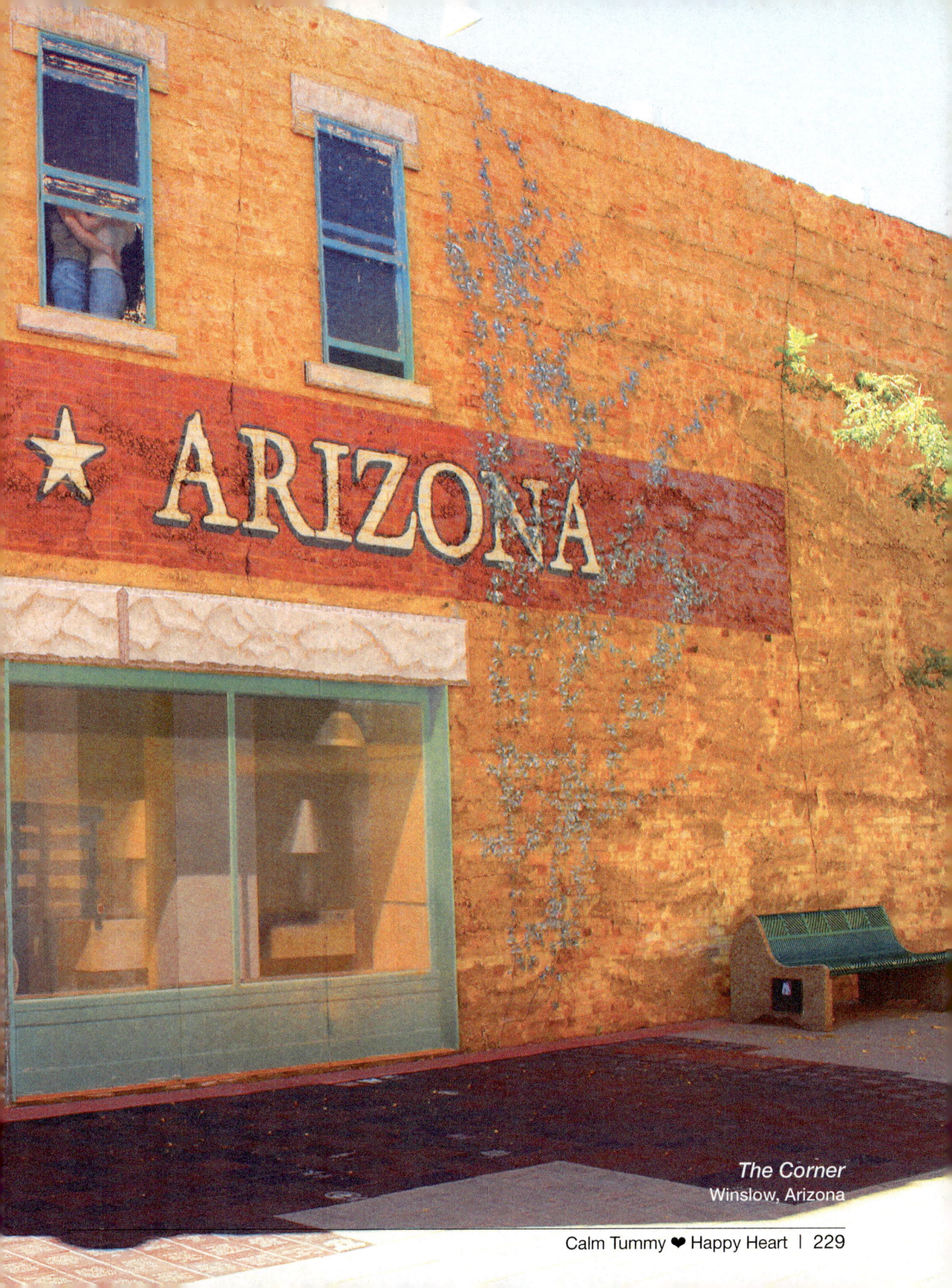

The Corner
Winslow, Arizona

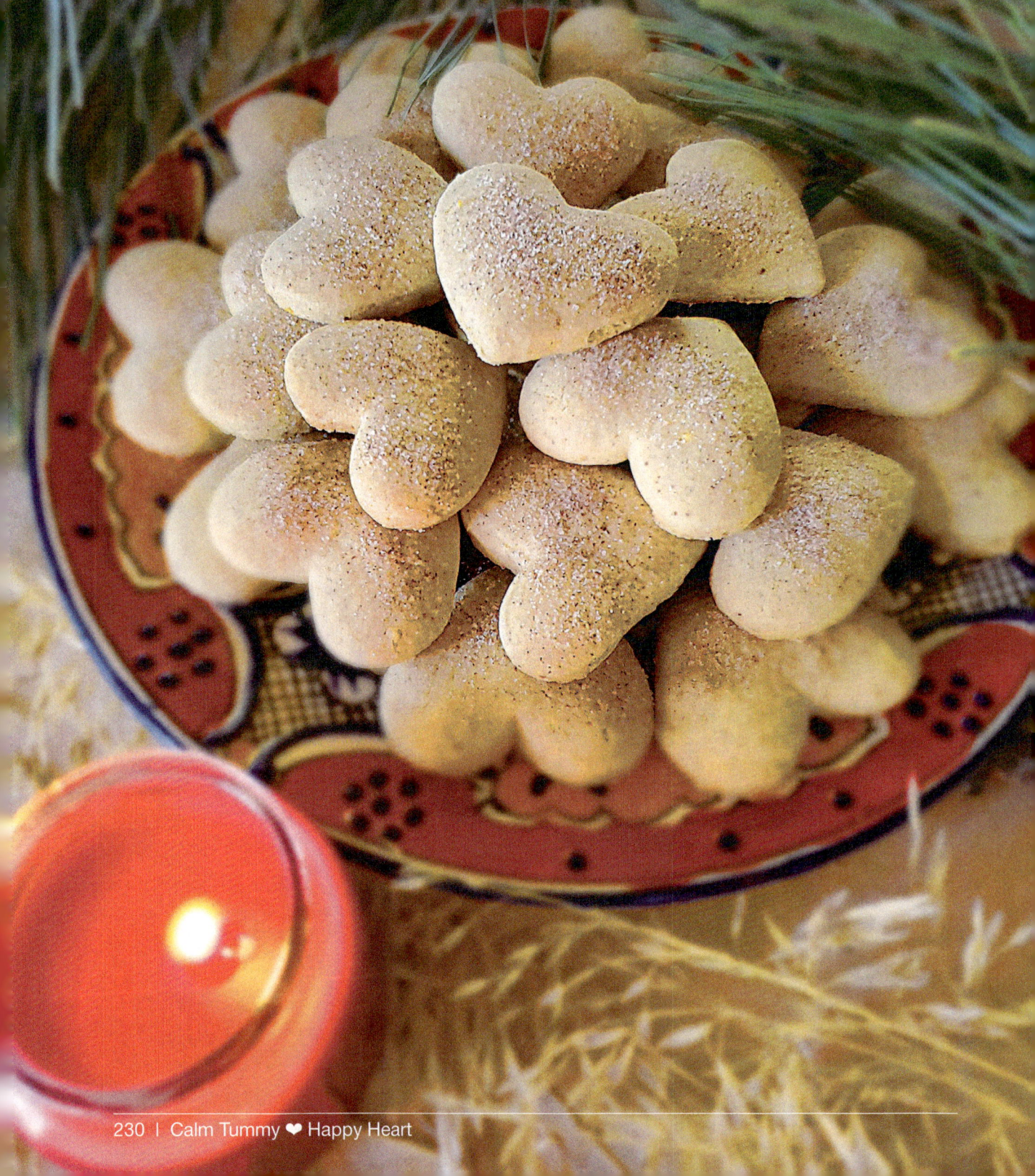

Desserts

- **Vanilla Flan with Caramel Sauce**

- **Todos Mis Mananas Para Ti Cake
  with Vegan Cinnamon Buttercream Frosting**

- **Tres Leches Cake**

- **Bizcochitos**

- **Taos Brownies**

- **Cornmeal Dusted Meringues with Candied Poblanos**

Food brand names are sometimes listed within a recipe, and this means they are Monash Certified.
For more brand options we use and love, please visit **FodifyIt.com**

Monash Note: Although chiles (chillies) are generally low in FODMAPs, some people with IBS may be
sensitive to the capsaicin they contain. Capsaicin is a natural compound that gives chiles their spicy
quality. You may need to limit how much chile you eat if your IBS symptoms are triggered by spicy food.

Vanilla Flan with Caramel Sauce

LOW FODMAP ❤ IBS FRIENDLY ❤ GLUTEN-FREE ❤ DAIRY-FREE

Where is the statue of the person who first decided to mix eggs with cream, sugar and vanilla, then bake it with caramel sauce? There must be one somewhere, in recognition of their genius to create such a delicate, creamy dessert.

This dairy-free version uses almond milk and canned full-fat coconut milk and I promise that it is as flantastic as the conventional dairy version. Please note - this recipe requires 8 hours or overnight refrigeration.

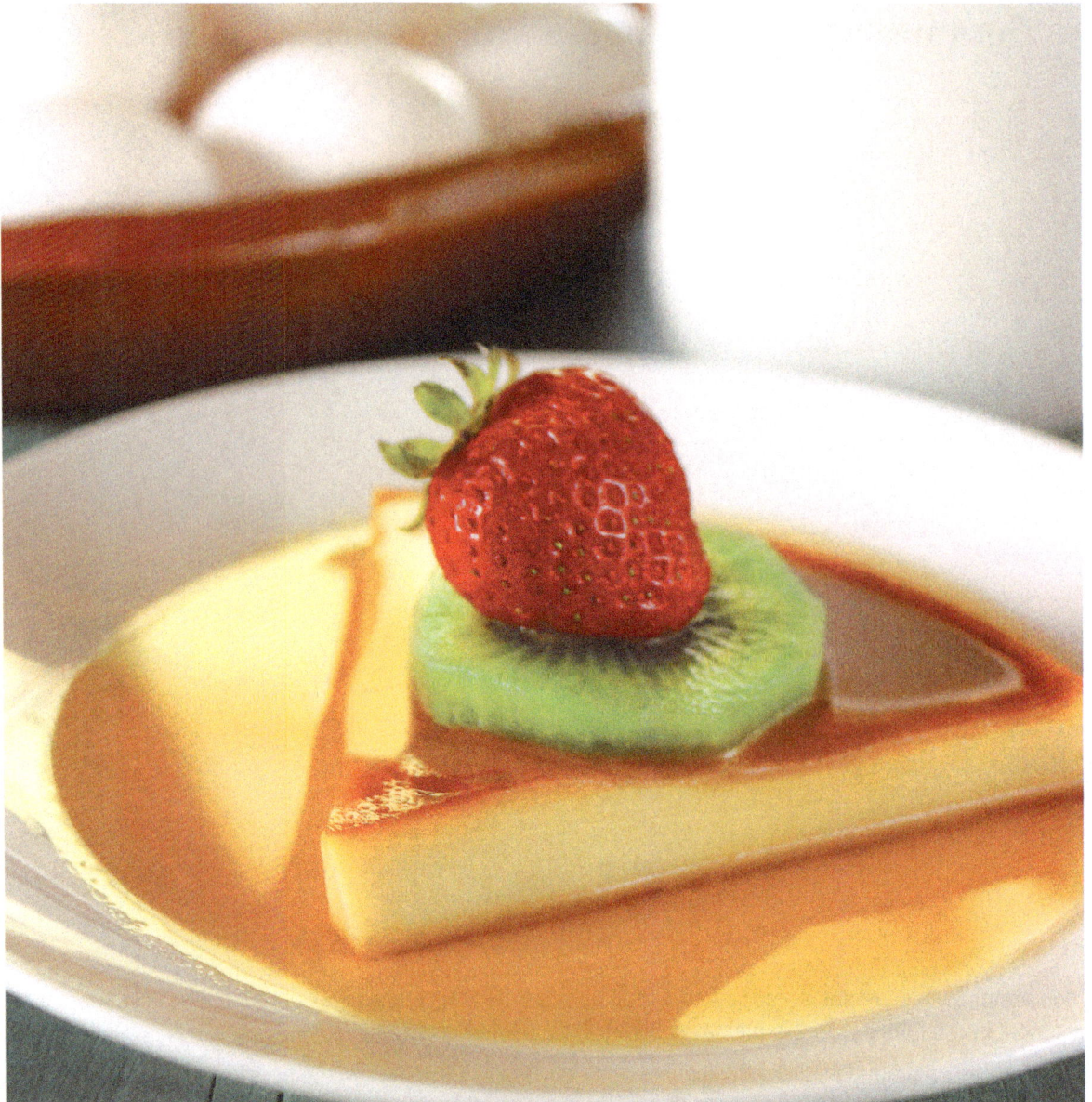

MAKES 6 SERVINGS
CARAMEL INGREDIENTS

1/2 cup (100 g) sugar

3 tablespoons (45 ml) water

9-inch (23 cm) flan mold or metal pie tin

Large rimmed baking pan that the flan mold will fit inside for a water bath

FLAN INGREDIENTS

3 large eggs plus 2 large egg yolks, room temperature (save the extra whites for tomorrow's omelet or meringue)

1 cup (240 ml) plain, unsweetened almond milk, room temperature

3/4 cup (180 ml) canned full-fat coconut milk for cooking, containing no inulin, well-stirred, room temperature

1/2 cup (100 g) sugar

1 tablespoon (15 ml) vanilla extract (essence)

Pinch fine sea salt

Method: Preheat oven to 325 F / 163 C

Caramel: Pour the sugar and water into a medium saucepan over medium high heat. Swirl the pan for 1 to 2 minutes until the sugar dissolves. Let the sugar water simmer gently and cook undisturbed for 3 minutes. As the color begins to turn a light honey color, gently swirl the pan 3 times, then allow the caramel to continue to simmer until it turns medium-dark amber, but not dark brown. Be sure not to stir or swirl too much or it will crystallize and seize up. This step should take about 7 minutes.

Place the flan mold inside the rimmed baking pan. Pour the hot caramel into the mold. At this stage the mixture is lava hot so be very careful to not touch, splatter, or dip your finger in for a taste. Using heavy oven mitts, tip the mold back and forth to coat the bottom with caramel, and slightly up the sides. Return it to the baking pan and let cool for 10 minutes.

Flan: Pour the flan ingredients into a blender and purée for 2 minutes. Pour through a fine mesh metal strainer over the caramel. It may make a loud crack! sound that is perfectly normal if the caramel is still warm when the cold liquids are added. Place in the oven. Pour hot water into the larger baking pan, surrounding the mold in 1/2-inch (1.25 cm) deep water. This will create steam for a creamy, tender flan.

Baking times will vary according to your oven and the pan you use. Bake for 25 minutes and check by inserting a knife into the flan, but not all the way through to the caramel as this will leave a mark on the top of the flan when it's turned out onto a platter. When the knife comes out clean and the center of the flan is only slightly jiggly, it is done. If still soupy, bake 5 to 10 more minutes. (There have been cold winter days when I have cooked mine for 50 minutes).

Remove from the oven and use heavy mitts to lift the mold from the water bath. Allow to cool for 20 minutes, cover with plastic wrap and refrigerate 8 hours to overnight.

When ready to serve, run a knife around the edges of the mold to release the flan. Invert onto a rimmed serving platter to contain the caramel. Slice and serve as is, or topped with a kiwi slice and a strawberry.

Todos Mis Mananas Para Ti Cake with Vegan Cinnamon Buttercream Frosting

LOW FODMAP ❤ IBS FRIENDLY ❤ GLUTEN-FREE ❤ DAIRY-FREE

When you serve this chocolate Mexican olive oil cake, your sweetheart will whisper in your ear "All of my tomorrows belong to you," hence the title. It's truly decadent and proof that where there is cake there is love.

Most Southwestern restaurants offer a spicy chocolate cake with warm cinnamon and cayenne that get your taste buds and circulation going. They're a Valentine's and everyday special treat.

This LoFO version offers a gluten-free, vegan cinnamon buttercream frosting, but if you'd prefer to skip the frosting, a light brushing of warm extra virgin olive oil on top of each slice is a traditional finish. Or simply use a heart-shaped stencil and sprinkle the top with a light dusting of confectioners' sugar.

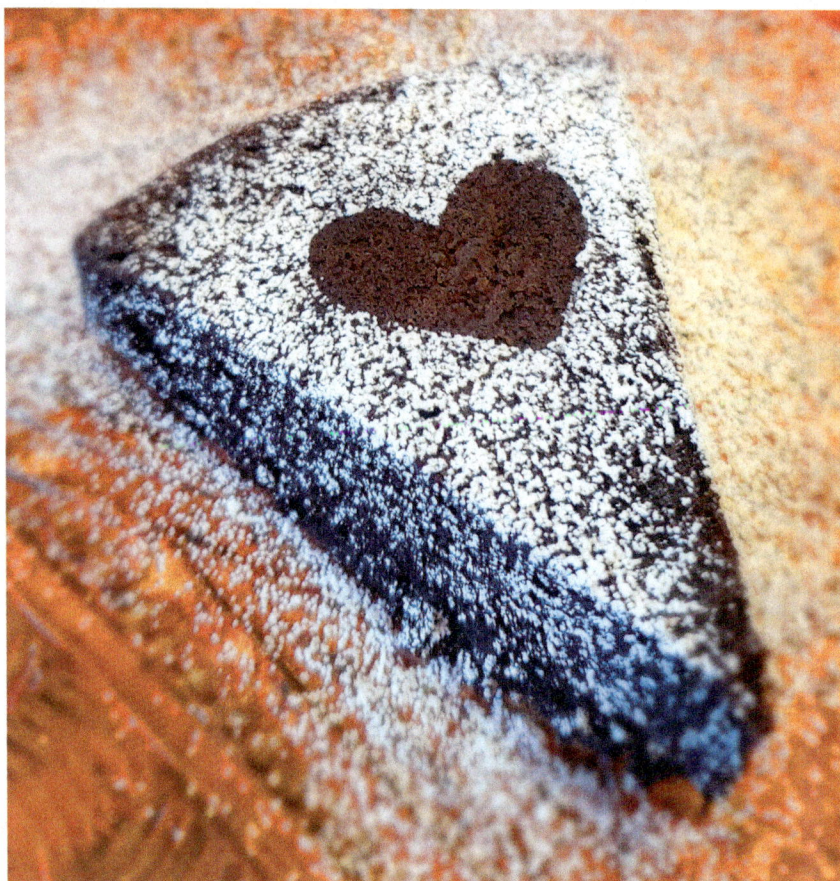

MAKES 8-10 SERVINGS
CAKE INGREDIENTS

3 large eggs

1 cup (200 g) sugar

1/2 cup (120 ml) extra virgin olive oil

3/4 cup (180 ml) plain, unsweetened almond milk

2 heaping teaspoons (4 g) instant coffee granules

2 teaspoons (10 ml) vanilla extract (essence)

1 3/4 cups (258 g) low FODMAP gluten-free all-purpose baking flour, containing xanthan gum (page 55)

1/2 cup (43 g) Dutch-processed cocoa powder, containing 70% cocoa minimum

2 teaspoons (4 g) ground cinnamon, plus more to taste

1 teaspoon (4 g) gluten-free baking powder, if you are following a gluten-free diet

1/2 teaspoon (1 g) cayenne powder, plus more to your taste

1/4 teaspoon (1 g) fine sea salt

VEGAN BUTTERCREAM FROSTING INGREDIENTS

1/2 cup (112 g) dairy-free butter alternative, room temperature

2 teaspoons (10 ml) vanilla extract (essence)

1 teaspoon (2 g) ground cinnamon

1/4 teaspoon (1 g) fine sea salt

3 cups (375 g) confectioners' sugar

2 to 3 tablespoons (30 – 45 ml) plain, unsweetened almond milk, room temperature

Method: Preheat oven to 350 F / 177 C

Cake: Coat a 9-inch (23 cm) round cake pan with cooking spray oil and line the bottom with a circle of parchment paper.

Using the whisk attachment on a stand mixer, beat the eggs and sugar for 2 minutes. Slowly drizzle in the oil. Mix in the milk, coffee and vanilla.

In a medium mixing bowl, whisk the flour, cocoa powder, cinnamon, baking powder, cayenne and salt.

With the stand mixer set on low, gradually add the flour mix to the wet ingredients. Scrape down the sides of the bowl with a spatula. Set the mixer to medium speed and beat for 1 minute to fully incorporate.

Pour the batter into the cake pan. Bake 20 minutes. Insert a toothpick in the center. If it comes out clean, the cake is ready. If not, bake 3 to 5 minutes longer. You don't want to over-bake, as this will dry out the luscious moist texture.

Let the cake rest for 5 minutes. Turn out onto a wire baking rack, remove the parchment and allow to cool completely.

Buttercream Frosting: While the cake cools, clean the mixing bowl and switch to the paddle attachment. Beat the butter alternative, vanilla, cinnamon and salt for 2 minutes. Continue mixing until there are no lumps.

(continued on the next page)

(continued from previous page)

On low speed, gradually add 1 cup (100 g) of the confectioners' sugar then speed up the mixer to fully incorporate. Add 1 tablespoon (15 ml) milk and continue mixing and alternating the sugar and milk until you have a lovely, soft yet firm buttercream frosting. Each time you add more sugar, set the mixer on low to avoid a pop-up snowstorm poof! in your kitchen. If the consistency is too thin, add a bit more powdered sugar. If too thick, add a bit more almond milk.

Frost the cake with an offset spatula, or use a piping bag to create a more polished look. Keep cool in the fridge until ready to serve.

Fresh strawberries add a nice touch, if desired.

Olive oil cake will keep in the fridge for up to 1 week when tightly wrapped in plastic or an airtight container.

Tips: Sensitive to chile heat? Omit the cayenne. The result will still be deliciously decadent.

Fresh organic orange zest sprinkled onto the frosting adds a bright finish.

Using a hand mixer rather than a stand mixer will take a bit more time to fully mix the ingredients.

Monash Note: Chiles contain capsaicin that may trigger heartburn and abdominal pain in some people with IBS. Limit intake if IBS symptoms occur after ingestion of spicy foods.

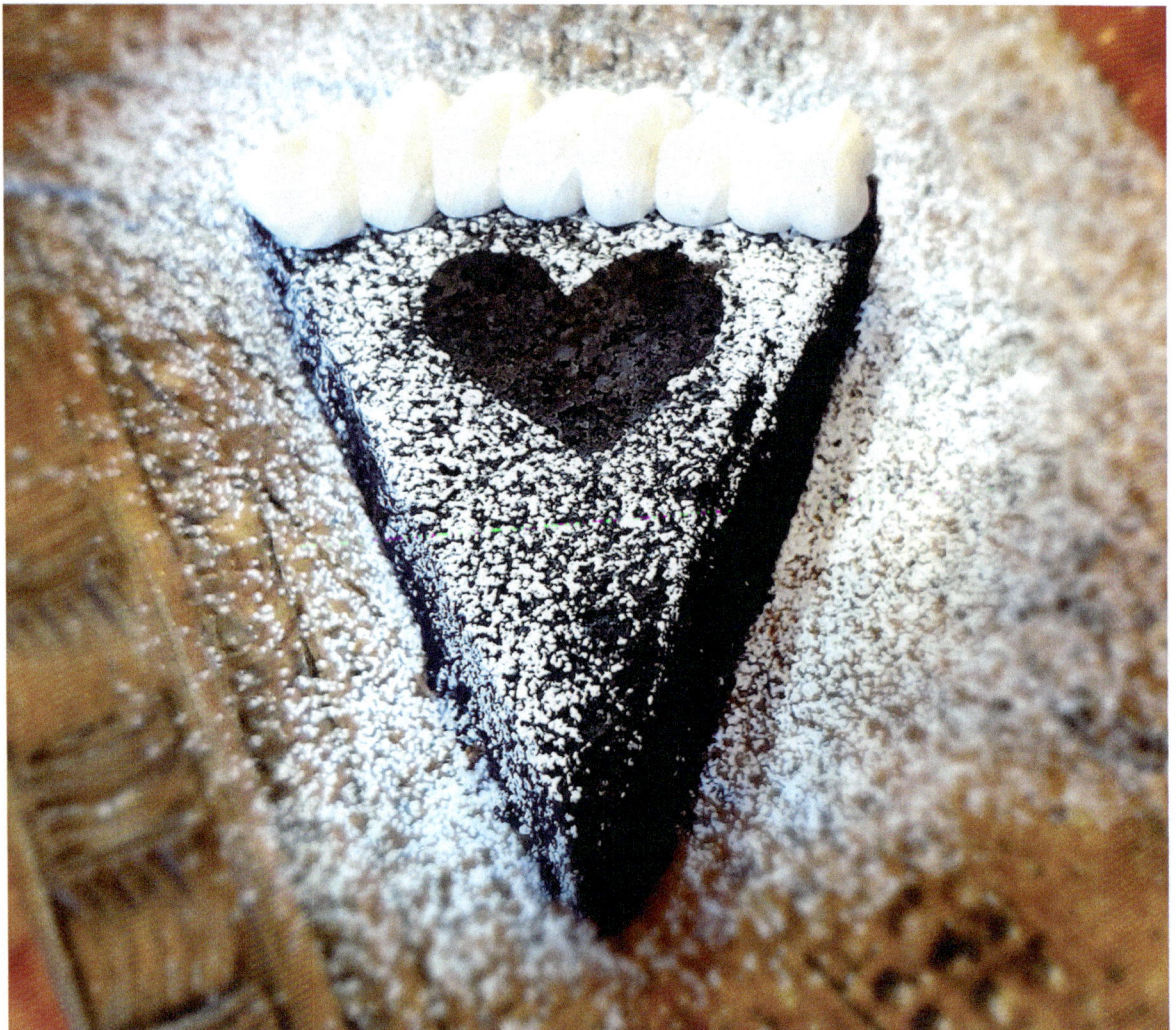

Tres Leches Cake

LOW FODMAP ❤ IBS FRIENDLY ❤ GLUTEN-FREE ❤ DAIRY-FREE

Italy has tiramisu. The Southwest has Tres Leches Cake. For special occasions and definitely Cinco de Mayo, a Tres Leches or two or ten are definitely on the buffet.

The low FODMAP diet is not dairy-free, but I have chosen to create a dairy-free version for those if us who are sensitive to lactose.

Tres Leches means "three milks." This is not for the milks that are baked into the batter, but rather the mixture of three different milks that is poured over the baked vanilla cake to saturate it. It is meant to have a pudding-like quality. Traditionally, the milks are heavy cream, sweetened condensed milk and evaporated milk.

That's a lot of dairy, and some brands include high FODMAP high fructose corn syrup in their sweetened condensed products. You will find that the dairy-free milk swaps for this recipe create an equally mouth watering Tres Leches that will become one of your most requested desserts.

The steps are: Bake the cake; heat the three milks; poke holes in the top of the cake; pour the milks over the top to soak; refrigerate 4 - 6 hours or overnight; plate with fruits and berries. One more thing – don't count on any leftovers!

This recipe requires chilling in the refrigerator 4 to 6 hours, or overnight.

(continued on the next page)

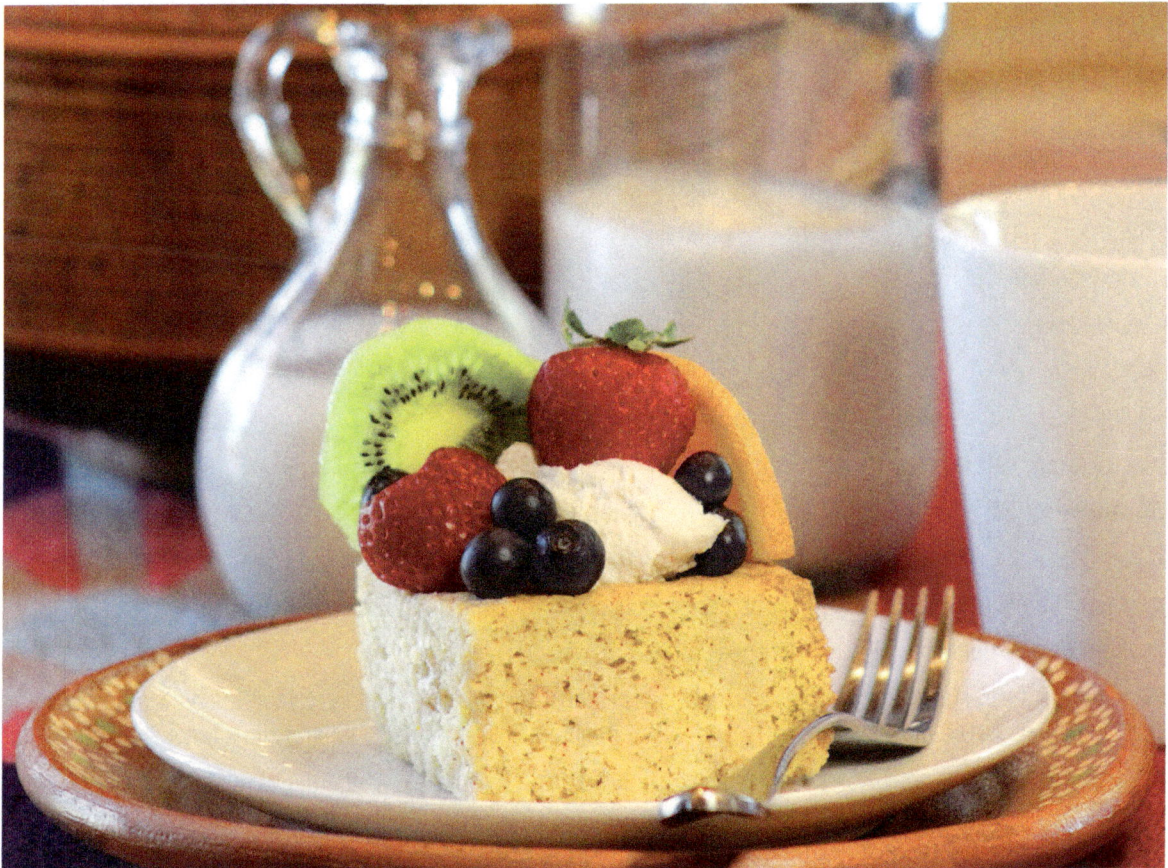

(continued from previous page)

MAKES 12 SERVINGS
CAKE BATTER INGREDIENTS

3 cups (444 g) low FODMAP gluten-free all-purpose baking flour, containing xanthan gum (page 55)

1/4 cup (30 g) cornstarch

2 teaspoons (2 g) ground cinnamon

1 teaspoon (4 g) baking powder; use gluten-free if following a gluten-free diet

1/2 teaspoon (2 g) baking soda

1/2 teaspoon (2.5 g) fine sea salt

1 cup (240 ml) canned full-fat coconut milk for cooking, containing no inulin, well-stirred, at room temperature

1 tablespoon (15 ml) vanilla extract (essence)

8 large eggs, separated, at room temperature; reserve 1 yolk for later in the recipe

2 cups (400 g) sugar

1 cup (224 g) dairy-free butter alternative, at room temperature

Zest of 1 orange

MILK INGREDIENTS

3/4 cup (180 ml) plain, unsweetened almond milk

3/4 cup (180 ml) canned full-fat coconut milk for cooking, containing no inulin, well-stirred

3/4 cup (180 ml) unsweetened macadamia milk

1/4 cup sugar (50 g), plus 2 tablespoons (24 g) more if you like a sweeter cake

2 teaspoons (10 ml) vanilla extract (essence)

1 large egg yolk, reserved from egg whites used in cake batter

TOPPING INGREDIENTS

12 strawberries, cut into fans

12 peeled kiwi slices

12 orange slices

1/2 cup (80 g / 36 individual) fresh blueberries, optional

3/4 cup (90 g) dairy-free whipped topping, see Tips, optional

Method: Preheat oven to 350 F / 177 C

Cake: Coat a 9 x 13-inch (23 x 33 cm) cake pan with cooking spray oil.

In a medium mixing bowl, whisk the flour, cornstarch, cinnamon, baking powder, baking soda and salt.

Measure out the coconut milk and stir in the vanilla.

In a separate mixing bowl, using a hand mixer or stand mixer with whisk attachment, beat the eggs whites on high until they have stiff peaks but not dry, about 2 -3 minutes. Spoon the fluffy whites into a bowl and set aside.

Wipe out the same mixing bowl with a clean cloth. If using a stand mixer exchange the whisk for the paddle attachment. Add the sugar and butter alternative. Beat on high for 5 minutes until fluffy. Scrape down the sides of the bowl with a spatula as needed. Add 2 egg yolks and orange zest. Beat for 2 minutes until fully combined.

On low speed, alternately add the dry ingredients and vanilla milk, in 3 batches, increasing to medium high speed once everything is added to avoid splatters. Beat on high for 1 minute (this timing will vary greatly between hand mixer and stand mixer). Gently fold in the whipped egg whites, in 3 batches, using a spatula to fully combine. Be careful not to over mix, which will deflate the whites.

Pour the batter into the greased baking pan and level the top evenly with a spatula. Bake 35 minutes and check to see if the top is golden brown. When a toothpick inserted into the center comes out clean, it is done. If not, bake 5 more minutes and check again. Remove from the oven and let cool for 10 minutes. Use a wooden skewer or fork to poke holes in the top, almost to the bottom, 1/2-inches (1.25 cm) apart. Set aside.

Milk: In a medium saucepan, whisk together the milks ingredients and 1 reserved egg yolk. Bring to a low boil and stir for 5 minutes, but do not let it come to a rolling boil. Pour evenly over the cake and around the edges. Cool for 30 minutes, cover with plastic wrap and chill in the fridge for 4 to 6 hours or overnight.

Assembly: Serve each slice with fruits and berries. Top with 1 tablespoon dairy-free whipped topping.

Tips: The flour used for this recipe is a gluten-free 1 to 1 baking mix containing rice flour, potato starch, sorghum flour, tapioca flour and xanthan gum. It does not contain bean flours, baking powder or baking soda. I've added extra cornstarch for a lighter consistency. See page 55 for more about flour blends.

The butter alternative sticks i use are a non-GMO, vegan vegetable oil combination with water, salt, natural flavor, pea protein, sunflower lecithin, lactic acid and annatto extract for color.

The canned dairy-free whipped topping used is made with almond milk, coconut cream, sugar, less than 2% mono and diglycerides, natural flavor, pea protein, xanthan gum, carrageenan, propellant and nitrous oxide.

By leaving the cake in the pan the milks continue to soak into the sponge. When turned out onto a platter, the milks seep out, which is part of the charm! This cake is a party pleaser, in which case I recommend transporting in the pan.

Use the leftover yolks for Hollandaise or a frittata.

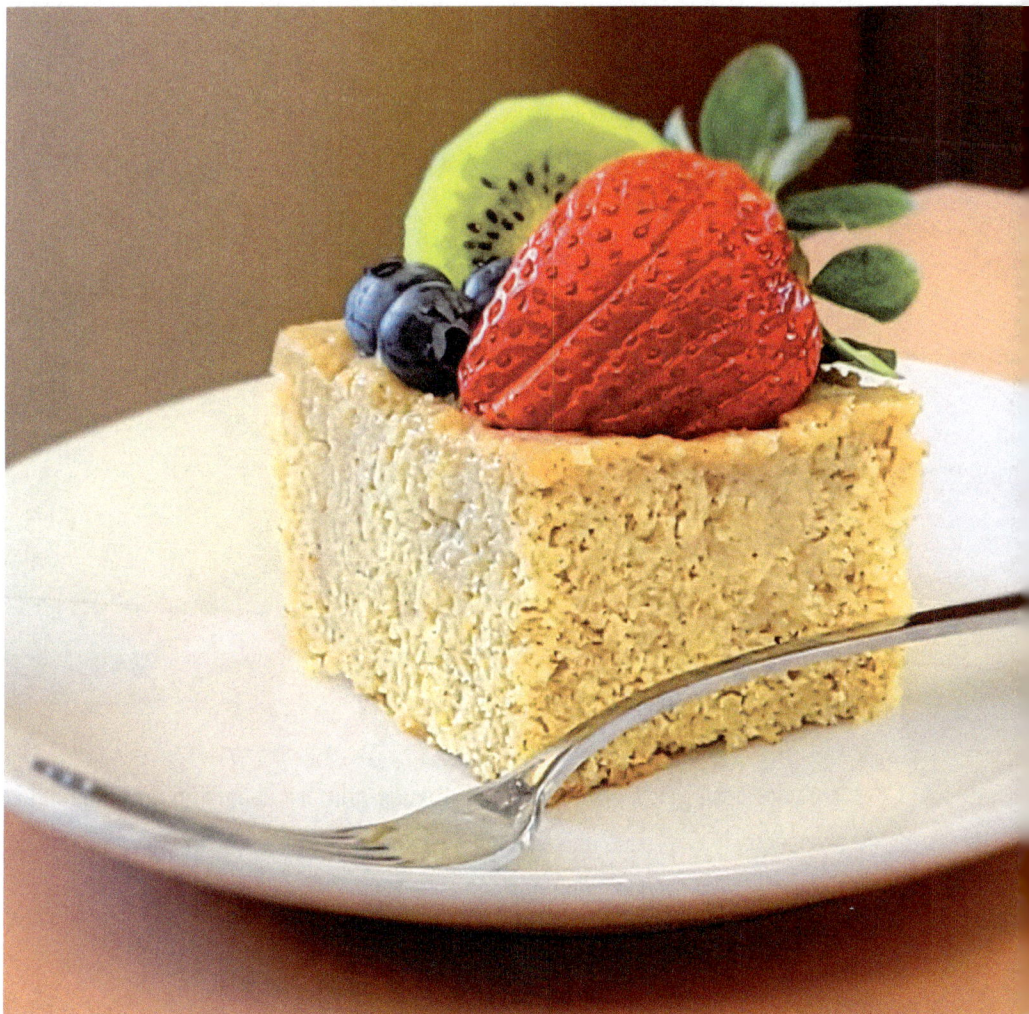

Bizcochitos

LOW FODMAP ❤ IBS FRIENDLY ❤ GLUTEN-FREE ❤ DAIRY-FREE

New Mexico's official state cookie, the Bizcochito, is also a holiday and special occasion treat enjoyed throughout the Southwest. The smell of sugar cookies with cinnamon, anise and orange lets us know the holidays have arrived. They're wonderful as is, or sandwiched with a melted 70% cocoa mass bittersweet chocolate.

This recipe requires 1 hour and 30 minutes chill time in the fridge before baking.

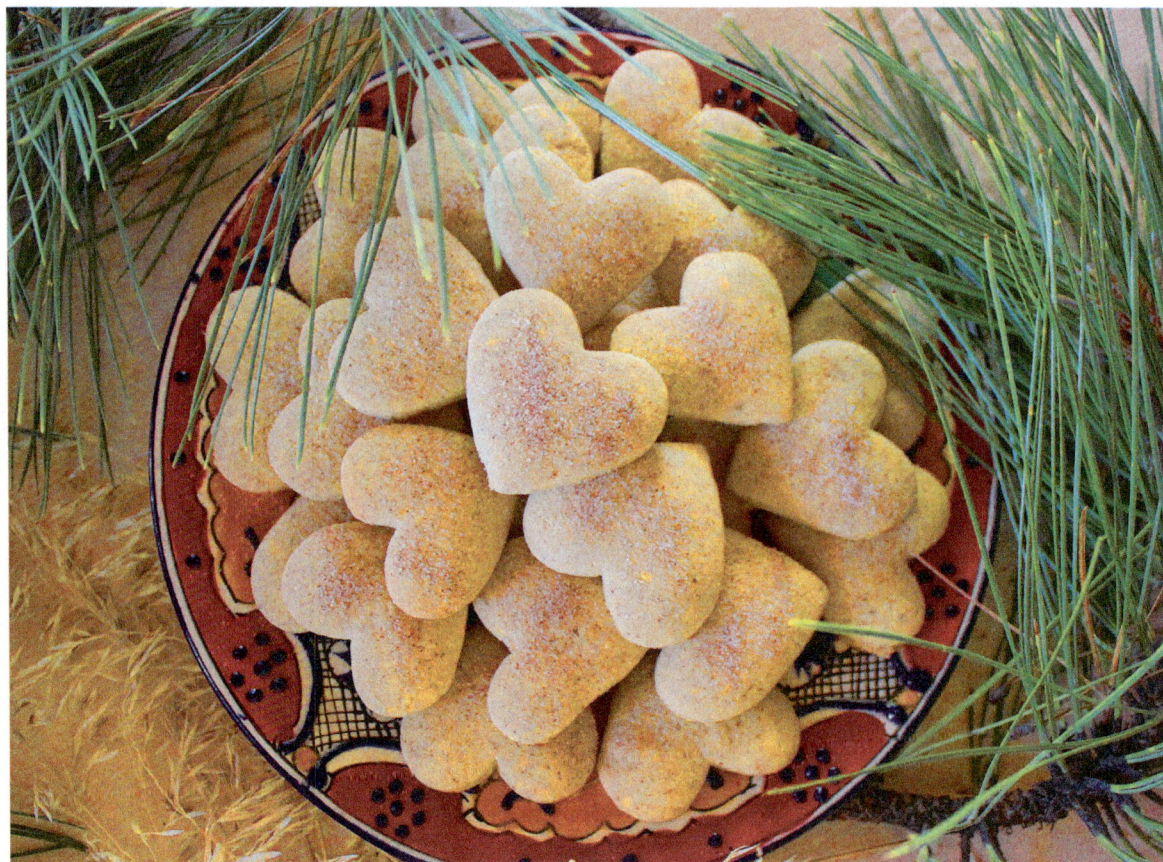

MAKES 44 COOKIES FOR 22 SANDWICH COOKIES – 2 PER SERVING
(using a 2-inch (5 cm) heart cookie cutter)

INGREDIENTS

1 3/4 cups (258 g) low FODMAP gluten-free all-purpose baking flour, containing xanthan gum (page 55)

2 teaspoons (4 g) ground anise seeds (use a coffee grinder for whole anise seeds)

1 teaspoon (2 g) ground cinnamon

1/4 teaspoon baking powder; use gluten-free if following a gluten-free diet

1/4 teaspoon fine sea salt

1/2 cup (112 g) plus 2 tablespoons (28 g) dairy-free butter alternative, softened but still cool to the touch

1/2 cup (100 g) sugar

1 large egg, room temperature

2 tablespoons (30 ml) plain, unsweetened almond milk, at room temperature

1 tablespoon (15 ml) fresh squeezed orange juice

2 teaspoons (10 ml) vanilla extract (essence)

Zest of 1 large orange

Cinnamon sugar topping of 6 teaspoons sugar and 1/2 teaspoon ground cinnamon, mixed

Method: Whisk the flour, anise, cinnamon, baking powder and salt in a medium bowl.

Beat the butter alternative and sugar in a stand mixer using the paddle attachment, or medium-sized mixing bowl with hand mixer for 5 minutes on high, scraping down the sides of the bowl as needed. Add the egg, milk, orange juice and vanilla. Mix on high for 3 minutes until fully incorporated.

Gradually spoon in the dry ingredients in 3 batches, first on low speed as you add and then on medium high to mix. Once all is blended the dough consistency will be very soft.

Form the dough into a flat 1-inch (2.5 cm) thick disk, wrap tightly in plastic and chill in the refrigerator for 1 hour 30 minutes.

Preheat the oven to 375 F / 190 C

Cover a baking sheet with parchment paper and coat lightly with cooking spray oil.

Roll 1/2 of the dough out on a gluten-free flour-dusted surface to 1/4-inch (.63 cm) thickness. Keep the dough you are not rolling in the fridge, wrapped. Cut into shapes with your cookie cutter (I use a 2-inch / 5 cm heart). If your kitchen is warm or it's a hot day outside and the dough becomes soft, just pop it back in the fridge for 10 minutes, then continue to roll out.

Stir the sugar and cinnamon together in a small bowl.

Place the shapes on the cookie pan, evenly spaced apart, and lightly sprinkle the tops with cinnamon sugar. Bake for 7 to 8 minutes or until they are a light golden color. Place on a wire baking rack to cool. Repeat for remaining cookies.

They are delicious as is and perfect for serving with a hot cup of ginger tea. If you'd like to take the extra step of making them into chocolate filled sandwich cookies, I highly recommend it and the added step is so easy!

FOR SANDWICH COOKIES

You will need 1/2-ounces (70 g) 70% minimum cocoa mass bittersweet chocolate. Some baking chocolates contain a bit of dairy that many people with IBS are able to tolerate. If you use this type or a dairy-free baking chocolate be sure that it is 70% cocoa minimum and contains no high FODMAP ingredients.

Place the chocolate in a small microwavable bowl and melt for 30 seconds. Stir. Micro 20 more seconds. Stir. If not completely melted, try 5 more seconds and stir.

Let sit too cool for 5 minutes. Using a butter knife or tiny spoon, spread a thin layer on the flat side of a cookie, just to the edges. Sandwich with another cookie and place on a serving platter. Repeat for the remaining cookies. Use any leftover chocolate to drizzle over the tops in a random striped pattern, using a back and forth motion. Sprinkle remaining cinnamon sugar over the soft chocolate.

Sandwich cookies will keep up to 3 to 4 days in the refrigerator in an airtight container, stacked with wax paper separating the cookies.

Taos Brownies

LOW FODMAP ❤ IBS FRIENDLY ❤ GLUTEN-FREE ❤ DAIRY-FREE

There is nothing so calming and grounding than watching snow fall on the brown adobes of Taos, New Mexico. On evenings such as these, we sit by a roaring kiva fire, share a blanket, and indulge in these rich brownies that are tender, fudgy and spicy. First, you taste the chocolate and cinnamon. Then the cayenne delivers delectable warmth.

Tolerances for cayenne heat vary. Some are able handle it to the point that it would take three hours for them to blow a cup of coffee cool. Others prefer to omit it all together. In our family, the brownie cayenne gauge goes something like this …

1/2 teaspoon = a little warm, nice	1 1/2 teaspoons = kicking in!
1 teaspoon = feeling it	2 teaspoons = kapow!!

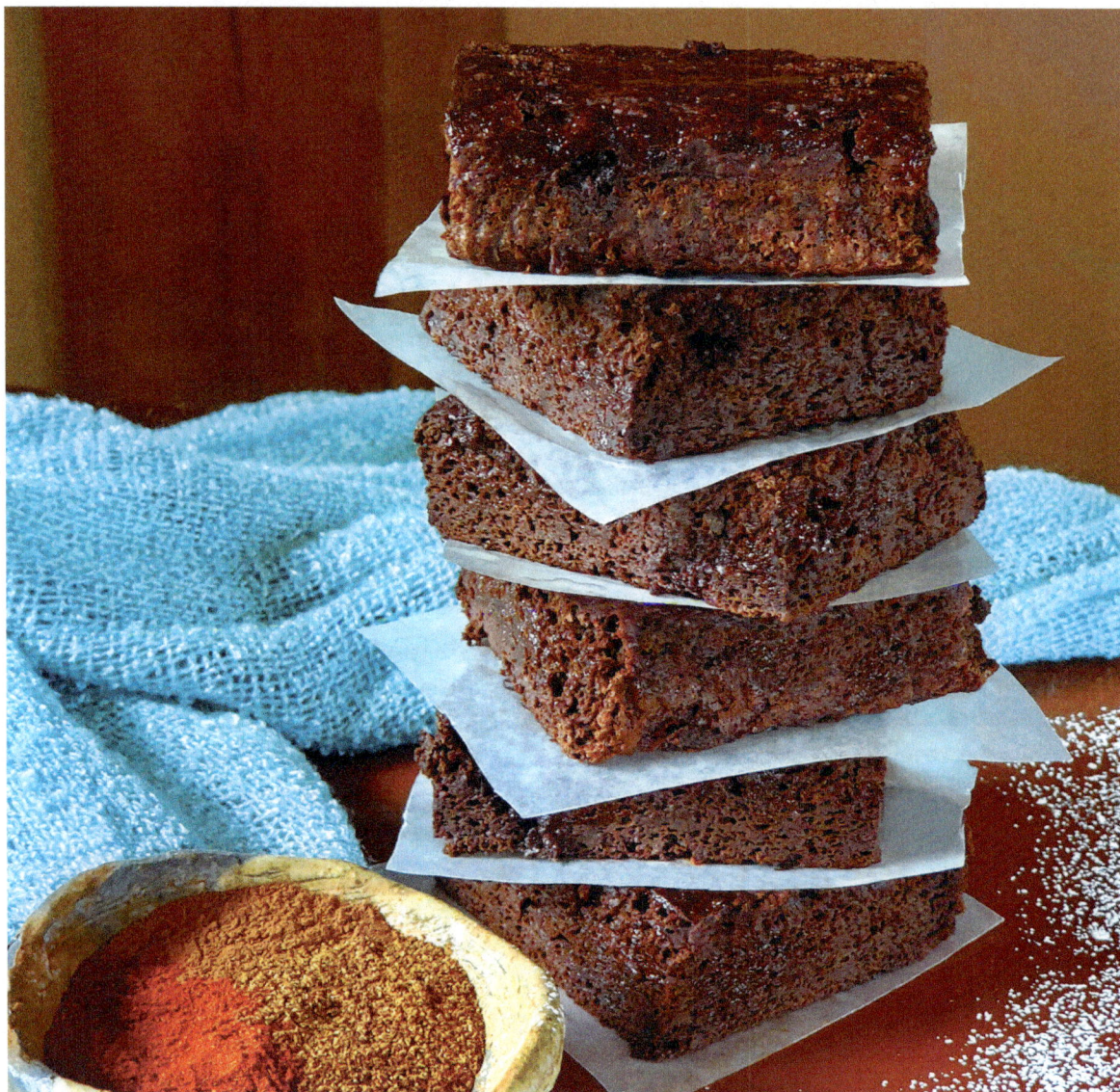

MAKES 9-12 SERVINGS
INGREDIENTS

1 1/4 cups (185 g) low FODMAP gluten-free all-purpose baking flour, containing xanthan gum (page 55)

1/2 cup (43 g) Dutch-processed cocoa powder, containing 70% cocoa minimum

1 tablespoon (6 g) ground cinnamon

1/2 to 2 teaspoons cayenne (I generally use 1 teaspoon)

1/2 teaspoon fine sea salt

3/4 cup (180 ml) plain, unsweetened almond milk

1/2 cup (120 ml) canned full-fat coconut milk for cooking, containing no inulin, well-stirred, at room temperature

3 large eggs, at room temperature

1 tablespoon (15 ml) vanilla extract (essence)

1/2 cup (112 g) dairy-free butter alternative

4-ounces (113 g) bittersweet chocolate, 70% cocoa mass minimum, fine chopped

1 1/4 cups (250 g) sugar

Confectioners' sugar for light dusting

Method: Preheat oven to 350 F / 177 C

Lightly coat a 9x9-inch (23 x 23 cm) baking pan (metal brownie pan) with cooking spray oil. Cut a piece of parchment to line the pan, leaving 4-inch (10 cm) overlaps on two sides for easily lifting the brownies out of the pan after baking. Crease the parchment into the inside edges as best you can. Lightly coat the paper with cooking spray oil.

Whisk the flour, cocoa powder, cinnamon, cayenne and salt in a large mixing bowl.

In a separate bowl, whisk the almond milk, coconut milk, eggs and vanilla.

Melt the butter alternative and baking chocolate in a small saucepan over low heat. Do not allow to boil. When the chocolate has just completely melted, remove from heat and let cool 5 to 10 minutes to room temperature. Slowly drizzle into the egg mixture, whisking continuously.

Pour the wet mixture into the dry ingredients and stir to combine. Add the sugar 1/4 cup at a time, folding and stirring to thoroughly mix. Spoon the batter into the baking pan and spread out evenly.

Bake 25 minutes. If the center is still jiggly, bake 5 more minutes and check again. Ovens vary from kitchen to kitchen. You want the consistency of inserting a toothpick to show moist crumbs still clinging. My oven bakes them perfectly at 30 minutes.

Remove from the oven to cool completely, about 30 minutes. Lift out, using the parchment as handles, onto a cutting board or work surface. Cut into 9 to 12 squares. Dust lightly with confectioners' sugar.

Tips: Some baking chocolates contain a bit of dairy that many people with IBS are able to tolerate. If you use this type or a dairy-free baking chocolate be sure that it is 70% cocoa or more with no high FODMAP ingredients. For party buffets, cut them into 1-inch (2.5 cm) pieces for a tray of bite-sized treats.

Stored in an airtight container, brownies will keep up to 7 days in the fridge.

Monash Note: Although chiles (chillies) are generally low in FODMAPs, some people with IBS may be sensitive to the capsaicin they contain. Capsaicin is a natural compound that gives chiles their spicy quality. You may need to limit how much chile you eat if your IBS symptoms are triggered by spicy food.

Cornmeal Dusted Meringues with Candied Poblanos

LOW FODMAP ❤ IBS FRIENDLY ❤ GLUTEN-FREE ❤ DAIRY-FREE

The beauty of these meringues is that they are dusted with yellow cornmeal that toasts as they bake to form crunchy shells with soft centers. The candied poblanos are not too sweet and the lime juice gives a brightness with every bite.

It's best to make these the day you plan to serve. They can be stored overnight in an airtight baggie or container but I find that the consistency becomes chewy.

The poblanos require roasting and prepping to remove the skins, so be sure to plan accordingly.

MAKES 4 SERVINGS
MERINGUES INGREDIENTS

4 large eggs whites, at room temperature

3/4 cup (150 g) sugar

1 teaspoon (5 ml) vanilla extract (essence)

2 teaspoons (5 g) cornstarch, gluten-free if you are following a gluten-free diet

Pinch fine sea salt

1 tablespoon plus 1 teaspoon (12 g) low FODMAP medium grind whole grain yellow cornmeal

CANDIED POBLANOS INGREDIENTS

2 large (360 g total) poblano chile peppers

1/4 cup (50 g) sugar

Juice of 1 lime

Method: Preheat oven to 275 F / 140 C

Line a half-sheet rimmed baking pan with parchment paper; lightly and evenly coat with cooking spray oil.

Using a stand mixer with whisk attachment or a hand mixer, beat the whites slowly at first, then increase to high speed until they form soft peaks. Add the sugar 1 tablespoon (12 g) at a time on high speed. Add the vanilla, beat 30 seconds. Sprinkle in the cornstarch and salt. Beat for 1 minute. Test that the meringue forms a stiff peak that holds shape when held upright with the whisk or beaters. If too loose, beat on high until you have the consistency of shaving cream that holds its form.

You can pipe the meringues with a pastry bag, however, I love the rustic look of using a spoon to drop and shape them onto the parchment in 3-inch (7.6 cm) diameter rounds, spaced evenly apart. Try to get them as poofy high as you can, as they will deflate a bit during baking. Use a spoon to press a small well into the tops. This is to hold the candied poblanos.

Once all 8 rounds are in place, dust 1/2 teaspoon of cornmeal over each.

Bake for 1 hour. Turn the oven off and leave them in the closed oven for 1 1/2 hours as they dry and become crunchy on the outside and fluffy smooth on the inside.

While the meringues are baking, prepare the poblanos as shown on page 46 to char, steam and remove the skins and seeds. Once you have those beautiful, skinless green fillets, cut them into thin strips, then chop back and forth, side to side into a mince.

In a small nonstick skillet, add the poblanos, sugar and lime juice. Heat to medium low and stir as it begins to bubble. Cook and reduce for 3 - 5 minutes or until the consistency becomes jammy, but not too thick or sticky as it will thicken more when refrigerated. Place in a bowl, cover with a lid or plastic wrap and place in the refrigerator until ready to assemble the meringues.

To Plate: Place 2 meringues on a dessert plate. Spoon candied poblano in the center wells. Repeat for the remaining meringues.

Tips: Taste your poblanos for heat levels. They are generally mild, but every once in a while you will get a slightly hot one. I like to buy 4 or 5 and select the mild ones. Any leftovers freeze nicely in a tightly sealed freezer baggie after they have been roasted (page 46), with the skins left intact until thawed and ready to prep and use.

If poblanos are not available, use Green Chiles such as Hatch, Anaheim, Colorado Green or Chiles Verde Del Norte.

Candied Poblanos are also a fantastic topping for LoFO vanilla or lemon-lime ice cream, LoFO cheesecake, pancakes and for topping frosted cupcakes.

Meringues are also delicious when topped with fresh strawberries, blueberries, kiwi and passion fruit.

Monash Note: Although chiles (chillies) are generally low in FODMAPs, some people with IBS may be sensitive to the capsaicin they contain. Capsaicin is a natural compound that gives chiles their spicy quality. You may need to limit how much chile you eat if your IBS symptoms are triggered by spicy food.

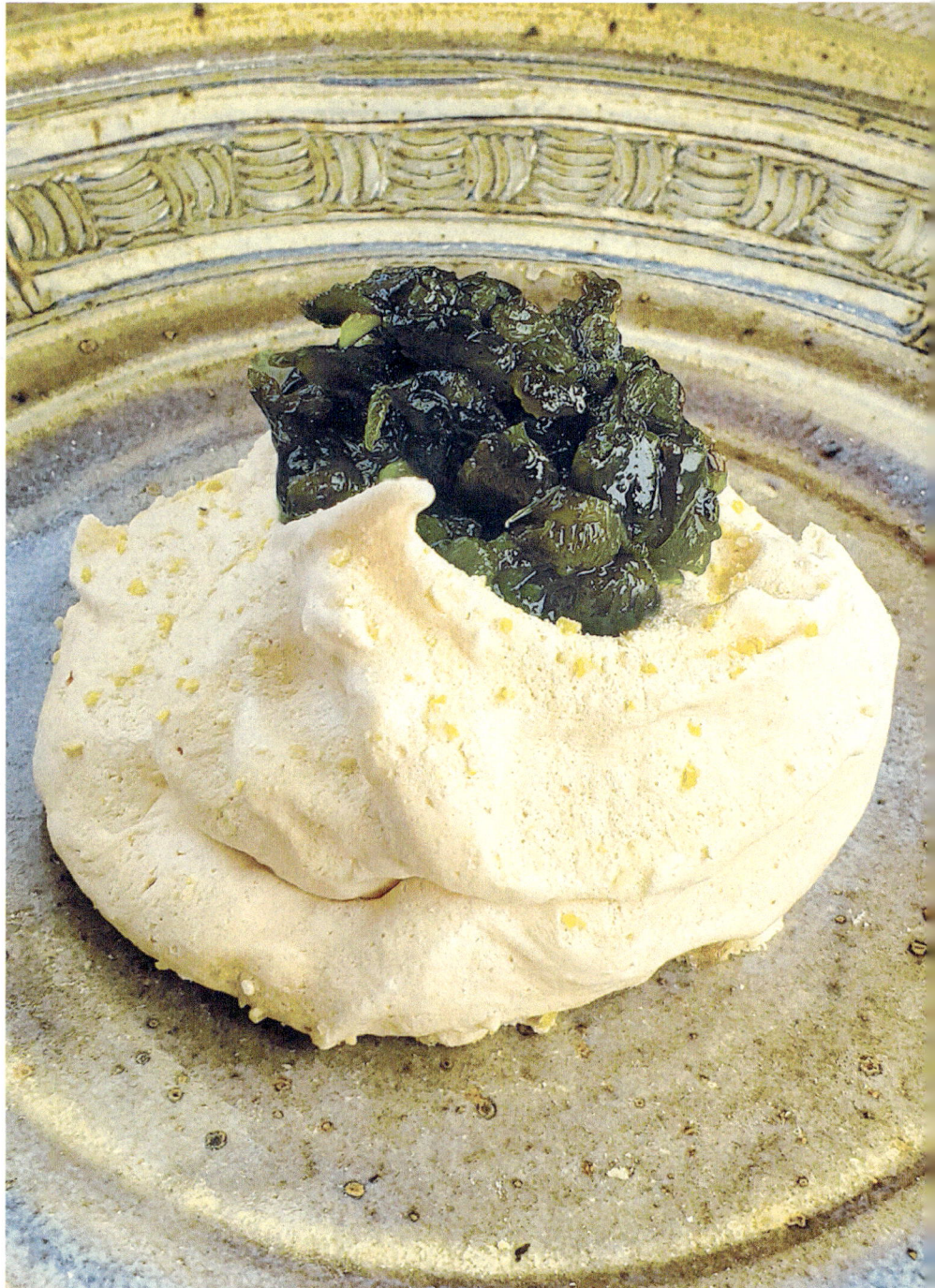

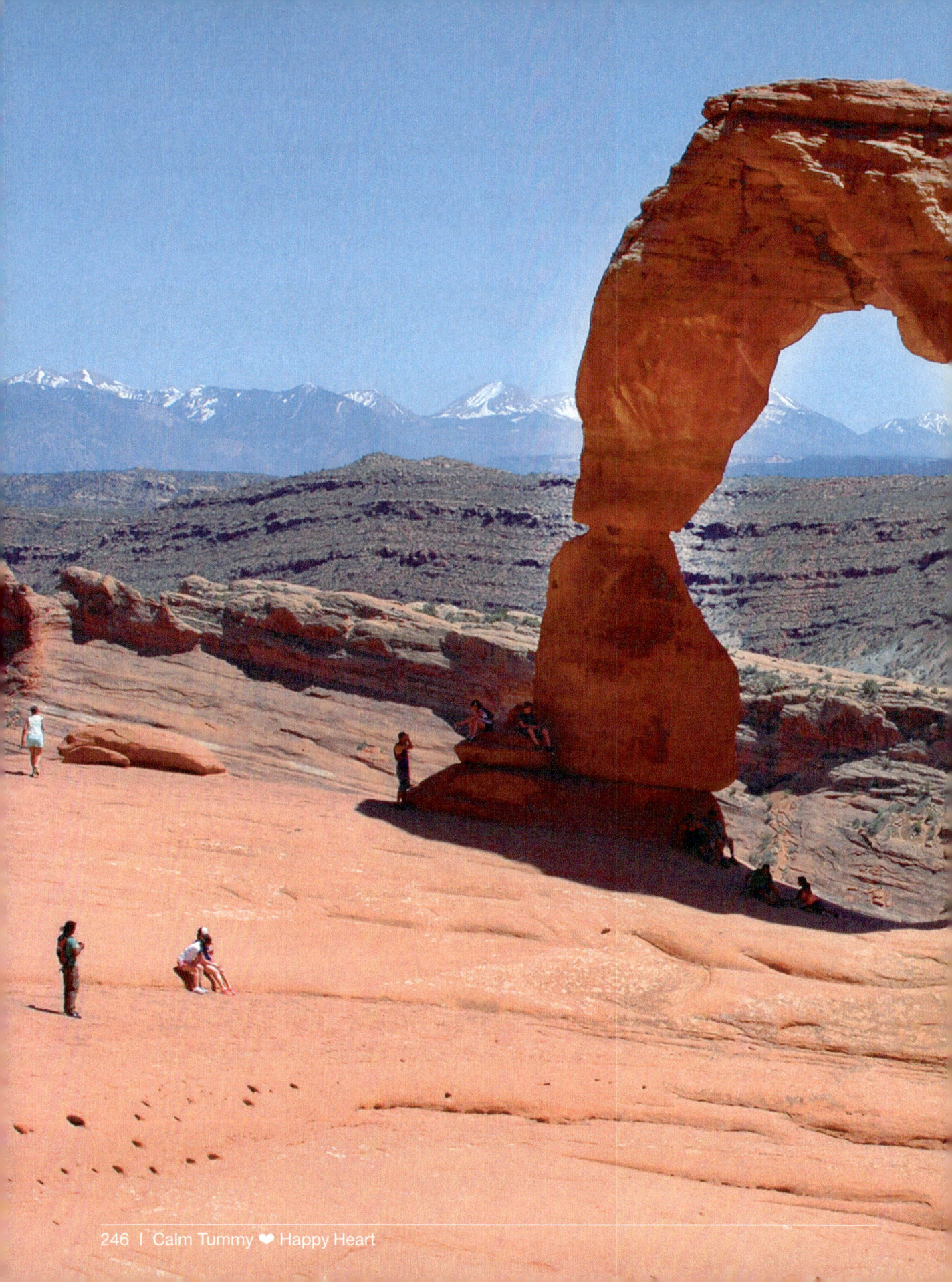

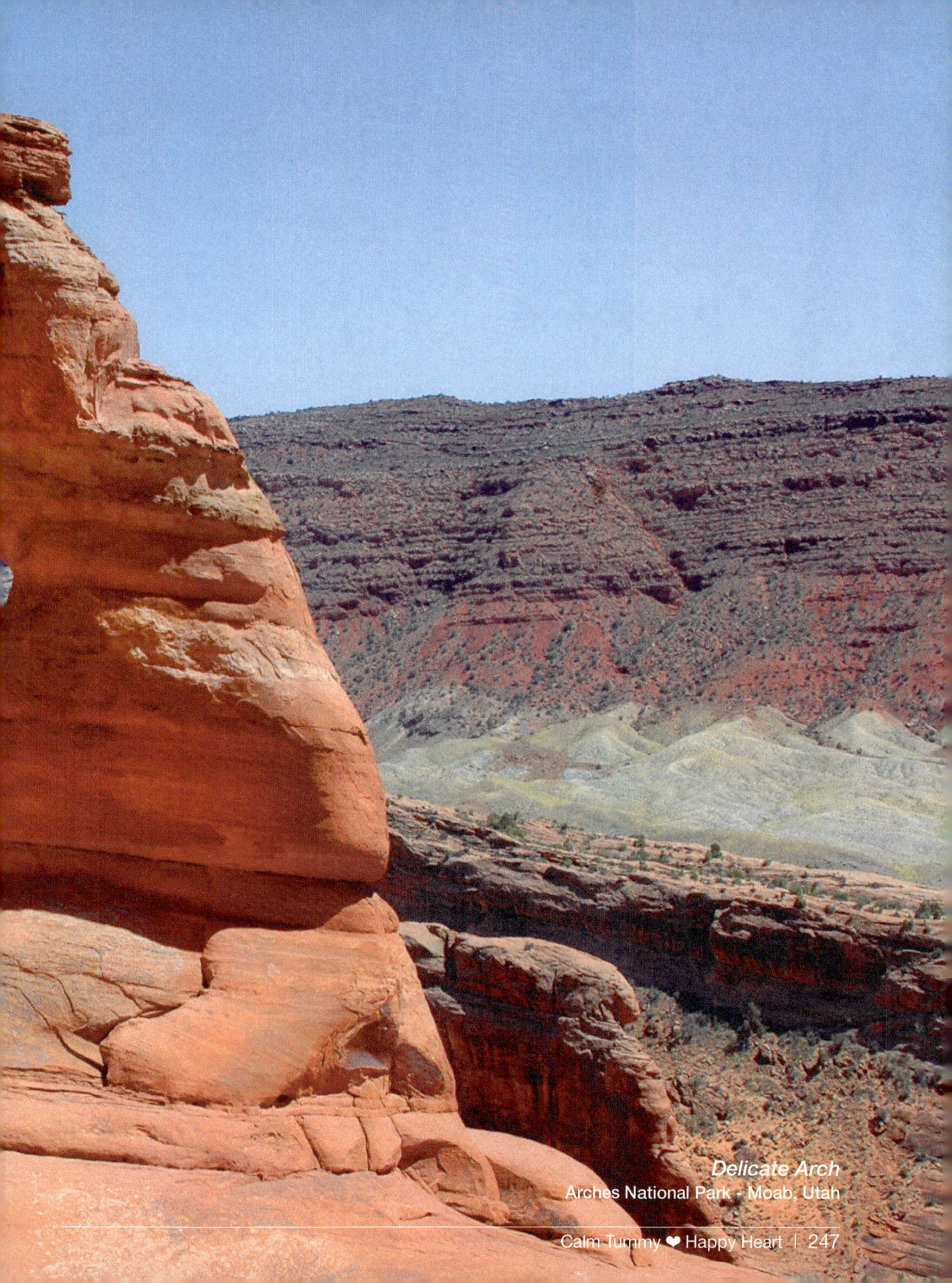

Delicate Arch
Arches National Park - Moab, Utah

Beverages

- ❤ **Sangria Rosa**

- ❤ **Mexican Hot Chocolate**

- ❤ **Horchata with Orange Essence**

- ❤ **White Wine Margarita Pitcher**

- ❤ **The Roswell with Alien Olives**

- ❤ **Roasted Poblano Bloody Mary**

- ❤ **Tea-quila Cocktails**

Food brand names are sometimes listed within a recipe, and this means they are Monash Certified. For more brand options we use and love, please visit **FodifyIt.com**

Monash Note: Although chiles (chillies) are generally low in FODMAPs, some people with IBS may be sensitive to the capsaicin they contain. Capsaicin is a natural compound that gives chiles their spicy quality. You may need to limit how much chile you eat if your IBS symptoms are triggered by spicy food.

Note: Monash advises that alcohol is an irritant to the gut. A limited intake is advised and only consume alcohol with food. **Please drink responsibly.**

Sangria Rosa

LOW FODMAP ♥ IBS FRIENDLY ♥ GLUTEN-FREE ♥ DAIRY-FREE

Sangria is a wine punch that is traditionally mixed with red wine, fruits and berries, and sometimes a liqueur. I enjoy serving this combination with an oaky chardonnay mixed with pure cranberry juice, a splash of brandy, fresh strawberries and orange. And don't forget the cinnamon stick – it adds a warm spicy note that balances the citrus and cranberry, making it all the more unique!

This recipe requires overnight refrigeration.

MAKES 6 SERVINGS

INGREDIENTS

1, 750 ml bottle of a good oaky chardonnay

1/2 cup (120 ml / 4-ounces) pure, unsweetened cranberry juice that is not apple juice based, nor contains high fructose corn syrup or other high FODMAPs

1, 1-ounce shot (30 ml) brandy

6 medium (78 g) strawberries, hulled and sliced

1 medium (130 g) orange, sliced thinly crosswise or into wedges

1 tablespoon (12 g) sugar

1 cinnamon stick

2 tablespoons (30 ml) maple syrup, plus 1 tablespoon (15 ml) extra if needed

Method: Place all ingredients, using 2 tablespoons maple syrup, in a large pitcher and stir to mix. Place the lid or plastic wrap over the pitcher and refrigerate overnight.

Stir and taste for sweetness. You may want to add more maple syrup, a little at a time. Serve over ice. Cheers!

Tips: Many juices including cranberry are apple juice based, so be sure you are using pure cranberry juice.

When selecting a chardonnay, I do not buy a pricey bottle because it's going to be mixed into a punch. Rather, I use a moderately priced wine that I would be comfortable bringing to a casual get-together.

Note: Monash advises that alcohol is an irritant to the gut. A limited intake is advised and only consume alcohol with food. Please drink responsibly.

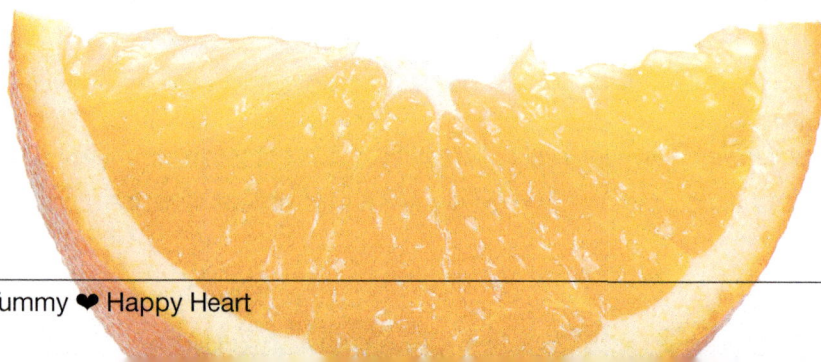

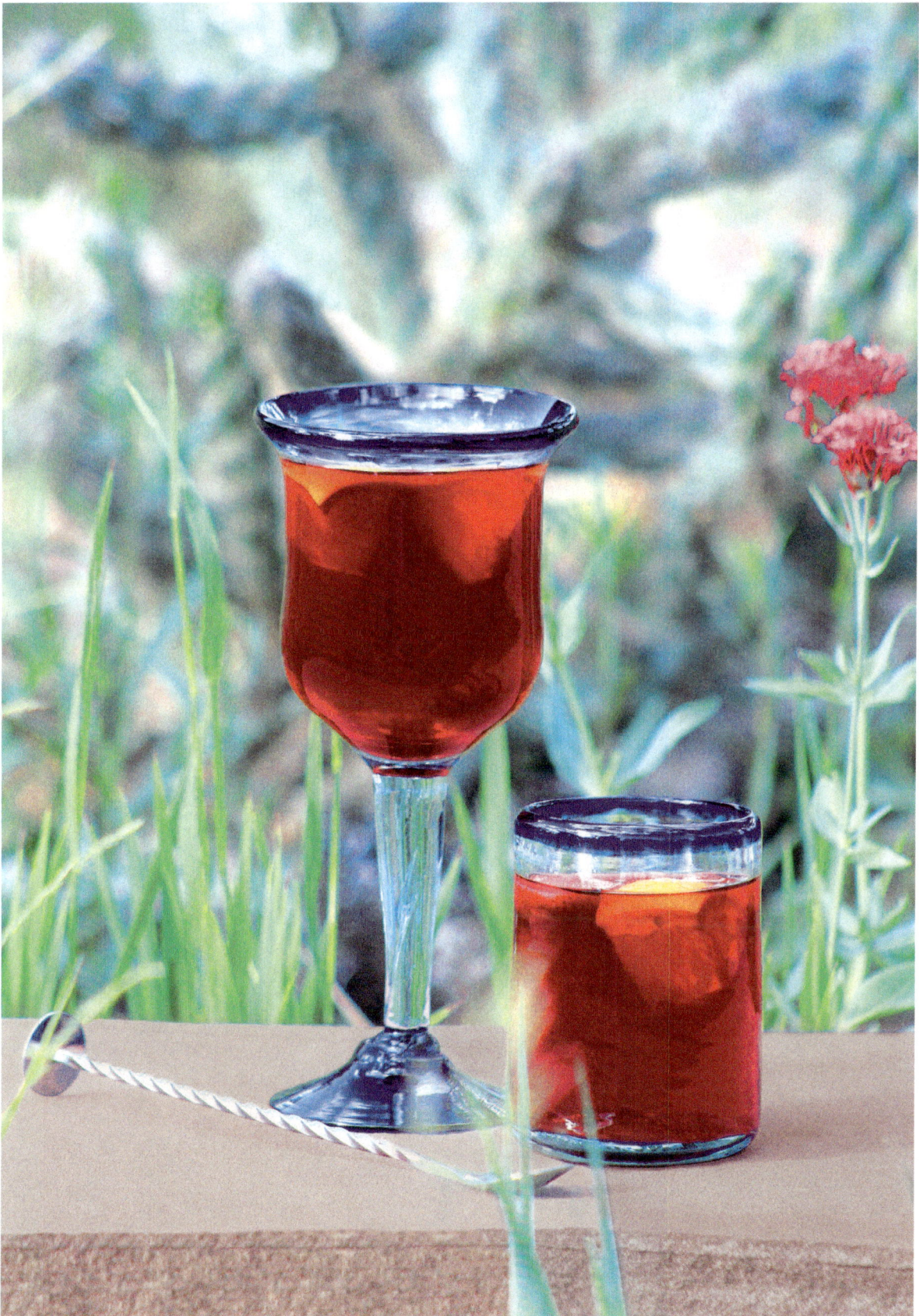

Mexican Hot Chocolate

LOW FODMAP ❤ IBS FRIENDLY ❤ GLUTEN-FREE ❤ DAIRY-FREE

Beyond the comfort of drinking a hot, milky chocolate beverage that sweetens your day with the first sip, Mexican Hot Chocolate also has a lovely maize (corn) flavor from the masa. I highly recommend using Mexican chocolate tablets if they are available to you. The texture is a rustic grainy sugary cocoa, and the flavor is quite intense.

MAKES 2 SERVINGS

INGREDIENTS

1 cup (240 ml / 8-ounces) water

2 cups (475 ml / 16-ounces) plain, unsweetened almond milk

2 tablespoons (30 ml) canned full-fat coconut milk for cooking, containing no inulin, well-stirred

1/2 cup (63 g) gluten-free masa harina

1/2 cup (80 g) medium packed light brown sugar

2-ounces (46 g) Mexican chocolate tablets, 70% cocoa mass minimum, rough chopped, or the equivalent of bittersweet chocolate

1 cinnamon stick

1/2 teaspoon (1 g) pure mild red chile powder (containing no onion or garlic, the ingredients should list only: red chile. On the Monash App this is called Chilli (chili) red, powdered.

Method: Pour the water, almond and coconut milk into a medium saucepan. Bring to medium heat. Add the masa, sugar, chocolate, cinnamon and chile powder. Stir until thickened, about 5 minutes. If too thick, add a bit more almond milk. Remove the cinnamon stick and pour into mugs. Serve immediately.

Tip: Some baking chocolates contain a bit of dairy that many people with IBS are able to tolerate. If you use this type or a dairy-free chocolate be sure that it is 70% cocoa minimum and contains no high FODMAP ingredients.

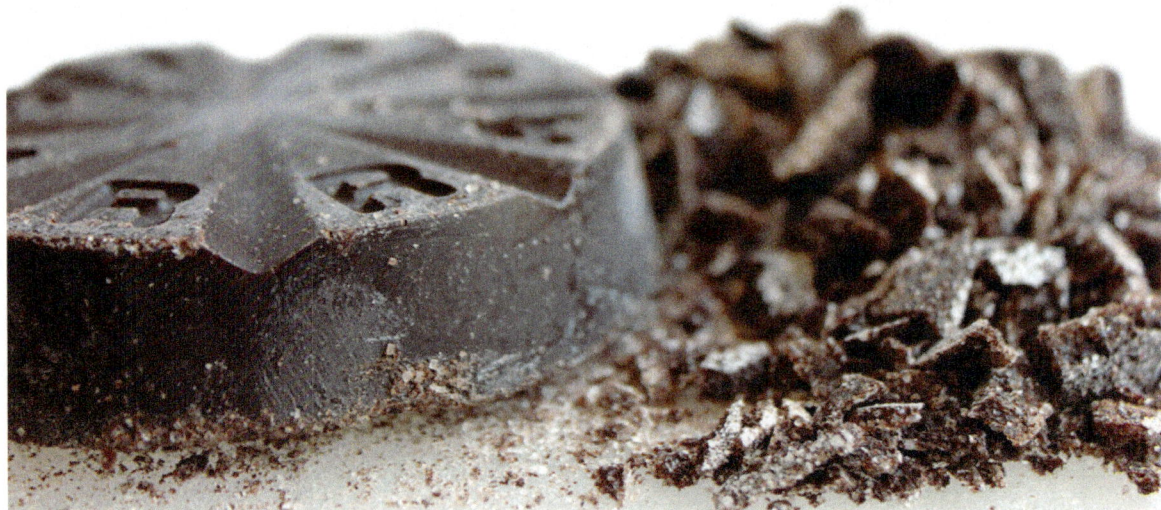

Horchata with Orange Essence

LOW FODMAP ❤ IBS FRIENDLY ❤ GLUTEN-FREE ❤ DAIRY-FREE

Horchata is a delicious white rice-based drink flavored with cinnamon and vanilla. Ingredients soak overnight in water to infuse. The next day requires a quick mix of the remaining ingredients, then poured over ice for refreshing chilled sipping on a warm afternoon. Adding orange zest gives it a bright citrus note. I do suggest using an organic orange if possible as you will be consuming the zest; non-organic might be treated with pesticides.

MAKES 4 SERVINGS
INGREDIENTS

1 1/2 cups (278 g) white rice, organic if available

3 cups (700 ml / 24-ounces) water

Zest of 1 orange, organic if available

1 1/2 teaspoons (3 g) ground cinnamon, or 2 cinnamon sticks

2 1/4 cups (535 ml / 18-ounces) plain, unsweetened almond milk

1/3 cup (66 g) sugar

1 teaspoon (5 ml) vanilla extract (essence)

Method: Wash the rice in a fine mesh metal strainer under cold water until the water runs clear.

Add the rice, water, zest and ground cinnamon to a blender. If using cinnamon sticks do not add to this step. Purée for 1 minute. Stop the blender and using a long spatula, stir the bottom blade to loosen any rice that has settled. Purée another 30 seconds. If you have a small blender, do this in 2 batches.

Pour into a bowl. If you are using cinnamon sticks, add them now. Cover and refrigerate overnight.

The next day, remove the cinnamon sticks, stir the mixture and pour through a fine mesh metal strainer into a pitcher. Discard the solids.

Whisk in the almond milk, sugar and vanilla. Serve over ice.
Garnish with ground cinnamon or a cinnamon stick.
If the Horchata is too thick, add more plain,
unsweetened almond milk for desired consistency.

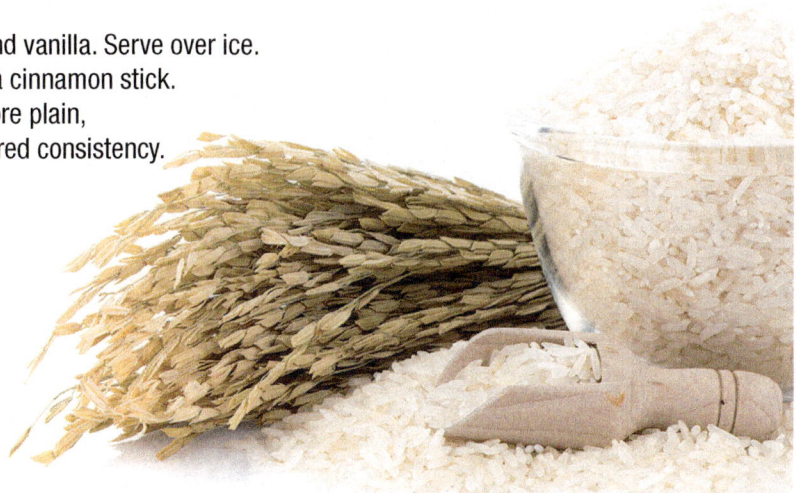

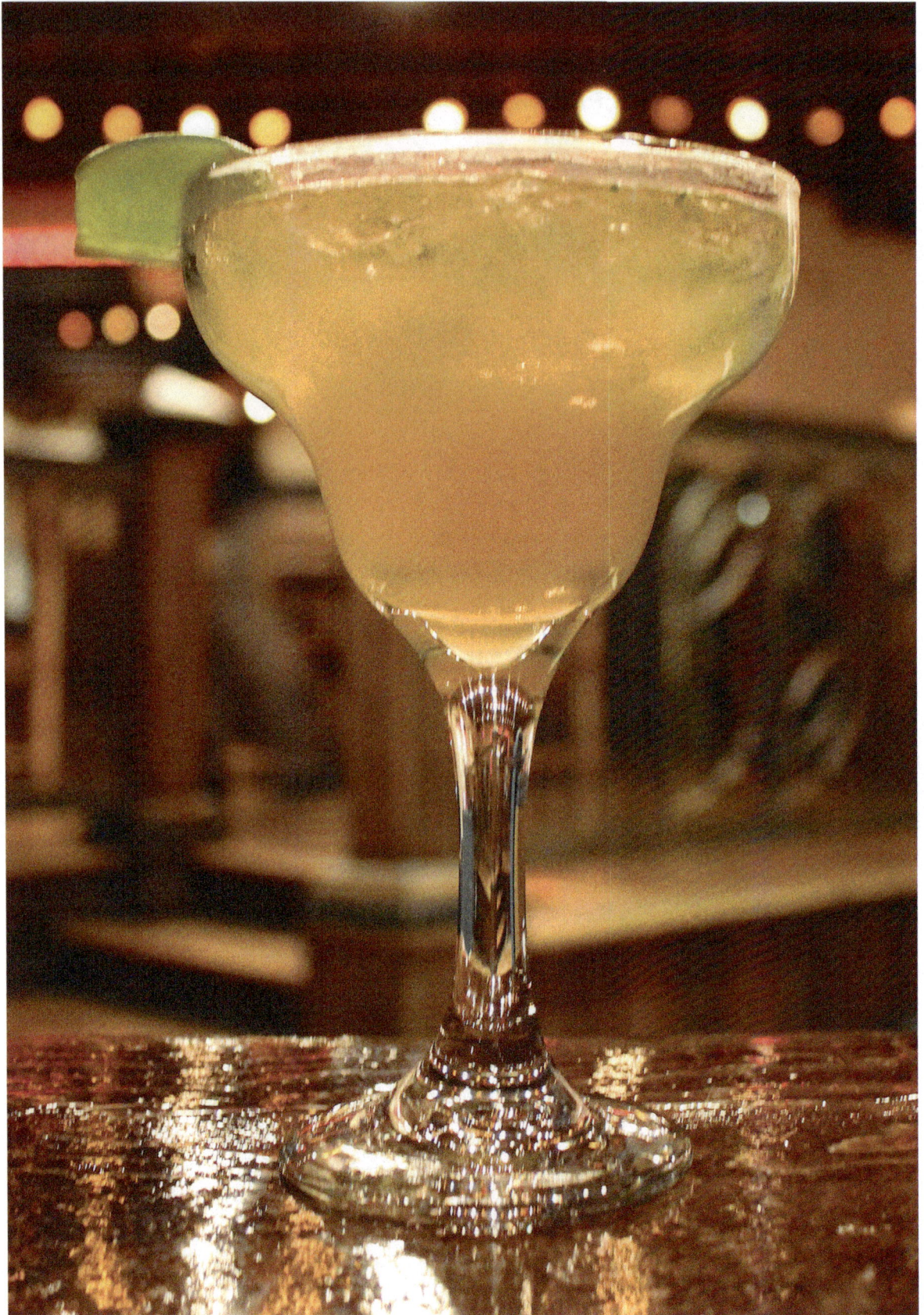

White Wine Margarita Pitcher

LOW FODMAP ❤ IBS FRIENDLY ❤ GLUTEN-FREE ❤ DAIRY-FREE

Meeting friends for margaritas is a big part of the Southwestern social scene. And while they are more often made with tequila, wine margaritas are oftentimes on the menu as a refreshing option. They taste like a delicious citrus wine punch.

Run a lime wedge around the rim of the glasses and then press into salt for that familiar celebratory flavor, and use a good bottle of wine, but not too fancy as this is a mixed drink.

MAKES 5 SERVINGS

INGREDIENTS

Margarita salt (a coarse grain salt with a flaky crunch), enough to cover 1/4-inch (.635 cm) deep in a small plate

3 lime wedges, for coating the glass rims

1, 750 ml bottle good white wine; an oaky chardonnay is great

Juice of 2 fresh squeezed limes

Juice of 1 large fresh squeezed orange (90 ml / 3-ounces)

1 1/2 tablespoons (21 ml) maple syrup

Crushed ice

5 lime slices with slit for placing on the glass rims

Method: Prepare 5 margarita glasses by pouring margarita salt onto a shallow plate. Run lime wedges around the rims of the glasses, then press the glass rims into the salt to coat.

Pour the wine, juice of limes and oranges, and maple syrup in a large pitcher. Stir to mix. Pour into the glasses, in equal amounts. Add crushed ice and garnish each with a lime slice. Serve immediately. Cheers!

Note: Monash advises that alcohol is an irritant to the gut. A limited intake is advised and only consume alcohol with food. **Please drink responsibly.**

The Roswell With Alien Olives

LOW FODMAP ❤ IBS FRIENDLY ❤ GLUTEN-FREE ❤ DAIRY-FREE

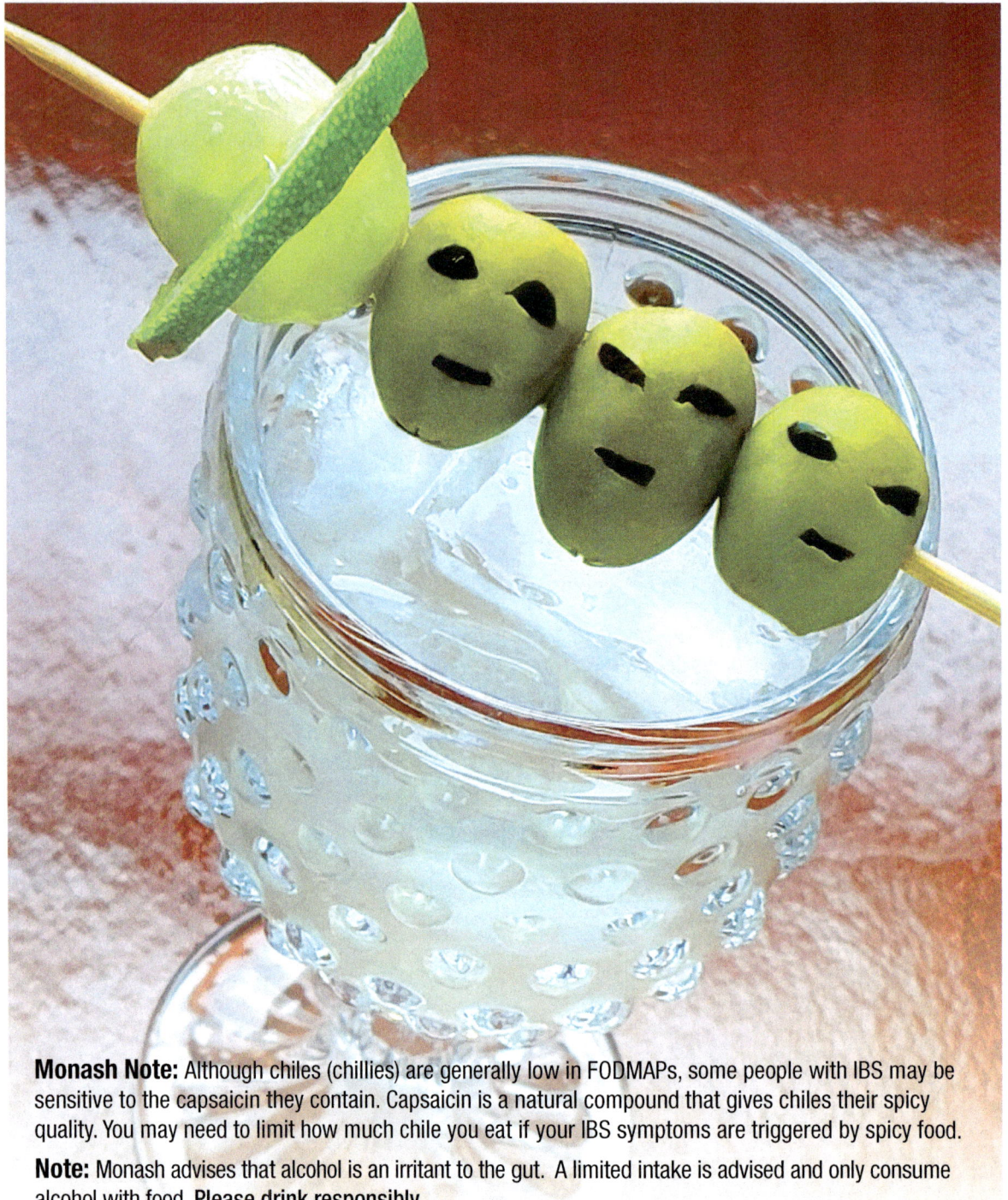

Monash Note: Although chiles (chillies) are generally low in FODMAPs, some people with IBS may be sensitive to the capsaicin they contain. Capsaicin is a natural compound that gives chiles their spicy quality. You may need to limit how much chile you eat if your IBS symptoms are triggered by spicy food.

Note: Monash advises that alcohol is an irritant to the gut. A limited intake is advised and only consume alcohol with food. **Please drink responsibly.**

The best time to visit Roswell, New Mexico is during an event when people from all over the world converge on this little town in east central New Mexico and go spaced out wacko (in the very best sense of the word) to celebrate the 1947 alien incident. Be prepared for lively conversation, inventive costumes and alien selfies on every street. Jim and I have been a few times and have yet to meet someone who has not seen something in the skies that they just cannot explain.

MAKES 2 COCKTAILS
INGREDIENTS

1/4 cup (60 ml / 2-ounces) good quality vodka

3/4 cup (180 ml / 6-ounces) sparkling water, or flat water if your tummy is sensitive to bubbles

Juice of 1/2 lime, plus 2 thin sliced circles of lime for Saturn garnish

1 teaspoon (5 ml) maple syrup

6 green Spanish olives, pitted

2 to 3 canned, pitted ripe black olives

2 cocktail skewers

4 melon ball cut-outs of a cucumber, cut in half crosswise

Crushed ice or ice cubes

Method: Mix the vodka, water, lime juice and maple syrup in a large glass and stir to mix.

Using a very sharp paring knife, cut the alien eyes and mouth impressions into the green olives. Use the knife point to press the eyes and mouth areas into the olive, as this is easier than pulling the tiny cut pieces out of the olives. Cut the eye and mouth shapes out of the black olives. Push them into the green olives to make the faces.

Place 3 alien olives on a skewer, then at an angle add half of the cucumber sphere, the lime slice, and the remaining cucumber sphere half to create a Saturn shape (use image as a guide).

Fill 2 highball glasses with ice to the rim. Divide the vodka mixture evenly into the glasses. Top with garnish skewer. If you want to have a little fun with your guests, skewer the Saturn ingredients and let the 3 little alien olives sink to the bottom of the glass. It's hilarious when people notice their beady eyes looking up at them.

Have a nice flight!

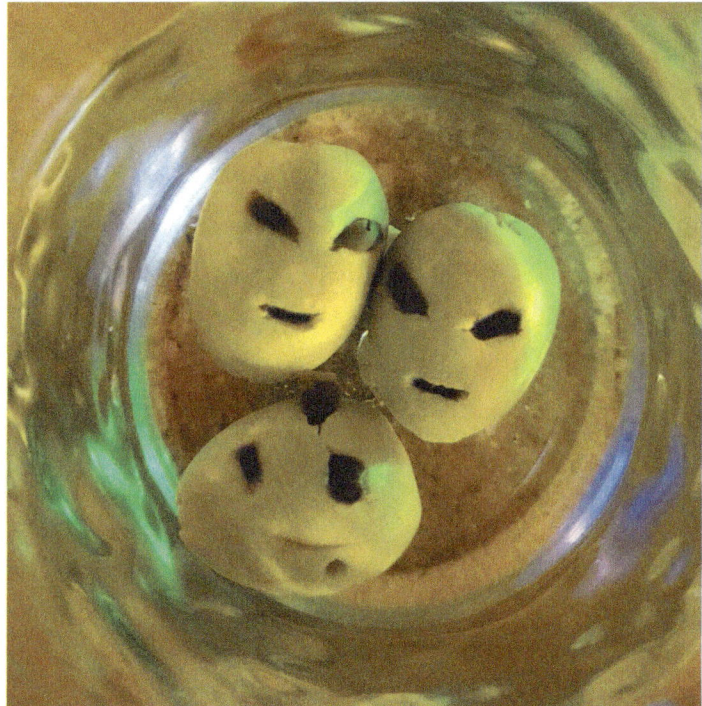

Roasted Poblano Bloody Mary

LOW FODMAP ❤ IBS FRIENDLY ❤ GLUTEN-FREE ❤ DAIRY-FREE

This fresh peppery cocktail calls for overnight infusion for the vodka, for a belly up to the bar hello! from the Southwest. Note: 1-ounce (30 ml) vodka per cocktail is a LoFO serving.

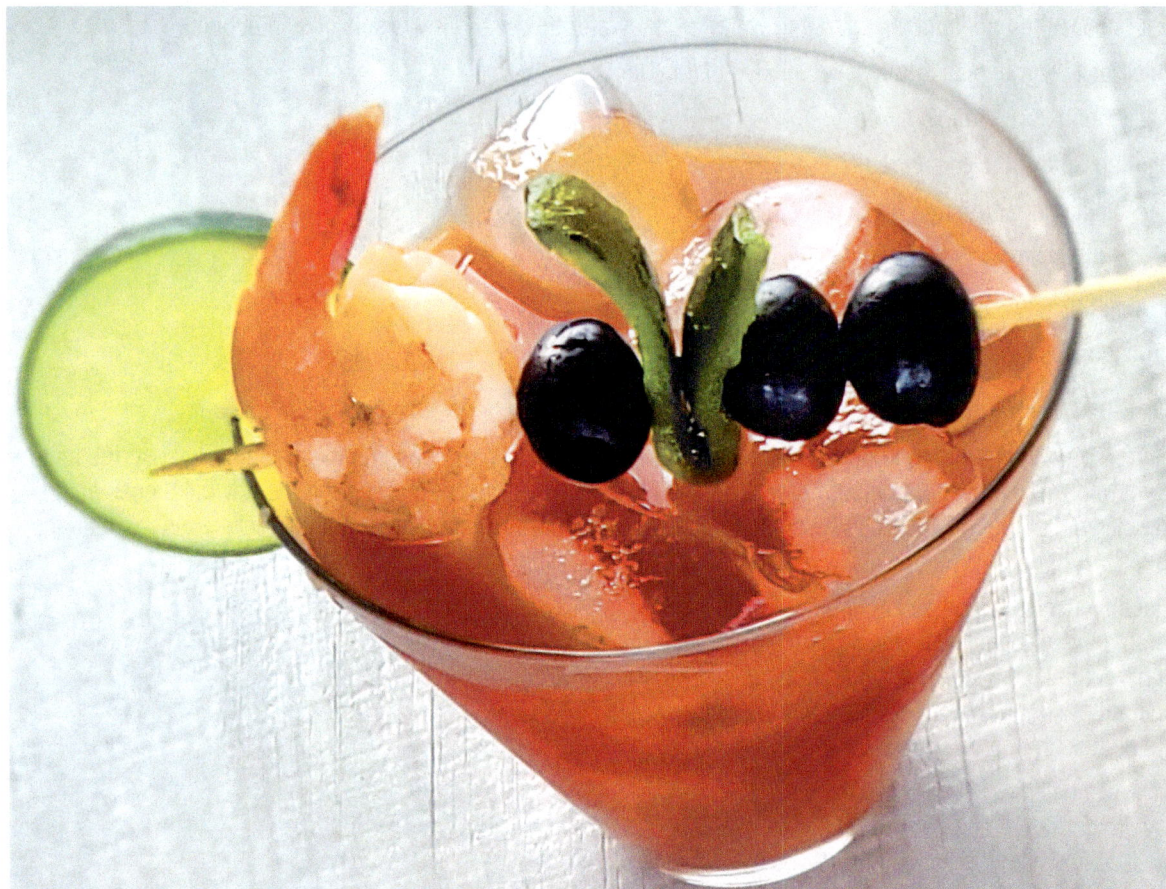

MAKES 4 COCKTAILS
VODKA INFUSION INGREDIENTS

1 glass bottle with wide top and lid, a small mason jar works well

1 medium (97 g) (4.6-inch / 11.7 cm) poblano pepper, roasted and prepped (page 46), you will only need half, sliced lengthwise into 4 strips (reserve the strips for garnish)

4-ounces (120 ml) vodka, your brand preference

MIXER INGREDIENTS

1 1/4 cup (300 ml / 10-ounces) plain tomato juice

3 teaspoons (15 ml) fresh lime juice

2 teaspoons (10 ml) Worcestershire sauce

1/4 scant teaspoon (1 g) fine sea salt

1/8 teaspoon fine ground black pepper

5 drops Sriracha hot sauce

GARNISH INGREDIENTS

4 cooked, peeled tail-on shrimp (optional)

4 lime rounds or wedges

8 - 12 canned ripe black or green olives, pitted

4 cocktail skewers

Method: Place the vodka and poblano strips in the wide-mouth glass jar. Infuse in the fridge overnight.

Place the mixer ingredients in a cocktail shaker or jar with lid and shake to mix. Fill 4 glasses with ice. Divide the mixer evenly in each glass. Add 30 ml / 1-ounce infused vodka to each glass. To garnish, skewer the olives, poblano strips and shrimp. Place 1 lime round on the glass rim. Serve immediately.

Tips: It's nice to have a full-batch bottle in the fridge for when friends pop by. Plus, the longer in the fridge – up to 4 to 8 weeks – the more flavorful it becomes. For a Full Bottle you will need:

2 medium (97 g each) poblano peppers, roasted and prepped (page 46), sliced lengthwise into strips

1, 750 ml bottle vodka

1 large glass bottle with a wide top and lid (the vodka bottle will have a narrow top making it difficult to place or retrieve the chile strips). Place the vodka and poblano strips into the bottle and keep in the fridge. Every few days, tip the bottle and shake lightly.

For Bloody Marias, use tequila in place of vodka. Silver and gold tequila have been lab tested as 1 shot (30 ml / 1-ounce) per proper serving.

Monash Note: Although chiles (chillies) are generally low in FODMAPs, some people with IBS may be sensitive to the capsaicin they contain. Capsaicin is a natural compound that gives chiles their spicy quality. You may need to limit how much chile you eat if your IBS symptoms are triggered by spicy food.

Note: Monash advises that alcohol is an irritant to the gut. A limited intake is advised and only consume alcohol with food. **Please drink responsibly.**

Tea-quila Cocktails

LOW FODMAP ❤ IBS FRIENDLY ❤ GLUTEN-FREE ❤ DAIRY-FREE

After a long day's hike through the San Juan Mountains of the southern Rockies, Tea-quila Cocktails over ice are a refreshing reward. Only 4 ingredients are required; green tea, tequila, lime juice and maple syrup.

My first choice of tea was chamomile because for years I'd been drinking it for it's anti-inflammatory and purported soothing abdominal pain qualities. I then learned that it's considered high FODMAP due to the fructans it contains, so I settled on pure green tea that is low FODMAP and has an earthy, grassy quality that goes well with tequila. If you are sensitive to caffeine, use a decaffeinated green tea.

This recipe requires about 45 minutes for steeping and chilling the tea, so if you make the tea one day advance and keep it in the fridge, you'll have the cocktails mixed in no time for your post-hike get together.

MAKES 4 COCKTAILS
30 ml / 1-ounce tequila per cocktail is a LoFO serving

INGREDIENTS
4 tea bags pure green tea

2 cups (473 ml / 16-ounces) water

Ice cubes

1/2 cup (120 ml / 4-ounces) silver tequila

1/4 cup (60 ml / 2-ounces) freshly squeezed lime juice, plus 4 round lime slices for garnish

1/4 cup (60 ml / 2-ounces) maple syrup

Method: Place the tea bags in a heatproof pitcher or measuring cup large enough to hold 2 cups (473 ml) water, plus space. Bring the water to a low boil in a teakettle or saucepan. Remove from heat and pour over tea bags; steep for 3 minutes. Remove the tea bags and cool for 15 minutes, then place in the fridge for 30 minutes or until completely chilled.

Assembly: Fill 4 glasses with ice. Mix the tea with the tequila, lime juice and maple syrup. Stir well. Pour equal amounts into the glasses. Garnish with lime rounds. Cheers!

Tip: Microwave the 2 limes for 12 seconds before squeezing to release more juices.

Note: Monash advises that alcohol is an irritant to the gut. A limited intake is advised and only consume alcohol with food. **Please drink responsibly.**

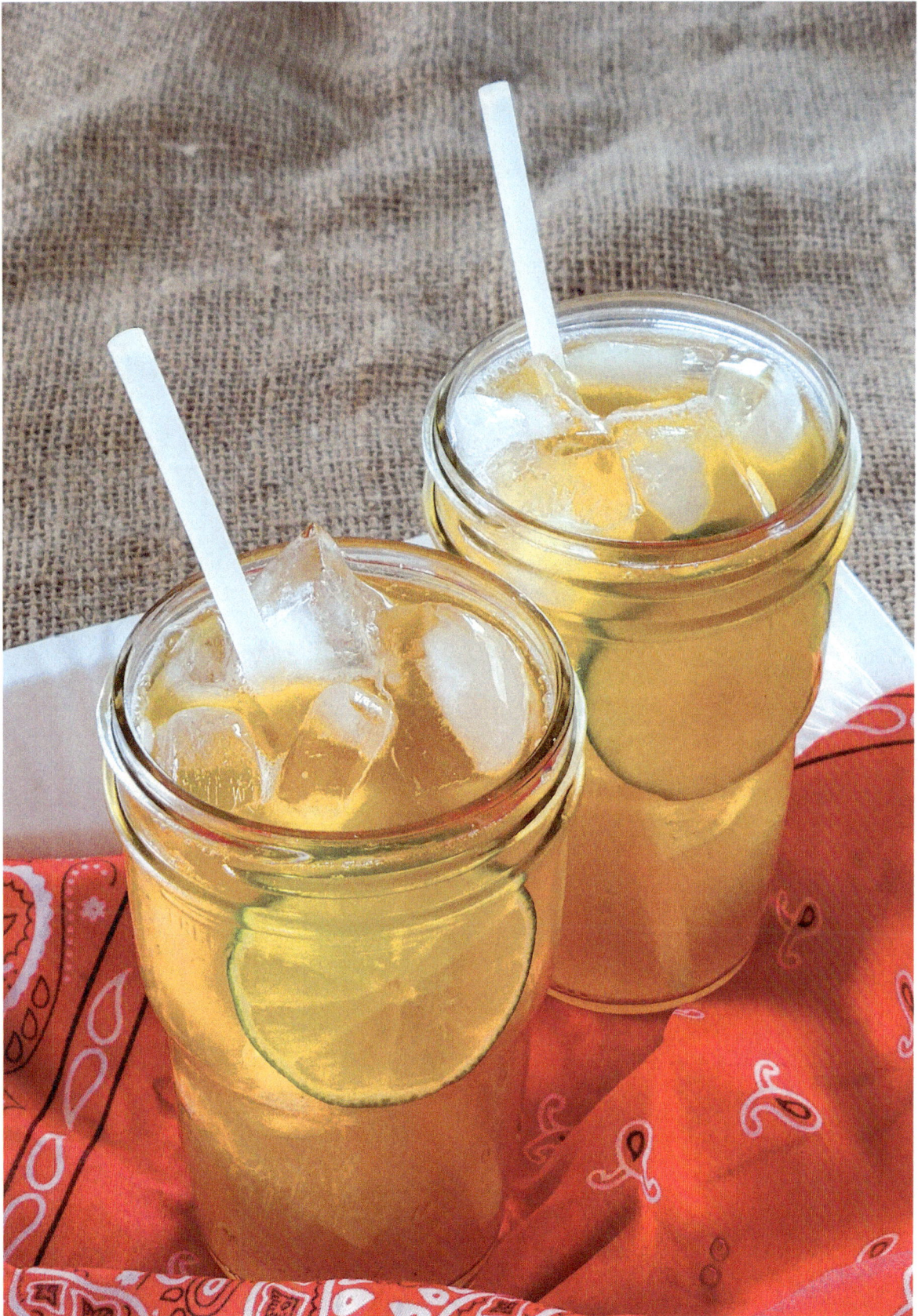

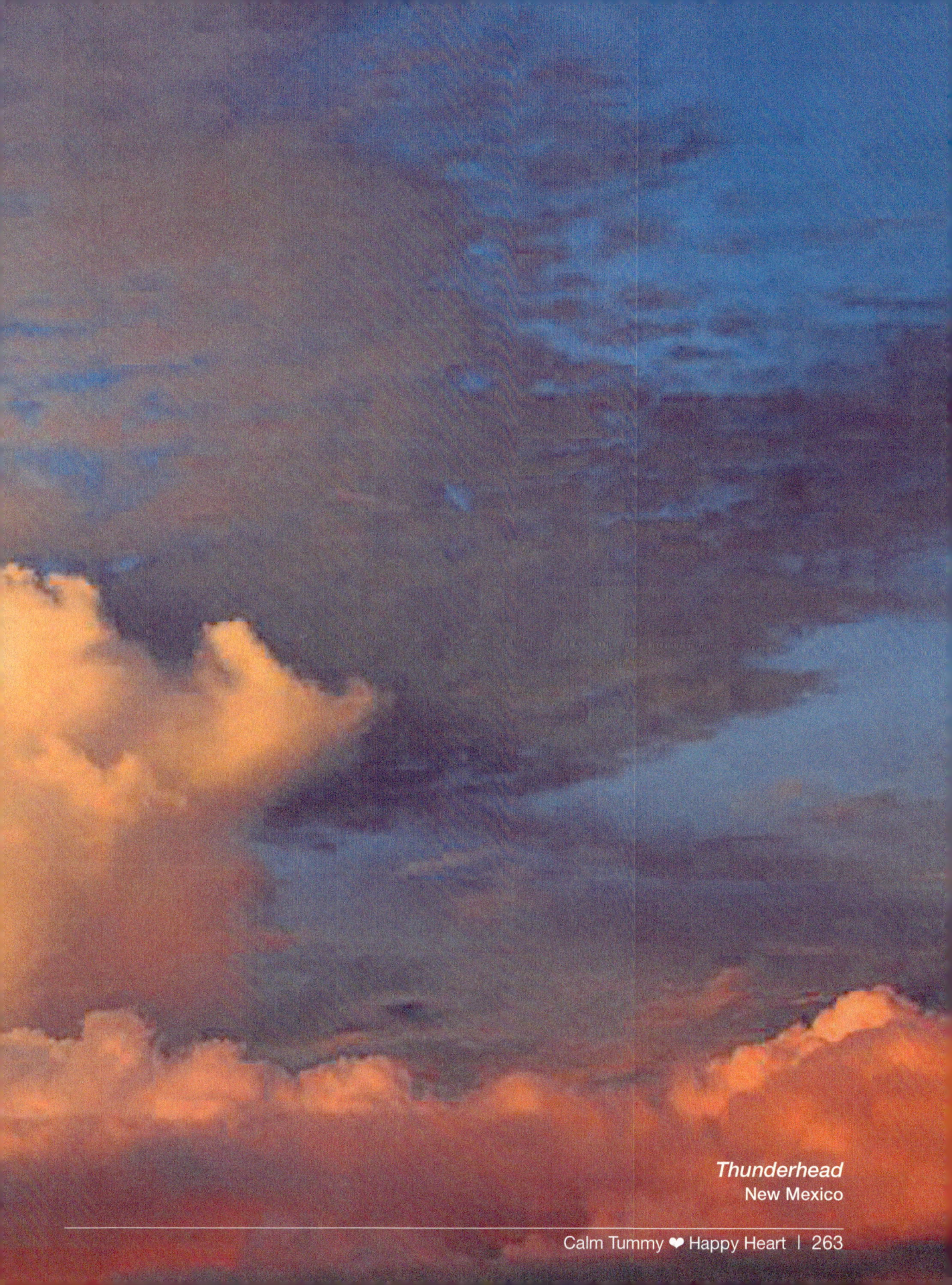

Thunderhead
New Mexico

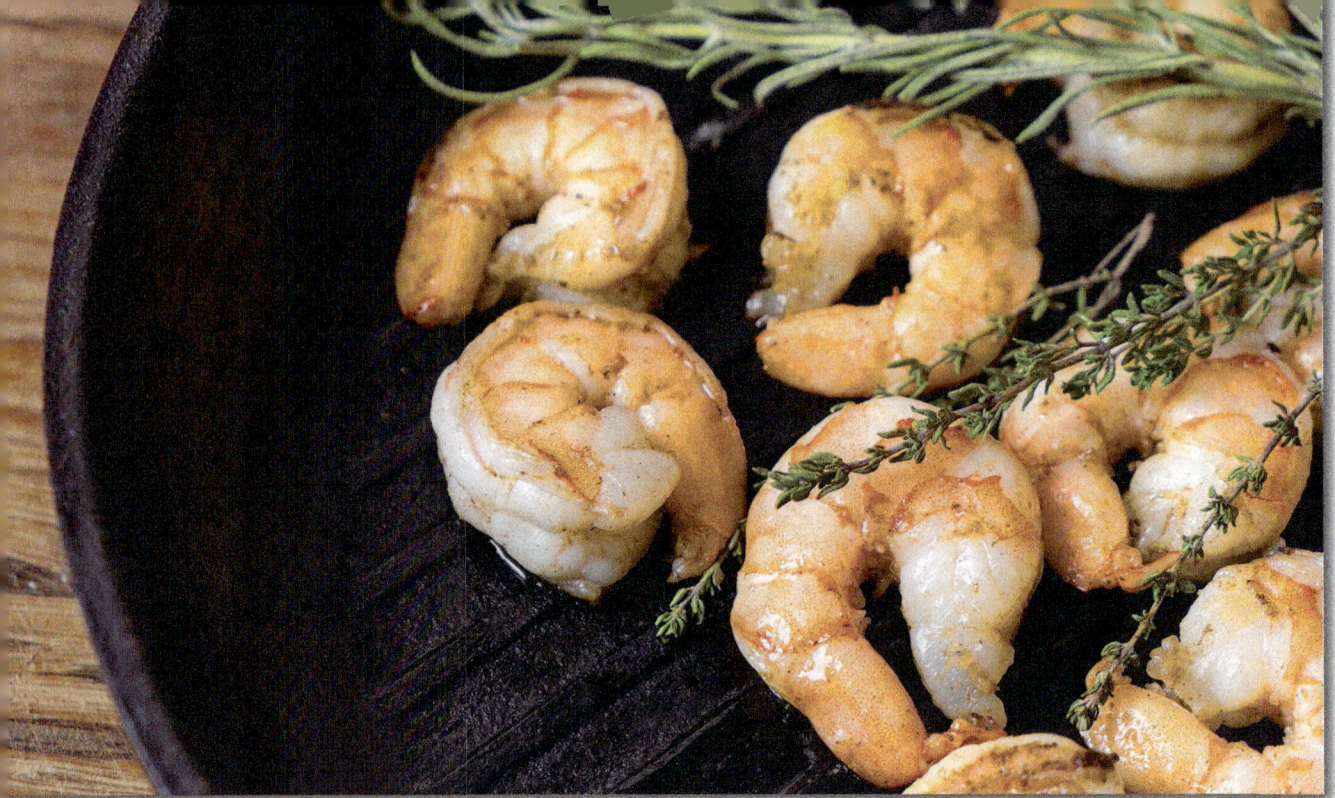

Problem Child Shrimp

Dinner invitations set off lots of alarm bells when I was establishing my low FODMAP diet. For a while I was hesitant to accept them because I felt like I would either be a burden by giving the host/ess my list of no and yes foods, or insult them by asking if I could bring my own food and beverage to their soiree. Then I realized it didn't have to be that way. I didn't have to miss out on my social life. Problem Child Shrimp is a story about how I learned to communicate my condition to people without making it such a big deal in my head.

PROBLEM CHILD SHRIMP & DINNER INVITATIONS

Jim and I had been looking to build a house in Mesa Verde country, but we wanted to rent a place and get to know the region before buying land. A wonderful couple made it possible for us to relocate to their ranch and be a part of the beautiful world they had created while we made our plans.

After our move-in, we were invited to their house for dinner. I had heard that our hostess was a wicked-awesome cook with a spice drawer that would make Diana Kennedy (the Julia Child of Mexican cooking) swoon. Her menus were thoughtfully planned out and this was not a bring-a-dish occasion.

Considering that most recipes begin with "heat oil in a pan and add onion and garlic," I felt that a pre-dinner email was the way to go. This is how it went …

ME: Hey there, we'd love to come over for dinner! 6:00 is perfect. Jim can eat anything. I should let you know that I have complex food sensitivities so if you don't mind I'd like to

Dinner Party Tips / Dining Out

bring a dish I know I can eat and share with everyone. Something that fits with your menu. Maybe a Romaine salad with grilled chicken? Lemme know. Can't wait!

HOSTESS: Bring your own food? No no no. Don't worry about it. I cook for people who have food allergies all the time. Send me your list of foods you can't eat and I will plan around it. No worries!

ME: Oh boy, I don't know if I want to put you through this. The list is waaaaaaaay long. But here goes – No Foods Are: onions, garlic, onion powder, garlic powder, chili powder and stocks with onion, garlic and celery. Most all dairy, gluten, wheat, apples, apple juice, asparagus, beans, stone fruits, some soy products, sauces thickened with wheat flour, high fructose corn syrup, peas, pears, artichokes, dried fruits. This is the abbreviated list, so … will my salad with grilled chicken fit with your menu?

HOSTESS: Wow. This is freaking me out. I don't think I can cook for you! My shrimp dish has garlic sauce. I can leave the sauce off for you. Can you eat plain boiled potatoes? Apples and apple juice, really? This is a new one. What is the common denominator here? What can you eat?

At this point I looked to Jim in the living room and said "She says my food list is freaking her out." And he laughed that cute, soft chuckle that I know and love.

ME: You are cracking me up! Okay, I have a digestive thing that's complex and I swap out foods that are triggers for foods that calm everything down. And it's working! Please don't feel that you have to go out of your way on my account. Yep, I can eat plain boiled potatoes. If all right with you I can bring: grilled chicken that's been marinated in extra virgin olive oil, lemon juice, pure red chile powder, cumin, coriander, s&p. Chopped Romaine, tomatoes, blanched carrots, quinoa, the green parts of scallions, radishes, sweet potato, olives, piñon nuts, avocado, with an oil and vinegar dressing. Also, if I do eat a NO food it's not a medical emergency like a peanut allergy or Celiac Disease. Not to worry about that. In that sense I'm lucky.

HOSTESS: BYOF please! :)

That Saturday we showed up for dinner with my salad. Our hostess had prepared a lovely platter of sumac garlic shrimp, along with a sexy black rice dish with roasted veggies. As I reached for the salad, she swooped a plate of plain grilled shrimp and potatoes in front of me with "Here you go! Problem Child Shrimp!" We all burst out laughing. I was eternally grateful to her for joking and making me feel completely welcome and not a burden at all. We had a terrific evening and I now have the endearing nickname Problem Child. I love it.

I find that the more at ease and open I am with people about my condition, they are not only understanding but also have food allergies or sensitivities themselves, or know someone with a GI condition. By contacting people in advance there are no surprises because we've already worked it out.

DINING OUT AND CALLING IN ADVANCE

This also applies to dining out. I contact the restaurant during off-peak hours, let them know when I plan to dine with them, ask if a certain dish can be made without onion or garlic, and if it's okay if I bring my own salad dressing, salsa or bbq sauce because of my "complex crazy food sensitivities." The lighter the tone with my requests, the better the response: "Can you believe, I can't eat apples? I know! Or peaches. But kiwis and pineapple, now we're talkin'." The chef or general manager make a note of my request, the dinner is hassle-free, I let them know how much I appreciate their efforts that make it easier to dine out with my friends, and that I'm a fan for life.

DINING OUT & EASY GO-TOS

Caesar Salads

In the IBS community, a Caesar Salad with a few swaps is considered to be a dependable go-to. This is how the order typically goes …

"Hi. I have some food sensitivities and would like to make a few changes to your Caesar, would that be all right? Great, thank you. Instead of the garlic dressing, may I have oil and vinegar? No croutons and light on the parmesan cheese (or no cheese). May I add chopped tomato? Great. And I'll have the plain grilled chicken (or fish) on the side. Thank you."

Even better is a bbq joint with a Caesar, and meats that are slow smoked with a salt and pepper rub. Oftentimes bbq pit experts prefer to cook their meats without a chili powder/garlic/onion rub, and the customer is offered bbq sauces to top as they like. In which case your FODified Caesar request can be topped with plain pulled pork, chicken or brisket. It's a dream to find these places and there is usually a plain baked potato on the menu.

Mexican Restaurants

My go-tos are the Fish or Shrimp Tacos. This is because the ground or shredded beef and chicken fillings are pre-marinated and contain onion, garlic and most likely chili powder (taco seasoning). Whereas the fish and shrimp are made to order.

My order request: corn tortillas, plain grilled shrimp or fish, no sauce or seasonings. With cilantro, chopped tomato, shredded carrot, avocado, light on the cheese (or no cheese), and lime wedges. This is when my small travel cooler (that I carry around with me everywhere) comes in handy. I stock it with my own LoFO pineapple salsa, Pico de Gallo and lots of other condiments and snacks. (See list at the end of this chapter).

Asian Restaurants

My go-tos are Royal Shrimp or Chicken with Vegetables because the sauces (in U.S. Asian restaurants) oftentimes do not contain onion or garlic and the veggies only require a couple swaps.

My order request: plain white rice (not fried rice), sauce with no onion or garlic (always best to check), swap the broccoli for zucchini. Baby corn, water chestnuts and bamboo shoots are fine. No MSG. (Note: some people with IBS can tolerate broccoli florets. MSG is a personal sensitivity I have, not a FODMAP issue).

When a restaurant is jam-packed and special orders slow the kitchen line, I sometimes write out my request with a note thanking the chef for making changes that will keep me healthy, with a few bucks or a fiver attached depending on the rush hour they're dealing with. I'm happy to say that nine out of ten times, the chefs come out to meet with me, we have a nice chat and I get the opportunity to thank them again. If a server is kind and understanding, I leave a nice tip.

IT'S NOT ALWAYS SMOOTH DINING

Not all special requests are met with a smile, particularly when I haven't called in advance. Some servers and chefs are offended by changes to their carefully curated menus. If their policy states "no changes permitted" I comply, do my best to eat around trigger foods, or order the Caesar with dressing on the side.

There have been occasions when a server has smacked my plate on the table and said, "There! There is your chicken skewer with no sauce, no yogurt, no onions. Plain!" When someone blatantly lets me know they're insulted by my order (and I probably didn't call ahead btw) my gut instinct tells me – do not eat the food. Because the server's attitude came from the kitchen that prepared it and I don't trust that. So I send it back, wait for others at the table to finish their meals, and afterwards grab a Caesar Salad from someplace else. Plate slamming is never okay, and I'm fine with sipping my tea and searching my phone for the closest Caesar or low FODMAP accommodating sandwich shop while I wait.

Thankfully, in the last decade huge progress has been made in food allergy and sensitivity awareness in the U.S. through articles in mainstream newspapers, health columns, magazines and online blogs / sources. I have noticed that servers are more understanding and educated about why some people need to change a few things with their orders and we're not just picky eaters. More restaurants are offering gluten-free and dairy-free options that always make me want to hug the servers, staff and everyone in the kitchen. I don't, but the overjoyed temptation is definitely there!

Food brand names are sometimes listed within a recipe, and this means they are Monash Certified. For more brand options we use and love, please visit www.**fodifyIt**.com

Monash Note: Although chiles (chillies) are generally low in FODMAPs, some people with IBS may be sensitive to the capsaicin they contain. Capsaicin is a natural compound that gives chiles their spicy quality. You may need to limit how much chile you eat if your IBS symptoms are triggered by spicy food.

THINGS IN MY DINING OUT / TRAVEL COOLER

Plain, unsweetened almond milk

LoFO salsa or Pico de Gallo

LoFO bbq sauce

LoFO green chile sauce

LoFO salad dressing

Corn tortillas

Gluten-free LoFO sliced bread or ciabatta

Butter alternative, dairy-free

Canned Spanish or ripe black olives

Hard boiled eggs

LoFO mixed nuts

LoFO snack bars

LoFO taco seasoning

LoFO gluten-free crackers

Maple syrup

Apple cider vinegar

Blanched carrots

Pineapple

Shredded chicken, frozen

It's a small-ish cooler, so I don't carry all of these foods with me all the time. But these are the general options that make travel and dining out all the more enjoyable.

Wishing you a calm tummy and happy heart! ❤ Amy Laura

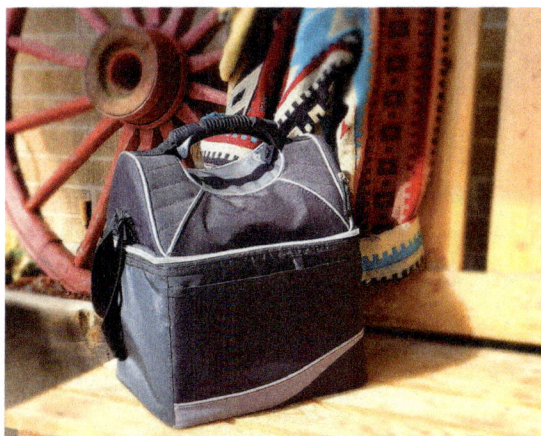

Fermentable Oligosaccharides, Disaccharides, Monosaccharides And Polyols

◄ HIGH FODMAP   **LOW FODMAP ►**

QUICK REFERENCE LIST

Swaps are a part of the beginning Elimination Phase of the diet when you remove/minimize high FODMAP foods and replace them with low FODMAP serving amounts. Always check the Monash University Low FODMAP Diet Smartphone App for proper serving amounts, tips and newly tested food updates.

Swaps are per your tolerances. FODMAPs are completely serving size related and many of the foods listed below under high FODMAP indeed have low FODMAP serving sizes such as apples at 2 teaspoons (25 g) per serving. While the diet is not dairy or gluten-free, some dairy and wheat swaps have been included in this list for people, like me, with sensitivities to them.

HiFO FOOD EXAMPLES	LoFO SWAPS
Apples, cherries	Kiwis, oranges, cantelope
Beans	Canned brown lentils, pozole (hominy)
Cheese Sauce	Cheesy Béchamel Sauce with Large Flake Nutritional Yeast (page 65)
Garlic	LoFO Garlic-Infused Oil (pg 50)
Green Chile Sauce	LoFO Green Chile Sauce (pg 60)
Honey/Agave Syrup	Maple syrup
Mango	Papaya
Mexican Restaurant Style Rice	LoFO Mexican Rice Version (pg 111)
Onion	Chives, green parts of scallions and leeks, properly Onion-Infused Oil (pg 50)
Red Chile Sauce	LoFO Red Chile Sauce (pg 62)
Refried Beans	No Beans Refried "Beans" (pg 114) or a side of hash browns with no onion or garlic
Regular Cow's Milk	Plain unsweetened almond milk, canned full-fat coconut milk for cooking containing no inulin, unsweetened oat or macadamia milk, lactose-free cow's milk if you eat dairy
Sour Cream	Plain dairy-free, unsweetened coconut yogurt, or lactose-free sour cream, if you eat dairy
Taco Seasoning	LoFO Taco Seasoning (pg 48), or purchased equivalent
Wheat Bread	Low FODMAP gluten-free breads, sourdough bread if tolerated
Wheat Flour	Low FODMAP flour mixes, see About Low FODMAP Flours (pg 55)
Wheat Flour Burrito Wraps	LoFO gluten-free burrito wraps
Wheat Flour Tortillas	LoFO gluten-free white corn tortillas

For brand options we use and love, please visit fodifyit.com

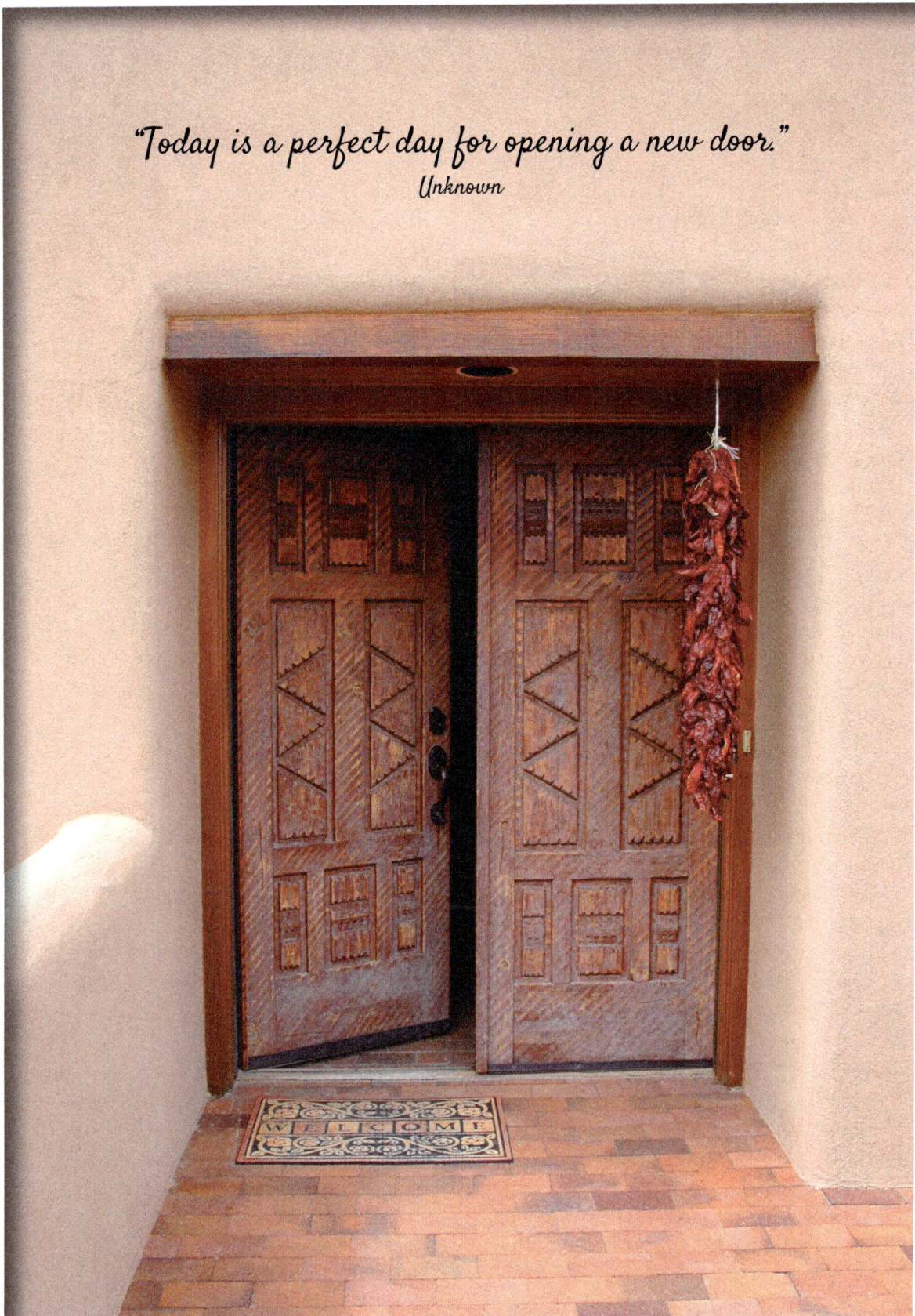

"Today is a perfect day for opening a new door."
Unknown

Index

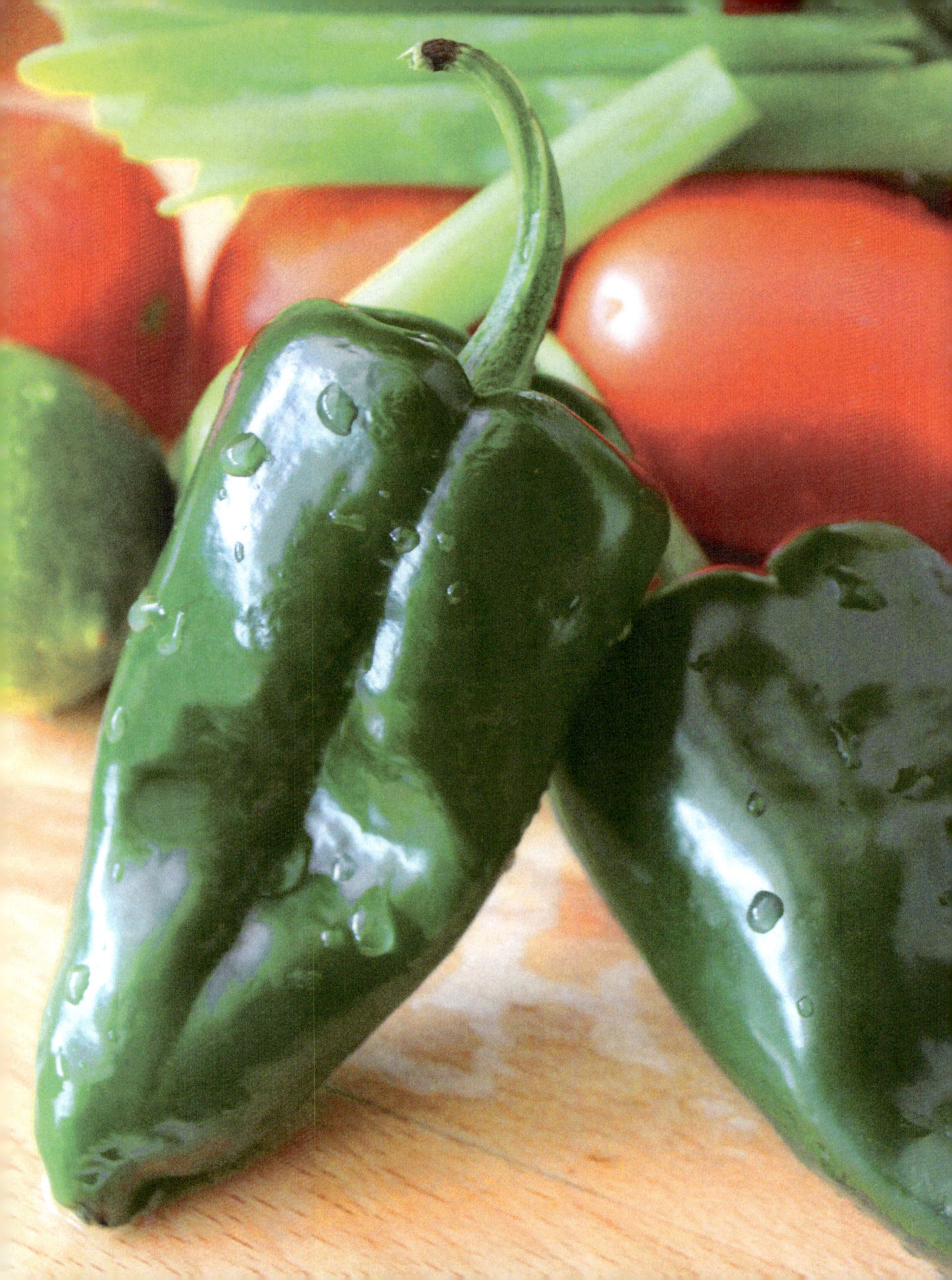

Printed in Great Britain
by Amazon

11616062R00160